Lockdown Therapy

This fascinating volume explores – from the perspective both of analysts and their patients – how the COVID-19 pandemic quickly and unexpectedly created profound and lasting changes in the ways psychoanalysis is conducted, and what those changes mean for analysis moving forward.

The first part of the book is made up of interviews conducted by Stefano Carpani with authoritative authors in analytical psychology during the earliest phase of lock-down, centered on themes of the pandemic, lockdown, and how each individual was coping with the challenges those circumstances brought on. The second part features personal essays that further details the subjective experiences of Jungian analysts and therapists worldwide, comprising a collection of reflections on how COVID-19 affected and changed the way analysts work with patients. These reflections focus on the theoretical, clinical, technical, and also practical points of view, including clinical materials on transference and counter-transference considerations. The third part of the book is specular to the second and offers reflections from patients' perspective on how the pandemic changed their therapies and lockdown affected their experience of therapy. Patients have provided anonymous testimonies through their writing of how they experienced of the change of setting, mindset and related implications.

A comprehensive overview of an important and ongoing conversation, *Lockdown Therapy* is crucial reading for Jungian analysts and scholars, as well as other clinicians training in analysis, psychotherapy and counselling.

Stefano Carpani, M.Phil., M.A., is a psychoanalyst (CGJIZ and IAAP). He is the editor of *Breakfast at Küsnacht* (Chiron, 2020), *The Plural Turn in Jungian and Post-Jungian Studies* (Routledge, 2021), *Anthology of Contemporary Classics in Analytical Psychology: The New Ancestors* (Routledge, 2022) and *Individuation and Liberty in a Globalized World: Psychosocial Perspectives on Freedom after Freedom* (Routledge, 2022).

Monica Luci, PhD, Jungian and relational psychoanalyst (AIPA-IAAP and IARPP), works in private practice in Rome. She is the author, translator, and editor of publications on the themes of trauma, displacement, collective violence, sexuality, and gender, among which are the monographs *Torture, Psychoanalysis & Human Rights* (Routledge, 2017), and *Torture Survivors in Analytic Therapy: Jung, Politics and Culture* (Routledge, 2022).

"It is a great pleasure for me to acknowledge the excellent work done by the editors and all the contributors to this important book. The pandemic has changed us all and we need tools to understand how. It is my belief that this book will make a lasting contribution to the understanding of how the pandemic changed the Jungian world and how creativity and profound reflectivity could help us all in finding new ways to continue the work. I am sure that the book will be of great value to our Jungian community."

Misser Berg, IAAP President Elect

Lockdown Therapy

Jungian Perspectives on How the Pandemic Changed Psychoanalysis

Edited by
Stefano Carpani and Monica Luci

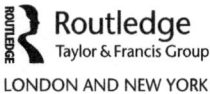

Routledge
Taylor & Francis Group

LONDON AND NEW YORK

Cover image: courtesy of Carlotta Carpani Ruano

First published 2023
by Routledge
4 Park Square, Milton Park, Abingdon, Oxon OX14 4RN

and by Routledge
605 Third Avenue, New York, NY 10158

Routledge is an imprint of the Taylor & Francis Group, an informa business

British Library Cataloguing-in-Publication Data
A catalogue record for this book is available from the British Library

Library of Congress Cataloging-in-Publication Data
Names: Carpani, Stefano, editor. | Luci, Monica, 1972- editor.
Title: Lockdown therapy : Jungian perspectives on how the pandemic changed
psychoanalysis / edited by Stefano Carpani and Monica Luci.
Description: Abingdon, Oxon ; New York, NY : Routledge, 2023. |
Includes bibliographical references and index. |
Identifiers: LCCN 2022013346 | ISBN 9781032210230 (hardback) |
ISBN 9781032200156 (paperback) | ISBN 9781003266402 (ebook)
Subjects: LCSH: Psychoanalysis--Methodology. | Psychotherapist and patient. |
Jungian psychology. | COVID-19 Pandemic, 2020---Influence.
Classification: LCC RC506 .L5448 2023 | DDC 616.89/17--dc23/eng/20220629
LC record available at https://lccn.loc.gov/2022013346

ISBN: 978-1-032-21023-0 (hbk)
ISBN: 978-1-032-20015-6 (pbk)
ISBN: 978-1-003-26640-2 (ebk)

DOI: 10.4324/9781003266402

Typeset in Times New Roman
by Taylor & Francis Books

This book is dedicated to the health care personnel who courageously faced and fought the emergency.

Contents

Contributors

Part 1

Paul Attinello, Ph.D. is a Jungian analyst in private practice and a senior lecturer at Newcastle University who has also taught at the University of Hong Kong and as a guest professor at UCLA. He received his PhD from UCLA and diploma as an analyst from the C. G. Jung-Institute in Zürich. He has lived and worked on four continents, has been involved in HIV groups and programs, creative and academic events and projects, and is co-founder of the Psychosocial Wednesdays video seminar series. He is published in essay collections, journals, and reference works, including the groundbreaking *Queering the Pitch: The New Lesbian & Gay Musicology.* He has written on contemporary music, the culture of AIDS, and philosophical and psychological topics.

John Beebe, M.D. is a North American Jungian analyst and author in practice in San Francisco, USA. He received degrees from Harvard College and the University of Chicago medical school. He is a past president of the C. G. Jung Institute of San Francisco, where he is currently on the teaching faculty. He is a Distinguished Life Fellow of the American Psychiatric Association.

Ursula Brasch, M.A. studied sinology, history, and politics in Freiburg and Tübingen, Germany. She is a training analyst and supervisor at the C.G. Jung Institutes of Zürich and Stuttgart, as well as a member of the Curatorium of the C.G. Jung Institute Zürich. She has engaged in many years of teaching and lecturing on analytical psychology, clinical psychology, and the I Ching.

Stefano Candellieri, M.D. is an Italian psychiatrist and psychotherapist based in Turin. Between 1993 and 2001 he worked at the Fatebenefratelli psychiatric hospital in Turin, where he held the post of assistant head of department, specialising in psychotic disorders and forensic psychiatry. Since 2001, he has been engaged exclusively in private work as psychiatrist and psychotherapist. He is, together with the psychologist Davide Favero, founder and director of the Centro Medico Psicologico Torinese. His current area of research is the intersection of psychoanalysis (with particular reference to the theoretical model of Antonino Ferro) and semiotics. On this last topic, he and Davide Favero wrote "Hyde Park – Officina di psicoanalisi potenziale," published by Moretti & Vitali in 2019.

Renate Daniel, M.D., studied medicine at the University of Heidelberg and specialized in the fields of psychiatry and psychotherapy. She is a Jungian analyst, training analyst/supervisor and Director of Programs at the C.G. Jung Institute in Zurich. She also works as specialist at the C.G. Jung Outpatient's Clinic in Zurich, and is a member of the Scientific Management Board of the International Society of Depth Psychology (IGT) and a member of the Scientific Advisory Board of the Lindau Psychotherapy Weeks (LPTW), held in Germany. She is the author of *Taking the Fear Out of the Night: Coping with Nightmares* (2017) and *The Self: Quest for Meaning in a Changing World* (2020)

Davide Favero, psychologist and psychotherapist, is a CIPA and IAAP Jungian analyst and psychodramatist. A former psychologist at Fatebenefratelli psychiatric hospital and Professor at the University of Turin, Faculty of Psychology, he is the founder and director of the Centro Medico Psicologico Torinese in Turin, along with psychiatrist Stefano Candellieri. He publishes articles in national and international journals and participates in congresses as a speaker, most notably at the International IAAP Congresses (Copenhagen 2013, Buenos Aires 2015, Kyoto 2016, Avignon 2018), the JAP International Conferences (Berlin 2014, New York 2017), the Tustin Conference (Boston 2014), the joint Conferences of IAAP and IAJS, (New Haven 2015, Frankfurt 2018) and the IPA Congress (Boston 2015). His main interest is the intersection of analytical psychology and related subjects, particularly referring to the Zeitgeist, the semiotics and the language.

Stefano Carpani, M.A., M.Phil. is an Italian psychoanalyst (trained at the C.G. Jung Institute, Zürich), sociologist (Cambridge and Manchester) and a Ph.D. candidate in the Department of Psychosocial and Psychoanalytical Studies from University of Essex. He graduated in Literature and Philosophy from the Catholic University of Milan. He works in private practice in Berlin (DE). He is the editor of *Breakfast at Küsnacht: Conversations on C. G. Jung and Beyond* (Chiron, 2020), *The Plural Turn in Jungian and Post-Jungian Studies: The Work of Andrew Samuels* (Routledge, forthcoming 2021), *The New Ancestors: Anthology of Contemporary Theoretical/Clinical Classics in Analytical Psychology* (Routledge, 2022); *Freedom after Freedom: Psychosocial Perspectives on Individuation and Liberty in a Globalized World* (Routledge, 2022).

Professor Verena Kast, studied psychology at the Universities of Basel and Zurich and trained as a psychoanalyst at the C.G. Jung Institute Zurich.

From 1973–2008 she taught at the University of Zurich. She has lectured internationally, and at the C.G. Jung Institute Zürich. She is past president of the Swiss Society for Analytical Psychology, and past president of the IAAP. She was chairwoman of the International Society for Depth Psychology, co-director of the Lindau Psychotherapy Weeks and president of the C.G. Jung Institute. She has written in the field of emotions, attachment and separation, but also symbolism. Her love belongs to the imagination and its development.

Monica Luci, PhD, is an Italian clinical psychologist and Jungian and relational psychoanalyst (IAAP&IARPP), working in private practice in Rome. She collaborates with NGOs and national and international institutions in the field of research, clinical evaluation and psychotherapy for vulnerable refugees, especially survivors of torture, war traumas and gender based violence, and unaccompanied minors. She speaks at national and international conferences and conducts training in academic and professional contexts. She is the author, translator, and editor of publications on the themes of trauma, displacement, collective violence, transcultural psychology, sexuality, and gender, among which the monograph *Torture, Psychoanalysis & Human Rights* (Routledge, 2017) and *Torture Survivors in Analytic Therapy: Jung, Politics and Culture* (Routledge, 2022).

Susan Rowland, Ph.D., is Chair of the Engaged Humanities and the Creative Life MA, earned her Ph.D. from the University of Newcastle and her MAs from the University of London and Oxford University. She was the first Chair of the International Association of Jungian Studies (IAJS). She is author of many studies of Jung, literary theory and gender including *C.G. Jung and Literary Theory* (1999), *Jung: A Feminist Revision* (2002), *Jung as a Writer* (2005), and also edited *Psyche and the Arts* (2008). Susan's work is not so much "about" Jung as an attempt to develop his special insights into myth, technology, the feminine, nature and the numinous for today's wounded world.

Professor Andrew Samuels is recognized internationally as a leading contributor to psychotherapy, counselling, analysis and depth psychology. Andrew is a Training Analyst of the Society of Analytical Psychology, in private practice in London, and was for many years Professor of Analytical Psychology at the University of Essex. He was Chair of the UK Council for Psychotherapy and (with Judy Ryde) founded Psychotherapists and Counsellors for Social Responsibility. His many books include (among others): *Jung and the Post-Jungians* (1985); *The Plural Psyche* (1989); *The Political Psyche* (1993); *Politics on the Couch* (2001); His latest books are *A New Therapy for Politics?* (2016) and *Analysis and Activism: Social and Political Contributions of Jungian Analysis* (edited with Emilija Kiehl and Mark Saban, 2016).

Murray Stein, Ph.D. is a Training and Supervising Analyst at the International School of Analytical Psychology Zurich (ISAP-ZURICH). He was president of the International Association for Analytical Psychology (IAAP) from 2001 to 2004 and President of ISAP-ZURICH from 2008 to 2012. He has lectured internationally and is the editor of *Jungian Psychoanalysis* and the author of Jung's *Treatment of Christianity, In MidLife, Jung's Map of the Soul, Minding the Self, Outside Inside and All Around* and *The Bible as Dream*. The first volume of his Collected Writings, titled *Individuation*, has recently been published. He lives in Switzerland and has a private practice in Zurich.

Part 2

Misser Berg is a Jungian Analyst trained in Denmark, London and Berlin 1985–1991. Individual Member of IAAP in 1992. Co-founder, member and past President of the Danish Society for Analytical Psychology. Member of the Training Committee at the C.G. Jung Institute, Copenhagen and Director of Training from 2005–2019. Co-founder, member and past President of the public Jung Society of Copenhagen. Member of the IAAP administration from 2010 and was in 2019 elected as President-Elect which means that she will be President of the IAAP from August 2022. Misser Berg has a private practice North of Copenhagen. She has published articles and book-chapters, and she lectures and examines in both Denmark and abroad.

Olivia del Castillo is a graduate and specialist in clinical psychology from the University of Barcelona. Since 1992 she has been an analyst for the Sociedad Española de psicología Analítica (SEPA), of which she was president and where she currently works as a didactic analyst and supervisor. She is also an overseas member of the Independent Group of Analytical Psychology (IGAP) in London. Olivia is actively involved in the dissemination and training of analytical psychology in Spain. She has written and published several articles about her experience and works in private practice in Barcelona and Madrid.

Dan Cross is a clinical psychologist with 16 years of experience working with individuals, couples and families in Edmonton, Canada. For the last several years, he has deepened a long-standing interest in Jungian psychology through studies at the C.G. Jung Institute, Zürich.

Renate Daniel—same as above

Roula-Maria Dib, Ph.D., is an assistant professor of English at the American University in Dubai, and editor-in-chief of *Indelible*, the university's literary journal. A creative writer and scholar in the fields of literature and Jungian psychology, her poems, essays, and articles have appeared in several journals. She has authored *Jungian Metaphor in Modernist Litera-ture* (Routledge, 2020). Her new poetry collection, *Simply Being*, will be published by Chiron Press in 2021. The themes that pervade her poetry usually revolve around different aspects of human nature, ekphrasis, surrealism, and mythology.

Daniela Eulert-Fuchs, Austria, M.D., G.P., is a paediatrician and neurope-diatrician; she has a psychoanalytic practice for adults, infants, children and adolescents in Vienna, Austria.

She is a training and supervising analyst for the Austrian Association of Analytical Psychology (ÖGAP). Active for many years in different psychotherapeutic and psychosomatic clinics and institutions, she has specialized in the work with infants and their caregivers. Daniela has a keen interest in exploring transference -countertransference dynamics and as well as in the influence of the analytical attitude in the analytic encounter.

Paolo Ferliga is an Italian Jungian psychotherapist and analyst, member of AIPA

(Italian Association of Analytical Psychology) and IAAP. He is a former Teacher of Philosophy and History, as well as Educational Psychology at the University Bicocca in Milan. He was trained in psychotherapy by Claudio Risé and in Sandplay Therapy by Martin Kalff and Maria Rosa Calabrese. He has published several books in the field of analytical psychology, included *Il segno del padre* and *Attraverso il senso di colpa*, and with Martin Kalff, *Old and New Horizons of Sandplay Therapy. Mindfulness and Neural Integration* (2022). He founded *Campo Maschile*, a research-action group exploring male identity, and chairs dream-related and active imagination workshops in Italy.

Roberto Grande M.D., is an Italian Child and Adolescent Psychiatrist, graduate and specialized in Turin, Italy. From 1983 to 1997 he acquired a training – personal and didactic – on Jungian group Psychodrama (Coirag). Diploma in Analytical Psychology for Adults, Children and Adolescents in 2015 at the CG Jung Institute, Zurich, where he is an Instructor and leads Lectures and Seminars. He worked as a clinician in Geneva (Switzerland), currently works in private praxis in Turin (Italy) as psychiatrist and psychoanalyst for adults, children and adolescents, dealing with psychiatric drugs if needed. The passion for human life brought him to write a book of novels about his clinical work, entitled: *The Chocolate Child – Stories of children and adolescents narrated by their psychotherapist*, (ed. Ponte alle Grazie—Mauri Spagnol Group, 2009). He is a IAAP member since 2015.

Tiffany Houck-Loomis, M.Div., Ph.D., L.P. is a licensed psychoanalyst and certified Jungian analyst in private practice in New York City. She is the author of *History Through Trauma: History and Counter-History in the*

Hebrew Bible (2018, Wipf and Stock Publishers); as well as numerous articles and book chapters published at the intersection of studies in gender and sexuality, psychoanalysis, religion, and trauma. Dr. Houck-Loomis serves as a Faculty Member of the Jungian Psychoanalytic Association in New York City.

Emilija Kiehl MSc. is a Jungian Analyst in practice in London. She is a training analyst and former Chair of the British Jungian Analytic Association, and senior member of the British Psychotherapy Foundation. She is Vice President of the International Association for Analytical Psychology (IAAP) and editor of a number of IAAP publications. She is a former book review editor for *Spring Journal* and current journal review editor for the *Journal of Analytical Psychology*. Before her training in Jungian Analysis, Emilija was a literary translator and contributor to cultural and informative journals in former Yugoslavia. Her published translations include works by Noam Chomsky, Harold Pinter, Arthur Miller, John Updike and others. She lectures, teaches and supervises in the UK and abroad.

Dr. phil. Milena Sotirova-Kohli was born and grew up in Sofia, Bulgaria. She received a M.A. degree in Japanese Studies at the University of Sofia and a M.S. in Clinical Psychology from Texas A&M University, College Station, USA. She earned a doctoral degree in psychology at the University of Basel, Switzerland, with empirical studies investigating the nature of the Jungian concept of the archetype as a form of implicit memory. After receiving her Diploma in Analytical Psychotherapy and Psychoanalysis from the C. G. Jung Institute Zürich, she works in a psychiatric praxis as a therapist in a delegated psychotherapy setting and as a therapist for group psychotherapy at the Psychological and School Psychological Services of the Kanton of Bern. She lives with her family in Bern, Switzerland.

Marianne Müller is a graduate of the C.G. Jung Institute Zurich (1996) and of the University of Bern (Master of Law 1981, Clinical Psychology 1998). She was president of the International Association for Analytical Psychology (IAAP) from 2016–2019, and president of the Swiss Society for Analytical Psychology (SGAP) from 2004–2010. She is a training analyst and supervisor at the C.G. Jung Institute Zurich, and Liaison Person for the IAAP Router Training in Greece. For many years she was the Regional Organizer for the IAAP Education Committee in Central Europe and has been engaged in training at many places. She works in private practice as analyst and mediator in Berne and Zurich.

John Merchant, PhD (Australia) is a Jungian Analyst in private practice in Sydney, a Deputy Editor of the *Journal of Analytical Psychology*, the former Chair of the IAAP's Research and Evaluation Working Group and an accredited supervisor with the Psychology Board (Australia). John supervises clinicians in Australia and overseas and runs adult education courses in Analytical Psychology at Sydney University. He has delivered professional presentations in Australia, China, Europe, New Zealand, UK and the USA. His publications include *Shamans and Analysts: New Insights on the Wounded Healer* (Routledge, 2012), plus chapters in *Psychotherapy and Counselling: Reflections on Practice* (OUP, 2015), *Research in Analytical Psychology* (Routledge, 2018), *Jung's Red Book for our Time* (Chiron, 2020) and the Jung entries in the online *Encyclopedia of Personality and Individual Differences* (Springer, 2018).

Prof. Jon Mills, PsyD, PhD, ABPP is a philosopher, psychoanalyst, and retired clinical psychologist. He is Honorary Professor, Department of Psychosocial and Psychoanalytic Studies, University of Essex, Colchester, UK; Faculty, Postgraduate Programs in Psychoanalysis & Psychotherapy, Gordon F. Derner School of Psychology, Adelphi University, NY; and Emeritus Professor of Psychology & Psychoanalysis, Adler Graduate Professional School, Toronto, Canada. Recipient of numerous awards for his scholarship, he is the author and/or editor of over 25 books in psychoanalysis, philosophy, psychology, and cultural studies including *Debating Relational Psychoanalysis: Jon Mills and his Critics* (Routledge, 2020); *Inventing God* (Routledge, 2017); *Underworlds: Philosophies of the Unconscious from Psychoanalysis to Metaphysics* (Routledge, 2014); *Conundrums: A Critique of Contemporary Psychoanalysis* (Routledge, 2012); *Origins: On the Genesis of Psychic Reality* (McGill-Queens University Press, 2010); *Treating Attachment Pathology* (Rowman & Littlefield, 2005); *The Unconscious Abyss: Hegel's Anticipation of Psychoanalysis* (State University of New York Press, 2002); and *The Ontology of Prejudice* (Rodopi, 1997). In 2015 he was given the Otto Weininger Memorial Award for Lifetime Achievement by the Canadian Psychological Association.

Tine Papič is a Slovenian Jungian training-analyst and supervisor. He studied computer and information science and philosophy at the University of Ljubljana and psychotherapy science at Sigmund Freud University Vienna and trained as a Jungian analyst in the router programme. He is currently president of the Slovenian Society for Analytical Psychology and a member of the steering group of the Analysis and Activism movement. He is also a co-founder, lecturer and organizer of the Jungian program at Sigmund Freud University Vienna Ljubljana branch and one of the founding members of Open Institute for Psychotherapy Ljubljana.

Heyong Shen, Ph.D., professor of psychology at CityU(the City University of Macao), Jungian analyst/IAAP, Sandplay Therapist/ISST, founding president of the Chinese Federation for Analytical Psychology and Sandplay Therapy, the main organizer of the International Conference of Analytical Psychology and Chinese Culture (1998–2018), speaker of Eranos

Conferences (1997/2007/2019), and the Fay Lecture (2018), chief editor for the Chinese translation of the Collected Works of C.G. Jung, and chief editor of the Chinese Journal of Analytical Psychology, the main organizer of the Garden of the Heart and Soul project.

Ruth Williams is a Training and Supervising Analyst of the Association of Jungian Analysts based in London. She is the author of *Jung: The Basics* (Routledge 2019). She is currently working on a second book on spirituality.

Nancy Robinson-Kime, Ph.D. is a Clinical Psychologist and Jungian Analyst in private practice for over 30 years. Her research includes developing a CD rom prototype on archetypal symbolism, and summary study guides to two lectures series by Edward Edinger on symbolism of the Old Testament and Apocalypse. She has presented at the Creativity and Madness conferences on archetypal themes in the work of Edward Munch in Oslo, Norway and Greek heroes in Athens, Greece and given public lectures on dream symbolism, and "The Problem of God: Transformation through Suffering." She has taught symbolism of fairy tales and Greek mythology at Art Center College of Design, Pasadena and various courses on Jung's Collected Works at the C.G. Jung Institut, Zürich. A founding member on the Board of Directors for the CG Jung Foundation Zurich, she currently lives in Zürich, Switzerland where she has a private practice.

Pia Skogemann's academic background is in Archaeology and Comparative Religion. She co-founded C.G. Jung Institute Copenhagen in 1980. She is active as a teacher, supervisor and currently (again) director of training. She joined the International Association for Analytical Psychology (IAAP) as an individual member in 1985. She was also a member of the IAAP executive committee 2001–2007 (involved with the developing groups, especially with the Router's exams; recently teaching at a supervisor course in Romania). Her papers and books have been translated in English or German: *Chuang Tzu and The Butterfly Dream* (1986); *Weiblichkeit und Selbstverwirklichung. Die Individuation der Frau heute* (1988); *Karolines Buch* (1989); *Where the Shadows Lie. A Jungian interpretation of Tolkien's The Lord of the Rings* (2009); *The Daughter Archetype* (2012)

Mark Winborn, PhD, NCPsyA, is a Jungian Psychoanalyst and Clinical Psychologist. Dr. Winborn is a training/supervising analyst of the Inter-Regional Society of Jungian Analysts and the C.G. Jung Institute in Zurich, Switzerland. He currently serves on the American Board for Accreditation in Psychoanalysis and the Ethics Committee of the International Association for Analytical Psychology, as well as the editorial boards of the *Journal of Analytical Psychology* and the *Journal of Humanistic Psychology*. He has presented papers at the past four Congresses of the International Association for Analytical Psychology (2010, 2013, 2016, 2019). His publications include *Deep Blues: Human Soundscapes for the*

Archetypal Journey (2011, Fisher King Press), *Shared Realities: Participation Mystique and Beyond* (2014, Fisher King Press), and *Interpretation in Jungian Analysis: Art and Technique* (2018, Routledge) as well as journal articles, book reviews, and chapter contributions.

Luciana Ximenez M.A., is a Clinical Psychologist, Master in Jungian Studies at PUC-SP, analyst in training at IJUSP, AJB and IAAP. Member of Lapa, archetypal psychology laboratory, founding member of Coletivo Aisthesis and coordinator of Thiasos, shared imagination workshop.

Part 3

The contributors to Part 3 will be kept anonymous.

Preface

The Covid-19 pandemic has had an immense influence on us all in the Jungian world, and documenting as well as understanding this is now, and in the years to come, a crucial task for our community. We have all had to adapt to profound changes whether being in places with lack of control or in places with strict lockdowns. The pandemic has forced us all to change our daily routines; most of us have been much more isolated than usual, and most of us could not see our patients physically in our clinics or meet with our colleagues at conferences, community meetings etc. Instead, the majority of us, more or less reluctantly, went online when analysing, supervising, and meeting with colleagues at online conferences and meetings. Jungian colleagues generously organised psychological aid for victims of the coronavirus which engaged a considerable number of Jungian analysts in helping infected patients, their families, as well as MDs, nurses and general medical staff involved in and affected by the Covid-19 crisis.[1]

The financial crisis following the outbreak of the pandemic challenged the economic situation for many of the IAAP societies and 2020 was a year of financial uncertainty for the IAAP as a whole. The IAAP Router Training Program was strongly affected because analysts, supervisors and teachers could not travel to the Developing Groups, so practically all work had to take place online. In order to preserve the frequency of the routers' analysis it became necessary to dispense and allow a larger number of online analytic sessions. Allowing online exams also became a necessity. Developing Groups were permitted to use their budget for a Zoom-Pro subscription and for professional AV-equipment so they could organise professionally held lectures and seminars with Jungian teachers from other countries.

All these decisions needed approval from the Executive Committee and, with the help of the IAAP lawyer, a legal way was found to approve online decisions. In spring 2020 two questionnaires were sent out: a questionnaire for all IAAP members about online analysis etc. and a questionnaire for examiners about online exams. The questionnaire for all IAAP members[2] revealed that a good number of analysts who had not used online analysis before the pandemic, now started to use it. The questionnaire also revealed that the lack of physical presence, interruptions due to poor connection, and difficulty finding a suitable room for online therapy were regarded to be the major disadvantages when using online analysis. Contrary to this, the possibility to continue therapy if the client and the analyst live far away from each other was regarded as a clear benefit. Also, the opportunity to work with the disabled, sick, mothers of new-borns, the minimized risk of infection, the avoidance of heavy traffic and expensive parking, the climate benefits, and the CO_2 saving were regarded as clear benefits. The questionnaire for examiners revealed that despite certain reservations with the changed situation, none of the respondents found that the result of the exams would have been different if it had taken place onsite. Both questionnaires supported the decision to dispense regarding analysis and exams within the Router Training Program, and they can now, when necessary, take place online. The pandemic has thus entailed both temporary and permanent changes within the IAAP. More online or hybrid arrangements have been adapted, as it became clear that e.g., online conferences allowed participation for many analysts and routers for whom it would not have been possible to travel to the planned conference site. Regular online meetings have been implemented within the IAAP administration; and Developing Groups continue, in addition to their local arrangements, to arrange online seminars and small conferences with both presenters and participants from other countries.

The Covid-19 pandemic has tested the whole Jungian community in a terribly difficult and painful way, but at the same time it has resulted in a considerable creativity in finding new solutions. The generous and very well-organised programs with psychological aid for victims of the coronavirus is an example of how Jungians can make a difference within our own field. It is an important part of our common Jungian identity also to be involved in psychological areas outside the traditional classical form and content.

We have by the pandemic been forced to leave our traditional comfort-zone and have reached out to other areas, practically, clinically, and theoretically. There has been a constant need to reflect on and understand the impact of the pandemic on our community as well as on each person involved. This has resulted in a comprehensive amount of articles[3] and conference presentations.[4] There have also been a number of (ongoing) research projects, supported by the IAAP. The research projects have primarily dealt with the influence on dreams during the pandemic.

The present book represents another very important research study, also supported by the IAAP, on how Jungian analysts as well as patients in analysis have personally been influenced by the pandemic; how they have reacted to this massive game-changing force, and what lasting changes it has brought about for them as well as for their theoretical, technical, clinical, and practical Jungian understanding. The first part of the book comprises a series of interviews with prominent authors of analytical psychology on how the Covid-19 pandemic including the lockdown has influenced them personally and professionally. The second part consists of personal essays from a number of analysts about experiences in their private practice and their reflections on how this has influenced and possibly changed their views on the clinical and theoretical aspects of their work. The third part brings important testimonies from patients in analysis on how the Covid-19 pandemic changed their analysis.

It is a great pleasure for me to acknowledge the excellent work done by the editors and all the contributors to this important book. Jungian theory is constantly evolving, but the pandemic has forced us to think faster and more focused on concrete physical challenges in order to continue our practice in entirely new, often unfamiliar ways. The pandemic has changed us all and we need tools to understand how. It is my belief that this book will make a lasting contribution to the understanding of how the pandemic changed the Jungian world and how creativity and profound reflectivity could help us all in finding new ways to continue the work that we all appreciate so much. I am sure that the book will be of great value to our Jungian community.

Misser Berg
IAAP President Elect

Notes

1 A further description of the psychological aid organised during 2020 in China, Italy and France can be seen at the IAAP website https://iaap.org/announcements/news/ and videos with interviews of key persons at https://iaap.org/media/ This generous work will be further documented in upcoming articles and research-projects.

2 The questionnaire to the membership: The use of online telecommunications by IAAP members (Data obtained during the Covid-19 pandemic) can be seen on the IAAP website, Members area: https://iaap.org/iaap-survey-2020/

3 A number of articles related to Covid-19 have been published in the *Journal of Analytical Psychology, 66*(3), June 2021

4 At the European Conference in Berlin (online), August 2021, several of the presentations dealt with various aspects of the Covid-19 pandemic.

Acknowledgements

Our gratitude goes to many. First of all to IAAP's President elect Misser Berg, and to IAAP' Academic Sub Committee, in the person of its Director, Prof. Pilar Amezaga, who recognized the importance of our project and decided to support it.

We are grateful to all the colleagues that accepted to contribute to this book in their own different capacities as interviewees, as analysts or patients writing on their own experience. Stefano Carpani thanks Carlo Alberto Fozzer and Ludmilla Ostermann for their editorial support for part 1 of this book.

We are thankful to Routledge, who decided to publish this book not academically pure and written *in media res*.

We would like to dedicate this book to the health care personnel who served during this unprecedented times risking their life and some loosing it.

Introduction
Stefano Carpani and Monica Luci

In early 2020, almost overnight, a sudden and massive spreading of a Coronavirus appeared as a pandemic, and brought profound and lasting changes in the ways we all live and work, in our inner and outer states, re-shaping radically the forms of our living together. Psychoanalytic practice was heavily affected by the pandemic, too, and this book focuses on this, offering a Jungian psychosocial analysis of what has been happening since then.

As we all know, under the mortal threat of the virus, some governments took measures to limit contagion with times of total lockdowns, and re-openings according to the rules of social distancing. The sudden and rigid containment measures transformed, almost overnight, our psychoanalytic practice from in presence to online for a significantly long period of time. After more than a century the boundaries of analysis were completely reshuffled. The frame, the traditional *temenos* of analytic therapy, was unquestionably dissolved in a few days: the general ground rules about the physical setting of place and time, the basic stance of the therapist, the couch, the room with its objects (let's think of sand play therapy or children therapy), the fee and ways of payment, the rituals of an embodied meeting were completely swept up and we had to deal with distance meetings, the (un)privacy of double rooms (the analyst's and the patient's) at home, screens, technology failures, to adapt to new safety standards.

This book provides space for Jungian psychoanalysts' early reflections on what they experienced and on their process of personal and professional adaptation to the profound, sometimes dramatic, changes in their life and to substantive changes of analysis and psychotherapy during the early phase of the pandemic. It also offers a glimpse into their working through of relevant issues connected to their practice.

In these new settings, for many patients past traumas were relived more easily, some re-experiencing chaotic families, others remembering the insecurity of economic hardship and uncertainty, for others the conditions of confinement creating fertile ground for domestic violence and abuse. The boundaries between past, present and future became more permeable, and traumatic memories were there available to be worked through and eventually integrated. The space and time of the daily lives of patients and analysts were completely 'altered' and the analytic setting as well. This concurred to what this book describes as the *suspension of certainties* and a *crumble* of the sense of time and rhythm of our outer and inner world.

The Tragedy and the Bewilderment: *Psychoagogia* and this Book

It is impossible to deal with the changes psychoanalysis underwent without looking deeper and placing it into what has dramatically been happening worldwide since early 2020, when Coronavirus started to infect and kill hundreds of thousands of people, spreading in populations one after another, at a much faster speed than we could realize. The severe restricting measures taken by governments were justified by the number of those dead and infected, and in some cases were extremely pervasive. They had a huge impact on people's life, and profoundly changed the lives of citizens, affecting their mental functioning and health. Limiting the discourse to the Western life style, children could no longer go to school, to their sports clubs, to music lessons; adolescents could hardly meet their peers and let alone go to parties; adults were forced to severely limit social contacts, professionally, personally, and in leisure activities; families were forced to share the space of their houses constantly during day and night as the only safe space. The elderly suffered and are still partially suffering immensely from social isolation, sometimes even dying alone. The death of those who passed away of Covid-19 was deprived of the rituals of funeral and burial, leaving family and friends to deal with a sort of suspended and 'ambiguous loss'. The countries that did not take measures to limit contagion had impressive numbers of deaths and difficulty to bury bodies. Dramatic images are impressed in our eyes of exhausted health staff in hospitals harnessed from top to toe, encapsulated in white overalls and protective equipment to isolate themselves from the virus; and stacked coffins, and transported by military trucks, waiting to be buried in large new cemeteries. For some this death reality was and still is so unbearable that the denial that all this happened is the only way to deal with this frightening reality. In this way, the pandemic globally affected the 'social link', *philia,* in all its forms: in the family, in love, at work, within friends, in politics, in psychoanalysis and, essentially, in our minds – our inner world.

Born in this context, this book looks like a collective mural that has been painted by many Jungian analysts that were interviewed in spring 2020 about the tragedy we were collectively living and who accepted to write short essays on how they felt in that exceptional circumstances, and how they adjusted their practice according to a new external and internal setting. The book has even the ambition of providing some flavour of the perspectives of patients, with a few contributions. And it is also a recollection on how analysts and analysands returned (or didn't) to in-person meetings with masks and disinfectants (or without), dealing with fear of contagion, trust and ways to handle all the related powerful emotions and ethical problems.[1]

The intuition beyond this book is that the method, the approach, the soul of analysis might have changed and under the influence of this huge global event. If and how this happened in each case can be different, and the editors' choice to include short essays from analysts and patients around the world is precisely to give this overall however-limited picture.

We ask for the reader's indulgence because this book was written *in medias res*, while the facts were unfolding. This has its merits and its defects.

One "defect" is that we wanted this book to be as personal as possible. For this reason, it is not scholarly or academic in the most strict and pure sense. It is dialogic and personal: a collection of interviews of people – an interviewer and an interviewee – in dialogue and short essays that have to do with *the personal* before any possible theorization on the topic. Although contributions here are certainly thoughtful and thought-provoking, the book wanted to offer space to emotions and intuitions, which reveal deeper truths in such emergency situations than well-crafted thoughts. And authors were free to address any topic they thought to be relevant in relation to this ongoing and continuously evolving situation.

One "merit" is that the interviews with some of the most influential Jungian psychoanalysts of the last generation (the so-called post-Jungians) were born out of necessity, i.e. guidance. At the time, the urgency was the need for *psychagogia*[2] by a group of wise wo/men, in an unprecedented historical time. This necessity of accompaniment – individual and collective – brought Stefano Carpani to interview Jungians during the early weeks of the pandemic, keeping in mind "how useful and effective perspectives derived from psychotherapy might be in the formation of policy, in new ways of thinking about the political process" (Samuels, 2001). Therefore, Carpani had the hopeful expectation that in such a difficult time Jungian analysts had "views to offer on social issues that involve personal relations" (Samuels, 2001: 2), reiterating the relevance of C. G. Jung's work today, as well as to the work of the post-Jungians and neo-Jungians (Carpani, 2021). These interviews became very popular[3] on You-Tube, which suggest that they worked as a sort of psychosocial tool to orientate and help people to cope with events. He interviewed these distinguished analysts, authors and thinkers, to ask them what was happening, how best to deal with the pandemic and what seemed a completely new phase of human history; and how best to survive *the suspension of certainties,* professional and personal, to which we were accustomed. The Jungians, each in their own way, provided their cues, certainly idiosyncratic but in which the reader can recognize and discern a common basic attitude, i.e. a Jungian *humus* toward the pandemic, the analysis and the world.

Many are the themes that are touched in this book, including: the psychological effects of lockdown and living in confinement; the question of illness and death; new beginnings; the theme of addictions and technology; the tasks for psychoanalysts; vulnerability and responsibility; personal reflections on how the restrictions affected the analytical work, but also very personal accounts of how the relationships with patients changed for good and for bad from the subjective perspective of the therapist. Other topics addressed are the mental attitude toward science, individuation and rhythm in the modern (accelerated/decelerated) society, the role of body in therapy, the analytic work online, even creative ways of surviving through poetry during the Pandemic.

Thus, the sense of this book is much wider than the "*zoomification* of analysis*,*" as some might suppose, although the problematic issues of 'distance and technologically mediated analysis' are a big part of the transformation of analysis and this is worth to be mentioned and discussed here. This debate about online work is not new, it has been going on for years and was characterized by high ambivalences and conflicting arguments.[4] However, as it always happens in individual and social emergencies, action comes first – reflection comes later. In one night many arguments and doubts had to be abruptly wiped away: the treatment by video or telephone was and, still in some regions is, often the only responsible means for many analysts, to continue the treatment especially in case of vulnerable patients or analysts (or some members in their families). Thus, we (almost) all adopted these changes, accepting them, willy nilly, as a necessity, trying to reflect while practicing them. In most of cases, the use of telecommunications allowed patients and therapists to 'co-create' a new frame for analytic work because, as Ogden anticipated some years ago (2005, p. 101), after all "The container is not a thing, but a process," although the possibility for all patients and therapists to access to this process without the support of the physical container in the traditional setting (Cwik, 2021) continues to be open to questions.

Some Tentative Reflections on Society and the Lessons of the Coronavirus

We believe that the ongoing evolving situation prevents us to deeply reflect on our recent experience. In fact, as we write, in winter 2021, there are new partial lockdowns established by governments as a consequence of new waves of mutations of the virus, and the constantly changing situation makes it hard to focus on the beginnings. Albeit refraining from providing 'strong' psychosocial readings of the reality we are still living, we think it is worth reaching some tentative considerations.

The Coronavirus pandemic is not the first worldwide plague psychoanalysis has gone through; however, we can assume with some degree of confidence that this event has unprecedented features. The speed of the spread of the virus, due to the high intensity of movement of people and goods in our globalized world, probably made it distinct from the multiple previous episodes of the plague and other epidemics of history, enormously increasing the impact of the infection and the depth of its permeation of the social life.

Many wished the pandemic to be nothing else then a bad dream: a nightmare. The truth is that it is still a reality for the majority of the world population, as we write. Renate Daniel (2016) underlined that we have nightmares when our soul is in distress and adds that, sometimes, a nightmare can be so intense that a physical reaction occurs. Can Covid-19 (with its lack of breath), therefore, be read as a nightmare humanity has to face? According to psychoanalysis nightmares can disappear only when its meaning is depicted. What is the ultimate meaning of the pandemic? Is Coronavirus a compensation? In case, of what?

Going beyond Bauman's theorization of *liquid modernity and society* (2000; 2007), with this pandemic we realized that the past decade could be called the *All You Can Eat Society* which is a "second-late modern" society[5] where the knowledge of *value* has been reshaped, and where the value of boundaries has been increasingly denied.

This second-late modern society seems to be a *bulimic* one, where it is possible to pay 9,99€ for dinner at a buffet restaurant and eat without limits, to vomit such meal and to eat again.[6] It is a society based on *24/7 hyperentertainment* (which – again – is without limit, hence endless) and where you can buy a T-shirt for 0,99€ without caring about the ethical implications of its cost and the consequences of such purchase.

The exploitation of natural resources, the systematic destruction of the ecosystems in which humans and animals live, as a function of limitless economic development, and of an unlimited, again, growth of the world population. After all, isn't the spill-over of viruses from animals to humans also the result of this systematic destruction of ecosystems and the consequent inappropriate contact with animals, besides our 'overeating' and mistreating them?, (Think of 'wet markets' supposedly the origin of the spill-over of Coronavirus).

The pandemic confirmed the already existent and change-resistant inequalities, one of which is that the most advanced countries were able to protect themselves and others didn't. That the most industrialized countries of the world were able to produce and offer free of charge vaccines to their population, while developing countries couldn't and still rely on the advanced ones for their supplies. Therefore, social inequality did not change, they even worsened. The gap between rich and poor, privileged and unprivileged is continuously widening. Mental health became a hidden emergency: evidence shows that the number of depressive disorders and other psychosomatic and mental illnesses have increased (Leuzinger-Bohleber and Blass, 2021). Domestic violence and sexual assaults, especially on women and children, reports state, are increased in frequency (Sacco et al., 2020). The systemic consequences are enormous: jobs are threatened, international supply chains were negatively affected, the social and economic consequences are still hardly assessable. The tensions in the societies, the paranoid splitting, social fragmentation, and susceptibilities to populistic and nationalistic seductions worldwide are unmistakable.

The pandemic proved that the lesson brought about by German sociologist Ulrich Beck, according to whom: "nature can be no longer understood *outside of society*, or society *outside of nature*" (Beck, 1992, p. 80) is still relevant. He thought that, "The principle of nation sovereignty, independence and autonomy is an obstacle to survival of humankind" and that the "'Declaration of Independence' has to be metamorphosed into the 'Declaration of Interdependence': cooperate or die!" (p. 38). And this, we propose, has to be on a global scale because of "the traumatic vulnerability of all and the resulting responsibility for all, including one's own survival" (p. 38). Beck even belived that, "Climate change may change the world for the better" (p. 48), if we are ready to act cooperatively. Inactions is fostered by deniers and often the deniers have also a nationalist mentality. Beck says "nationalism is particularly toxic" (p. 55), therefore he proposes a cosmopolitan perspective.

We, the editors of this book, believe that the pandemic, which exposed us all to profound uncertainty, can prove to be an opportunity for change and new beginnings. An opportunity to *decelerate*, to ponder and to realize that *Nature* wanted us to pass from the outer world to the inner one, from extroversion to introversion, then to the interior and the soul. To be able, later, to return outside and maintain an inner-outer balance.

A main "post-Covid challenge" seems to be that of moving from a world based on *hopes and expectations* of the linear world to one where *interiority and spirituality*, non-necessarily religious, returns to be contemplated, so that something new can really begin to sprout: creativity from the soul. In this sense, "authentic creativity" (creative fantasy) is what is lacking in a second-late modern society.[7] Creativity and creative fantasy help fluidity and pluralism and if fluidity, rather than individualization and liquidity, is fostered, there will be a chance to contrast anxiety, depression, suicidality, and, therefore, anomie. Anomie occurs when emotions are stuck, while, when one is able to "translate the emotions into images – that is to say, to find the images which were concealed in the emotions' (Jung, MDR), one becomes inwardly calmed and reassured" (Carpani, 2020b, p. 235).

Ágnes Heller, in her book titled *Dubitare fa bene?* (2017) underlines – quoting Kierkegaard – that philosophy begins with doubt, that the *sceptics* made of doubt the key against dogma, and that Descartes considered doubt at the centre of human existence. Therefore, she claims, doubting is equivalent to thinking and philosophers have always seen doubt as the foundation of an indubitable knowledge.

As of spring 2020 we have been living in a new context, that of the doubt and *the suspension of certainties*, i.e. the immovable certainties of modern life to which we have become accustomed in recent decades. A life made up of accelerations and the rush for success, in order to become some-one, instead of daring to investigate who we really are and what we really want. *The suspension of certainties* made us experience feeling and emotions that were hidden in our own Pandora's box and that suddenly and almost overnight were liberated by the lockdown.

The suspension of certainties, that was truly frightening for many, became – for those that dared to have the courage to look into their own Pandora's box – a space for reflection and for learning the art of patience.

In a second-late modern society, there is fresh need for renewed internal dialogue hopefully leading towards one's individuation (Carpani 2022). While we are aware of the risk to be perceived as näives and that Michel Houelle-becq's prediction – "the world will be the same, only some worse"[8] – might reveal itself true, our task as psychoanalysts and activists is to work for individual and collective change, even individuation. Ultimately, the pandemic begs the question: who are we? How do we want to live?

Going Back to the Psychological

What seems to be certain is that from a psychological perspective, "we have been living in a time of a massive *abaissement du niveau mental*, brought about by Covid-19" (Bryon 2021, p. 399). The *abaissement* is a prodrome of changes that can be positive or negative, but always functional to a new psychological adaptation to reality. Analysis needs adaptation to this new reality, too. Amid the pandemic, the practice of psychoanalysis faces new horizons, new boundaries, new openings. And it cannot ignore that its ethic is being at the service of the tragic experience of life, responding with responsible enacted therapeutic stance to it.

Reflecting on pandemic, Murray Stein in an online interview said,

> The image that comes to my mind is an *Umbra Mundi*, a world shadow hovering over us and infecting our psychic lives. I see this shadow spreading over the globe like a solar eclipse. The alchemical term for it is *nigredo*.
>
> (2020)

This

> depicts a period when life is full of confusion and bewilderment, disorientation, sickness of spirit and confrontation with the repressed shadows. During [such] liminal times the sense of direction is beclouded, one cannot move, the way is uncharted, unmarked [...] Old habits do not guide any longer. One is at a crossroads, confused and torn. Essentially, ego-consciousness has yet to work out a new relationship with the unconscious.
>
> (Schwartz, 2021, p. 523)

Donal Kalsched suggests that this experience with Sars-Covid-2 pandemic is to be linked to that of trauma, which simply refers to the fact that *"we all were given more to experience in this life than we can bear to experience consciously.*

This means that psychological defences will be necessary to help us survive experiences we cannot yet integrate" (2021, p. 444).

While writing, in Western countries the situation is more bearable thanks to massive campaigns of vaccination of the population. However, we are still in the process to re-opening our activities and social life to embodied social interactions. In addition, large layers of world population have not had access to vaccines yet. And in this kind of problem every person all over the world is only safe to the degree that everyone in the whole globe is safe. The virus does not discriminate, but its impact exposes deep weaknesses in the delivery of health services and the structural inequalities that impede access to them. We also see more systemic "side-effects" of the pandemic like the rise of hate speech, the targeting of vulnerable groups, and against the background of rising ethno-nationalism, populism, authoritarianism and a push-back against human rights in some countries. This crisis can provide a pretext to adopt repressive measures for purposes unrelated to the pandemic and can potentially cause other crises that are pandemic-related, albeit in non-obvious ways.

Kalsched reminds us, also, that in case of

an outer crisis like Covid-19 is metabolized by us psychologically, involving the imagination in the pathology of defence on the one hand or in the creative process of making deeper meaning on the other. The imagination can work either 'for' or 'against' us as we struggle to adapt to an outer crisis.

(2021, p. 447)

The paranoid thinking is always there, available for use when we are left to cower in fear in the presence of an invisible threat. In such circumstances, paranoia is defending people and today we see it in the denial of the pandemic by certain groups and in people who do not want to take vaccine for fear of being injected something dangerous, or something through which they can be controlled by the government or pharmaceutical industries, or some other power. We think this is 'imagination working against' or *archetypically.*

Going back to the main topic of our book, which is the practice and experience of analysis under such exceptionally new circumstances, an interesting and creative exercise of imagination ('imagination working for') is carried out by Kristina Schellinski (2021) in her article "Essential anxiety: Covid-19 in analytic practice." She found in an imaginative etymology of the word COVID the suggestion for a direction to follow: *CO* as 'together' and *VID* as 'see', in other words, *together we see.* We understand this as an invite to reconnection, at the same time our inner connection and connection with others; the reconnection to the Self and to others that create the possibility of 'soul making' together, amplifying our capability of making meanings comprehending ourselves and the world.

This intention is what humbly inspired this book fostering connections in our professional and personal experience because "*together we see,*" connecting to each other our ability to understand our experience is amplified.

Book Layout: A Reader's Guide

We suggest the reader pick the theme that is most appealing to them, instead of following a cover-to-cover reading approach.

The book is divided into three parts. The first part is entirely composed of interviews of authoritative Jungian analysts, conducted by Carpani, on a variety of themes related to the Pandemic during the earliest phase of lockdown. The second part is made up of essays, sketching out the subjective experience of Jungian therapists world-wide in relation to what was happening in their lives and practice. They reflect on diverse topics, especially how the Covid-19 pandemic and lockdown measures affected and changed the analytical work with patients. The third and concluding part is specular to the second. Some analysts in training agreed to write, anonymously, short essays to open a small window on the perspective of patients in analysis during these dramatic times. We asked these 'patients' to give testimonies of the experience of the change of setting, mindset and related implications. Unfortunately, not all the contributions we received in the end could be published, because of understandable changes of mind about the possibility of publishing such sensitive material.[9]

Here is a grouping of the themes at hand.

The Psychological Effects of a Lockdown

In her interview, Verena Kast underlines that anxiety and collective solidarity are aspects of the pandemic. She emphasizes the importance of accepting the crisis in general and facing anxiety by coming into contact with other people. The activation of imagination in the collective by sharing memories is key according to her. She wishes for a shift from autonomy towards humility and solidarity because the problem lies within the idea that people do not depend on each other. Murray Stein states that the unconscious is very active during times of crisis (like in lockdown) because when being inactive socially, psychic energy can regress and flow back into the unconscious and activate autonomous complexes. Stefano Candellieri and Davide Favero questioned themselves on what was happening at a psychosocial level, focusing not only on the most immediate level of the ongoing traumatic experience but also on the pre-existing critical social issues that the Sars-CoV-2 pandemic contributed to make more evident, such as individualism and anomie.

Illness and Death

Stein underlines that the fear of death is archetypal, and, as animals we instinctively want to live, but he sees in the pandemic an opportunity of talking of death, a topic so intensely avoided in the Western world. Paul Attinello – stating the necessity to take the fear of death very seriously – looks at our relationship to illness and death, the ways that panic or avoidance appear, and our personal and cultural and political assessments. Applying Susan Sontag's work *Illness as Metaphor* a disease that affect the lungs – as Covid-19 does – John Beebe stands for an illness of the soul. On this regard Beebe seizes the opportunity to discuss the complexity of metaphors and shares his experience as medical student when he learned how violently the body wards off illnesses – to the extent of dying from it. Renate Daniel talks about sleep as a state of unconsciousness (giving up control) and links this circumstance to the pandemic and death – a part of nature humankind fears deeply. She observes that we live in a society that is too concerned about the physical death and adds that Covid-19 – like giving up control in a dream – shows the limits of humankind's power to overcome nature.

New Beginnings

Beebe touches upon Jung's concept of extraversion and introversion and urges committed attention instead to defensive extraversion. For him it is a chance to take better care of oneself and each other. Stein suggests introversion to explore the inner world and become creative with the images that appear – like Jung himself did with the *Red Book*. Kast wishes for a shift towards humility and solidarity and sees the possibility of change and a good life after the pandemic. She expresses her hope for a critical mass within society that starts to make change happen. Ursula Brasch emphasizes the crucial nature of breathing and the symbolism of breathing as a connection between the outer and the inner world, between the body and its environment. She claims that this is deeply disturbed by the pandemic and asks whether the effect on life will be like a wake-up call, a point in time when real changes happen. For Susan Rowland, creativity is at the heart of who we are and being creative is only possible when we are not certain about everything. The Coronavirus, she states, functions as an invasion of the unknown psyche into our collective world and questions everything we knew. However, by giving up on certainties we are able to change and adapt. According to Andrew Samuels, change in a world of climate crisis and economic inequality is not easy. And that is where he sees therapists come in that insist on change and face the struggle together with progressive forces. He sees a basis for taking risks in the world, especially within the younger generations.

Addictions and Technology

Beebe recognizes that people went through a phase of hyperactivism, entertaining themselves with Zoom calls and online activities and he wonders if doing so they (we!) miss the opportunity to take a new perspective on the world. Candellieri and Favero reflect on the pervasive spread of digital tools and social-media, the emotional-cognitive dissociation of a human being on the one hand hyper-technological and on the other prey to primitive and pervasive emotional states. By using the example of the British physicist Stephen Hawking, Rowland speaks out for a new view on technology. She points at the Janus-face of technology: We use it, it uses us. Therefore, Rowland speaks out for a new view on technology, in which she sees also a chance for individuation.

The Task for Psychoanalysis

Kast underlines that out task is to be the advocate of dealing with the inner world that gains importance during lockdown. By doing so, change is possible. Attinello looks at the political and communicative chaos that appeared in the first month of the epidemic, linking it to different cultural and psychological interpretations, ultimately wishing to return to a basic ground of existential awareness around this crisis, which is also, unavoidably, a space for change. Samuels asks "does the coronavirus create a momentum that leads to change?" He states that it is by taking action that psychology can help transformation during a crisis like Covid-19. In doing so he reminds us of *Accogliere le ferrite di chi cura*, an initiative that the editors of this book (with Maria Giovanna Bianchi, Roberto Grande, Antonio Lanfranchi, Alessandra di Montezemolo, Eva Pattis-Zoja, Chiara Tozzi with the precious the support of Paola Cascino, and the generous availability of about 130 Italian analysts) formed to provide psychological help to Covid-frontline-workers in Italy free of charge. Brasch looks at the symbolism of breathing as a connection between the outer and the inner world, between the body and its environment. She suggests that this concept is deeply disturbed by the pandemic.

Vulnerability and Responsibility

Another theme that runs through the chapters of this book, is the link between vulnerability and responsibility. On this issue, Kast, underlines that the problem lies within the idea that people do not depend on each other, and the illusion that every single person has control on his or her own life. On the other hand, Samuels laments the words "We are all in this together" that came up shortly after lockdowns were enacted worldwide, it does not reflect the real situation: he points out that billions of people (including refugees) were not in the same position as those in the First World that can lock themselves into beach houses or cottages.

The Outer and the Inner World

Tiffany Houck-Loomis calls for a radical reconceptualization of the ethical responsibility of the analyst in and out of the office. Instead of the old analytic dictum, "The patient cannot go where the analyst has not gone," the patient should take the analyst where the analyst unknowingly needs to go but has not yet been able to go. Milena Kohli argues that the pandemic and the measures introduced to stop the spreading of the virus lead to slowing down of life and provide the possibility of the return to oneself, seeing in the current situation both a danger and a chance for Western society. Heyong Shen uses the I Ching images and the images of Chinese characters as threads to analyze the meaning of "suffering" and "anxiety," "compassion," and "transformation," four words that characterize our time of pandemic. Luciana Ximenez notices that the extreme search for consumption and production leads to pressures for similarity and demand for performance. The quarantine imposes a mandatory slow down, a "great introversion," an opportunity for us to go into the transformation cave. Ximenez questions if this demand for slowing down and deceleration may also be a form of pressure towards similarity. Dan Cross noticed a trend in which science is increasingly doubted or rejected in casual, off-handed ways. He analyzes one quotation representing this distrust (The quotation is "I was thinking that I should get vaccinated, but I'm not going to, because they [the vaccines] haven't been tested. This is just a big experiment on people. I'm not sure the virus is even real anyways. You know, science doesn't really know much.") as representative of this trend, and offers a psychological interpretation of the attitude of mind that it reflects. Roula-Maria Dib explores the soothing effects and boundary-breaking role of poetry during the recent times of global crisis. Her chapter looks at the therapeutic side of poetry, which manifested during the unfolding of a literary community.

Online Analysis

John Merchant reports on analysts' very personal responses to working online including the adjustment to online sessions as well as exhaustion and an overall finding that online work does not preclude a genuine analytic process. Tine Papič looks at how video technology influences the analysis (especially when analysands home is part of the analytical setting) and how to deal with the problems that might emerge while using it. Mark Winborn highlights the alterations that occur in the field when physical bodies are not mutually present, the reduction in analytic ritual and frame that occurs when analysis is mediated via computer and possible negative impact of these developments on future psychoanalysts and therapists. In Part 3, K.E.K. reflects on the phases of approaching and departing from the analytic hour as a ritual integral to the therapeutic phenomenon that shapes the analytical experience. This essay explores how this ritual "frame" that occurs in therapy helps to facilitate the desires, emotions, thoughts or intuitions that one is waiting to emerge in each session. M.S., also in Part 3, accounts for a personal reaction to lockdown measures, a gradual exit from a state of denial and an adjustment to the new situation. The chapter focuses on personal analysis, especially on transference dynamics and on a different meaning connected with the process taking place in the unconscious.

The Personal and the Professional in a Different Analytical Setting

Misser Berg describes reactions among her patients to when she had to close her clinic. She reflects on her own reactions and the gradual change in her attitude towards online work from a rather one-sided focus on the benefits of online work to a more balanced position. Olivia del Castillo delves into her experience of changes in the analytical framework. According to her, ethical doubts and the mourning for what was lost could not be ignored. Roberto Grande emphasizes the sensory limitation and therefore the value of it in the therapeutic relationship. He believes that, in order to get out of the pandemic and the climate risk, it is necessary to reflect on the irrational collective components that prevent better psychic and social functioning. Emilija Kiehl tells us that psychosomatic aspects of the interactive field cannot be "transported" from a shared physical space into cyberspace. In this new reality, new themes are entering the analytic space that occupy patients and analysts. Marianne Müller illustrates her professional experience as a psychotherapist, focusing on the setting, referring to the large number of younger clients who came into therapy during the pandemic. In the closing remarks, she specifically questions the analytic attitude in this time of the pandemic. Jon Mills in a most personalized narrative, reflects – having decided to retire from practice during the age of Covid-19 – on his career as a psychologist and psychoanalyst in his final days of terminating with his long-term analytic patients. His musings on the end of analysis, the client-therapist relationship, and mutual recognition are emphasized during the final session of therapy. Nancy Robinson-Kime reflects on the process of working online both before and during the pandemic, looking at the analytic container. The relationship between outer and inner, the concrete-material and psychological is discussed in various contexts: the analyst's office, the patient's home, etc. Her view of the analytic container expands from its concrete determinants into a psychological process of connecting and relating to psychic energy through whatever means possible. Pia Skogemann describes how in different cases the change of setting was worked though together with patients. She found much more complicated to handle the teaching of the candidates; learn how to use Zoom for teaching purposes and adapting the day schedule, overcoming the online fatigue and finding new ways of feeling together for the group while teaching and learning. Ruth Williams touches on the trauma of living in the period 'as if' it was a war. She reviews some of the practical ramifications which have flowed from the shifts which have been thrust on to practitioners as well as ethical concerns.

The Body in Online Analysis

Daniela Eulert-Fuchs, taking the unexpected and sudden termination of an analysis by a patient as a starting point, asks what impact the pandemic had on the analytic space, and in particular on patients with early relational trauma. She also questions whether the analyst's analytic ability may have been reduced due to her unconscious fear of the virus and reflects on the possible impact of this fact on the analytic process. Paolo Ferliga focuses on the changes that distance therapy generates in relation to the body which plays a very important role in the *co-transference*, the relationship between therapist and patient. After describing the problems generated by this situation, the author shows the role that mindfulness and active imagination can play in fostering communication and exchange in the analytic couple. In Part 3, J.F. explores the wonders of online therapy, focusing on embodiment and the ability to phantasize and float comfortably in space. She shows how she draws on body memory and the power of imagination when relating to the image of her therapist on a screen.

This journey through different themes of the book is not intended to be exhaustive.

Notes

1 Even today, while writing on the autumn 2021, many colleagues continue to work remotely, depending on how strongly the Pandemic is hitting their country, the rhythm of vaccinations or have decided to shut down completely their in-person-practice and moved to an online-only practice, or even retired.
2 *Psychoagogia* means "guidance of the soul" or "soul-leading." Socrates (in Plato"s *Phaedrus*, 261a) claims that, "Is not rhetoric in its entire nature an art which leads the soul by means of words, not only in law courts and other public assemblies, but in private discussions as well?"
3 Verena Kast's and Murray Stein's interviews on YouTube, alone, were viewed by more than 20,000 people.
4 Before this emergency we had authors emphasizing advantages of "technologically mediated therapy" (Branham, 2017) and authors who more definitively cautioned about the use of telecommunications in analysis, and those who tried to make an open-minded critical evaluation of both (Merchant, 2016; 2021).
5 "Modernity is the term used to refer to the ways of living, or social organizations, which appeared in Europe around the 17th century and extended their influence to most of the world. [...] an essential element of modernity is the notion of change and progress" (Carpani, 2004). "Modernity evolves into what Beck and Beck-Gernsheim (2002) call "reflexive modernization" or "second modernity," what Giddens (1990) calls "high" or "late" modernity and what sociologist Zygmunt Bauman (2000) calls "liquid" modernity. This is characterized by the intensification and speeding up of aspects such as reflexivity (Beck, Giddens, & Lash, 1994) and the reduction of space and time separation (Giddens, 1990)" (Carpani, 2022). "A second-late modern society is characterized by the acceleration and compression of the afore mentioned traits (enabling 24/7 connectedness) and could situate it's beginning with the launch of the first smart phone (iPhone) on June 29th 2007. Taking this into account, and in the extremization of Marcuse's 1964's view of the West as of an Advanced Industrial Society (1986), a second-late modern could also be termed *Electronic Accelerated Society*" (Carpani, 2022).

6 It is also an *emotionally bulimic society*, where people ingest an unprecedented amount of emotions daily, to later vomit them because they cannot deal (process) and digest them.

7 A "second-late modern society" or "second-late individualized society" – as Carpani underlines elsewhere (2022), followed the previous (second or late modernity) without a break. The start of this epoch can be traced back to the launch of the first iPhone in 2007, because the incorporation of this technology in our daily lives changed it radically in terms of how and when we are connected with others and the world. When looking at Giddens' (1990) claim that late modernity reduces the separation of space and time, second-late modernity does so even more. Also Umbach's and Huppauf's (2005, p.8) concepts of flux, change, and unpredictability become accelerated. This period, in the radicalization of Marcuse's definition of modernity as "advanced industrial society" (Marcuse, 1986, p. xv), can also be named "advanced electronic society" or "accelerated electronic society."

8 Translated from Italian. Retrieved from *Corriere della Sera*: www.corriere.it/esteri/20_maggio_04/houellebecq-cari-amici-mondo-sara-uguale-solo-po-peggiore-e512c852-8e40-11ea-b08e-d2743999949b.shtml

9 For the contributions published here, we were given permissions and they are anonymous.

References

Bauman, Z. (2000). *Liquid Modernity*. Cambridge: Polity.

Bauman, Z., (2007). *Liquid Times*. Cambridge: Polity Press.

Beck, U. (1992). *Risk Society. Towards a New Modernity*. London: Sage Publications.

Beck, U., and Beck-Gernsheim, E. (2002). *Individualization: Institutionalized Individualism and its Social and Political Consequences*. London: Sage.

Beck, U., Giddens, A., and Lash, S. (1994). *Reflexive Modernization. Politics, Tradition and Aesthetics in the Modern Social Order*. Cambridge: Polity Press.

Brahnam, S. (2017). "Comparison of in-person and screen-based analysis using communication models: A first step toward the psychoanalysis of telecommunications and its noise.." *Psychoanalytic Perspectives, 14* (2), 138–158.

Bryon, D. (2021). "Processing trauma in psychoanalysis in 'real' time and in dreams: The convergence of the past, present and future during COVID-19." *Journal of Analytical Psychology, 66* (3), 399–410.

Carpani, S. (2004). *The Formation of Narratives of Self-identities. A Study of the Turkish Community in Berlin*. Unpublished M.Phil. thesis. University of Cambridge.

Carpani, S. (2020a). *Breakfast at Küsnacht: Conversations on C. G. Jung and Beyond*. Asheville: Chiron.

Carpani, S. (2020b). "The Consequences of Freedom." In E. Brodersen and P. Amezaga (Eds.), *Jungian Perspectives on Indeterminate States: 'Betwixt and Between' Borders*. Routledge.

Carpani, S. (2021). *The Plural Turn in Jungian and Post-Jungian Studies: The Work of Andrew Samuels*. London & New York: Routledge.

Carpani, S. (2022). *Absolute Freedom: The I+I (Individuation + Individualization) as a Metanarrative of Self-Development in a Second-Late-Modern Society*. Unpublished Ph.D. thesis. University of Essex.

Cwik, A. J. (2021). "The technologically-mediated self: reflection on the container and field of telecommunications." *Journal of Analytical Psychology, 66* (3), 411–428.

Daniel, R. (2016). *Taking the Fear Out of the Night: Coping with Nightmares*. Einsiedeln: Daimon Verlag.

Giddens, A. (1990). *The Consequences of Modernity*. Cambridge: Polity Press.

Heller, A., (2017), *Dubitare fa bene?* Roma: Castelvecchi.

Kalsched, D. (2021). "Intersections of personal vs. collective trauma during the COVID-19 pandemic: The hijacking of the human imagination." *Journal of Analytical Psychology, 66* (*3*), 443–462.

Leuzinger-Bohleber, M., & Blass, H. (2021). "Editorial introduction: Psychoanalytic perspectives on the COVID-19 pandemic." *International Journal of Applied Psychoanalytic Studies, 18* (*2*), 109–120.

Marcuse, H. (1986). *One-Dimensional Man*. London: Ark.

Merchant, J. (2016). "The use of Skype in analysis and training: A research and literature review." *Journal of Analytical Psychology, 61* (*3*), 309–328.

Merchant, J. (2021). "Working online due to the COVID-19 pandemic: The hijacking of the human imagination." *Journal of Analytical Psychology, 66* (*3*), 484–505.

Ogden, T. (2005). "On holding and containing, being and dreaming." In *This Art of Psychoanalysis: Dreaming Undreamt Dreams and Interrupted Cries*. London: Routledge, pp. 93–108.

Sacco, M. A., Caputo, F., Ricci, P., Sicilia, F., De Aloe, L., Bonetta, C. F., Cordasco, F., Scalise C., Cacciatore, G., Zibetti, A., Gratteri, S., and Aquila, I. (2020). "The impact of the Covid-19 pandemic on domestic violence: The dark side of home isolation during quarantine." *Medico-Legal Journal 88* (*2*): 71–73.

Samuels, A. (2001). *Politics on the Couch*. London: Profile Books.

Schellinski, K. (2021). "Essential anxiety: COVID-19 in analytic practice." *Journal of Analytical Psychology, 66* (*3*), 534–545.

Schwartz, S. (2021). "COVID-19, precarity and loneliness." *Journal of Analytical Psychology, 66* (*3*), 517–533.

Stein, M. (2020, April 1). "'A World Shadow: COVID-19', interview by R. Henderson." https://chironpublications.com/a-world-shadow-covid-19/

Umbach, M., and Huppauf, B. (2005). *Vernacular Modernism: Heimat, Globalisation, and the Built Environment*. Stanford: Stanford University Press.

Part 1

Chapter 1

Spring and Imagination

Verena Kast

Verena Kast addresses the themes of anxiety and collective solidarity during the pandemic. The expert on crisis intervention emphasizes the importance of accepting the crisis in general and facing anxiety by coming into contact with other people: after all, it's a shared crisis. This interaction turns out be fruitful as soon as ideas of dealing with the crisis come up – even if we are left with the uncertainty about its end. At this moment, the activation of imagination by sharing memories is key. The task for psychoanalysts in particular is to be the advocate of dealing with the inner world which gains importance during lockdown because, by doing so, change becomes possible. She wishes for a shift from autonomy towards humility and solidarity. The problem lies within the idea that people do not depend on each other, that every single person controls his or her own life. In the last part of the interview, Verena Kast gives an outlook on the near future that is positive. She sees the possibility of change and a good life after the pandemic, not based on consumption but on being more at one with nature.

Stefano Carpani: Professor Kast, Dear Verena, good evening and thank you very much for accepting to talk to me in these, I would say, strange days.

Verena Kast: Good evening, Stefano. I'm happy to talk to you.

SC: My first question is: How are you and where are you?

VK: I am in my home. I'm isolated. I'm not going out, sure I'm going out for some walks, but not for shopping or something similar. So I am really isolated, but I have a good house and a nice garden and so I can walk in the house and around the house. I am fine for the moment, and I hope that I will stay fine also for the future, I hope

SC: We are both isolated. Most of the Western world is isolated. And this is the news. I would like to ask you another question, which you usually ask us when we do group supervision with you: how do you feel?

VK: This is a very important question. I have contradictory feelings: on one hand I love being at home. I like it to be at home. Everything is cancelled. OK, I have to attend some meetings online, but there is a lot of free time, it's a lot of time to deal with myself. On the other hand: when I think about what is going on in the world, about people who die, who get infected, but also when I think about all of

DOI: 10.4324/9781003266402-1

my colleagues who have not anymore so many clients because the clients are not coming, or if I see some musicians I know who lose their whole income, and we do not know how long it will last, and when I think of economics, then I feel very, very bad. And then I see the wonderful spring coming. Spring always means a lot for me, it is connected with genuine hope. And I think it's so important that I keep in my emotions both sides: one side where I'm really sad and I feel very much with these people who have really difficulties for the moment. And on the other hand I see the spring and that life is going on.

SC: Yes, it's interesting, spring and life is going on. But psychologically, what is happening psychologically? The virus is spreading and many Westerners thought, oh, it's in China, it will not come to us as it didn't come a few years ago. But now it's spreading globally. There is uncertainty, there is denial, big denial. That's why perhaps countries like Italy and Spain and France had to enforce the lockdown. There is even fear of how long the lockdown will be. What is the impact of this anxiety, panic, but also collective solidarity?

VK: Talking about the denial, we have a far-reaching crisis, and when people are in crisis, they have three possibilities. One possibility is the denial it does not exist. The other possibility: one is full of anxieties and helpless. And the third one is experiencing and facing anxiety. We accept it. We say we don't like it, but we accept it. And we try to make the best out of this situation. Denial is one way. If we have a crisis, we don't want to have the crisis. We deny it as a first reaction to calm ourselves first. I personally think that with this virus, our anxiety is very reasonable and high. Usually in our societies, the fear of death is repressed and now we have to face it. The fear is emerging and it's so hard and it's so impossible for us because we have the conviction that we can manage everything, that we are in control. And this small virus shows us that we only believe that we can manage everything, but this not correct. And this makes us very helpless. Even more reason to repress it. But not only, you mentioned the solidarity. And I'm really impressed by the solidarity I experience. I'm even impressed when I go for a walk. Everyone says, hello, how are you? We don't know each other and we shouldn't even speak to each other on our walks due to the problem of getting infected – but we talk a bit, it is warm, we are in the open, and we are connected.

SC: I think of the initiative in Italy and even here in Berlin, young people or younger people send messages to people that maybe cannot leave the house or elderly people. They offer to buy groceries for others. You are an expert on crisis intervention. Which are the possible scenarios, psychologically, for us as practitioners, as psychoanalysts? What is our job now? To comfort? To accompany? To survive? What do you think?

VK: I think there are different aspects. What the Italian colleagues are doing with their project to help people who are helping others and who are in despair, is really helpful. I think we have also – if we were asked – to tell people how we can deal with this crisis. One important aspect of dealing with the crisis is to accept that we have a crisis. And if I have a crisis, I am in anxiety. And for this I need the other, I need to contact others, it must not necessarily be physical contact.

Physical contact would be better, but we have to open up see other people, to talk to other people about our anxieties. It is a bit easier, because it is a shared crisis. When we are sharing our anxieties, new ideas are coming up for resolving the questions we have: how can we deal with the crisis, especially what are my resources, where I am strong and how can I face the problem of this crisis knowing that we do not know how long it will last. This is a huge problem because we are very good in managing crisis when we estimate it to last for some weeks. But when we don't know how long it will be, this bothers us a lot. But this is the same with some illnesses: we have to refer back to ourselves in all the uncertainty and ask ourselves what is the most important for me in the moment. And one very helpful aspect for dealing with the crises is the imagination. When you are caught in anxieties, you have only this kind of imagination of everything getting worse and will end in a catastrophe for sure. Sure: we have to be concrete and realistic. It is a very serious situation, but we have also the imagination of good things at our disposition, we have good memories creating hopeful wishes for the future. We should not forget.

And so some people just start and say, oh, I will be so happy when I again can go where I want, because I think all about this requirement that we shouldn't leave the houses, it's very difficult. But then we find out what was really important for us in normal life. And, in our imagination, we can imagine going away, going to the mountains, going to the lake, going to friends, going to dance. And we know from neuroscience that in the imagination, when we have these imaginations of joy, of inspiration, that this has also an impact on the body. And this has an impact not only on our mood, but it also has an impact on our immune system, helps to fight the virus. When almost everything is forbidden and we have to cut down this and this and this and this, we lose joy of life. We don't have a good mood and this is bad for the immune defence. And this is why I think it's very important what we experience at our phone calls – now we are doing phone calls all the time – we experience friends starting to say: do you remember last year at the same time what we have been doing, how we have felt? We have been enjoying this and this and this. These are all imaginations, memories; a memory can be for most people accessible, And out of those memories we create imaginations for the time after the crisis.

SC: I like this very much, and I realize I've been doing it with my daughters since they are forced to do home-schooling. We decided, to imagine every day, *imagine* what we will do to celebrate the end of this year. The first thing that came up between my three daughters and I, is to meet my baby-nephew Leonardo (their new cousin), who was born on March 8. For obvious reasons, we couldn't meet. Such a simple thing as this is impossible now. I really like what you suggested and it links to the idea of spring, of rebirth, of starting anew (which is really important for me).

I want to ask you now, what is the – possible – archetype of the coronavirus? For me it is reset: the absolute reset. Therefore, total restart. Perhaps even the end of the ego society, the society based on lust, entertainment or the superfluous.

VK: And especially on the outer world, everything happens in the outer world. And that's what the virus forces us to face: our being in the world, you know. And this is what could be our role as psychoanalysts; which is important when you say it is a kind of research. We have to say now: enough is enough, we have to change, we have to value more our inner world. This is what I like and what I think is difficult in the situation we are in, is that we are now referred to our inner world. But a lot of people are used to regulate their emotions in activities in the outer world, doing sports, in having parties and so on. Now the question is: how do I meet myself, can I meet myself?

SC: I totally agree. It's a time of new routines for parents home schooling their kids, parents who at the same time have to work from home. But I think it's also a time of pragmatism, responsibility and integrity. Yeah, hopefully a time to appreciate these three things. Anew.

VK: You're right. And it's also a time of modesty.

SC: This morning I was reading an article by Mary Watkins where she mentions James Hillman who wrote: *The ego must relinquish its propensity to overcontrol and dominate its tendency to attribute what is to itself. The ego must undergo a transformation in which it is humbled.*[1] Is it time to become humble, Verena?

VK: Time to be convinced that you can't control everything, to control everything means that we do not accept that we have anxieties, that we feel helpless, that we fear death. And now if we accept that we can't control everything, then we must connect with other people. We relate to others in the world and we have to cope the exceptional situation together; this is the kind of humility I mean and this is also the background of solidarity, of the huge solidarity, we can experience. It is not so much about autonomy; we have this idea that the ego has to be autonomous. It is perhaps becoming a little bit less because we feel, we need autonomy but we must be autonomous in respecting relationships. I'm not so sure. The priority of autonomy causes that we do not value the other enough and do not consider enough that we are dependent on each other. And I think at the moment when we when we accept that we are dependent from others, and they are dependent from us, we are much more careful, we are much more caring. We are much more appreciating each other. And I think this is perhaps what could become very important for ourselves and also for the ecological problem; that we have to be more caring. And this is would be also responsibility.

SC: Two days ago the French president declared the lockdown and said "we are at war". Why is the symbolism of war used so often nowadays? Usually, when a country is at war or makes a declaration of war, it is against an enemy. This is the first time in human history that the enemy is invisible. The South African president said every citizen is a soldier right now, and this makes me think of symbolism of *the hero.*

VK: But I think I don't like the metaphor of war. It's not war, its faith. Sure we fight, we fight the virus. But in war you can win; I think we can't win. We can find a vaccination, we can find some medicaments, but the virus is there and we know that other viruses will show up in the future. It is life. I don't like the metaphor of war.

SC: We said that this is a psychological, but I would say a psychosocial crisis, as well as a financial one. It is a psychosocial-financial catastrophe. People are losing jobs already and perhaps it will be worse than 2008. How do you see the next few years and what is the archetype behind all this that is going on?

VK: Well, I think it is the archetype of destruction and redemption and I think is it will take us some years until we have, again, a functioning economy and if we are wise, then we will consider the ecological problem. So I think it's really a moment where we can change something, perhaps even socially. This basic income for everybody we have been voting about in Switzerland and lots of people said this is not possible. Perhaps now it becomes possible. We don't know. So I think it's a question of adaptive regulation. And this would be the positive aspect of it. But it is very hard. And it will cost a lot, life time of a lot of older people. But I am quite an optimist, and I think sometimes life is really very hard and then it's not so hard, it is much easier. We fight, we arrange ourselves with the situation and important: we become creative. We have ideas. Take these Italians on the balcony with happy music. That's wonderful that there are such a lot of creative projects in the world. I'm quite sure, it will take time, but we will again have a good enough life, perhaps not in such a way as we had before. Not so much the same life as before, not so much this wanting to have everything, nor so much the sense of entitlement, but a life you can like and consider to be a good life, more responsible for nature. And I'm sure that we can achieve it. But for this, we have to fight.

SC: You as well as an expert on dreams and active imagination, on fairy tales and myth. Which myth or fairy tale comes to your mind, that could help us overcome those days? Because reading fairy tales to our kids or to our partners or just to ourselves is an act of creativity.

VK: I think it's OK to read fairy tales for kids: in each fairy tale, almost in each myth you can find a specific dynamic: something is terribly wrong. It's in a way a catastrophe. And then you have a protagonist who is doing something very important; he or she is very authentic and tries to resolve the problem. They want to overcome the misery, they break up – very often in despair, helpless. And then something new will happen. And I think this is how life is. But I wouldn't say that there is one specific fairy tale which is coming to my mind. And this is because it is such a global problem. It's not, in a way, a clearly defined problem, as for example situations, where the water of life is missing: people are depressed, and then you have to go for water of life. And before you get the water off of life, you are threatened by you are in danger of death. And so to be in danger of death is always a part of the way of the developing process of the fairytale. But what we have now, it's this is also why it is so difficult for us. We don't have models in our head because it's just too much. It's too global. But the search for the water of life is not that bad …

… If it helps, if we have stories, because the stories are working on our psyche and they are touching emotions, triggering imaginations and especially stories with a good ending are helping us at least to feel better.

SC: I like this, which links with the need to be creative, and to fantasize of a good ending. Also, following German sociologist Ulrich Beck (2016), I believe it is fundamental to realize that everyone is vulnerable as well as responsible right now.

VK: This are two very important points, yes everyone is vulnerable. We knew this before, but now it is felt in the body, it is embodied. To be vulnerable has been an idea we have been talking about philosophically. But now we feel the connected emotions. They are strong. We feel it, we can feel it in the stomach. But then we feel also love for life in the body. And this is the opposite.

SC: Yes, but also from a political point of view. I always like to quote Erich Fromm's *Escape from Freedom*, when he claims that when people are not able to hold the responsibility of freedom, they give it back to the politician who becomes an authoritarian one. This is threatening when looking at the rise of populist movements in Italy, Spain, Germany, England, Brazil and the US.

In Italy we have Salvini, leader of *La Lega*, who used to say: "Close all ports, don't let in the refugees". And now that the virus, that is not a refugee, is threatening, he says: "Open everything, open the economy, open the bars". It seems to me he is out of contact with what is really happening and he is just trying to use the virus for political reasons. I feel it is not the time for populism (and we will see in the next few month of these populist leaders will perform in relation to the pandemic). It's not the time for a declaration of independence and close to borders, but it's time for a *declaration of interdependence*. Because, as Beck (2017) underlined, we are all interdependent and connected.

VK: It is also not responsible what he's [Salvini] doing and other politicians are doing the same. Trump as well. They try to use the virus for their political ambitions. And this is not the point. This is what we have been talking about: inflation, about the ego, and it is just for the ego. But I hope that there is a critical mass of people who have understood what it means to go through this crisis and that they feel more responsible themselves. It's so easy to delegate everything to the politicians. And yes, I'm hoping for the critical one's because we all need a critical mass of people who are believing in something, who are doing something, and then things can change.

SC: Thank you very much Verena. I take your words as a warm invitation to be(come) creative.

VK: I hope so, too. All the best for you, Stefano. Thank you.

Note

1 This quote was shared by Stefano Carpani as a memory. Therefore it is not 100% accurate.

Bibliography

Beck, U. (2016). *The Metamorphosis of the World: How Climate Change is Transforming Our Concept of the World*. Cambridge: Polity

Fromm, E. (1941). *Escape from Freedom*. New York: Holt Paperbacks.

Watkins, M. (2014). *Hillman and Freire: Intellectual Accompaniment by Two Fathers*. Online at: https://mary-watkins.net/library/Hillman-and-Freire–Intellectual-Accompaniment-by-Two-Fathers.pdf

Chapter 2

Nature and Death

Murray Stein

The interview with Murray Stein focuses on the psychological effects of lockdown. Stein states that the unconscious is very active under such circumstances. The reason is that by being socially inactive psychic energy can regress and flow back into the unconscious, activating complexes that eventually lead to feelings of anxiety and anger. While he initially expected a baby boom due to the lockdown, the opposite is the case. Instead of Eros, Phobos and Deimos are taking the lead in society. Stein suggests introversion to explore the inner world and become creative with the images that emerge – like Jung himself did with the Red Book. To answer the question of the reason why especially Westerners are so afraid of death, Stein looks back in history and finds there was a shift in how individuals and society looked at death. Once theme to intellectuals like Sartre or Kierkegaard, today death is a topic that evokes strong emotions and panic. The fear of death is archetypal, as animals we instinctively want to live, but by thinking of death the thought about afterlife is not far. In the pandemic he sees a chance to reflect about death and afterlife anew.

Stefano Carpani: Doctor Stein, dear Murray, thank you very much for your time. How are you? I guess you are at home in Switzerland?

Murray Stein: That's correct, I'm presently at my home in the small village of Goldiwil, which is just outside Thun in the Bernese Oberland. We've been relatively content to remain here during the Pandemic. Of course, all the health concerns that occupy people everywhere in the world right now are very present here as well, and also in my work as an analyst and among my family members who live in the US and Canada.

SC: You say you're concerned. How do you feel, apart from being concerned?

MS: This varies depending on who I'm talking to or what I'm doing. I spend quite a bit of my time working with analysands and students online, and depending on where they are and what's happening with them, I can feel anything from very concerned for their well-being to reflective on the ways they're coping with the situation, inner and outer. For myself, I'm quite aware of the dangers of the virus to people my age.

DOI: 10.4324/9781003266402-2

SC: These days are forcing us into a lockdown. Where I am, Berlin, there is a partial lockdown. Where you are, in Switzerland, there is a partial lockdown, too. But there are many, many countries where there is a full lockdown. And so there are new routines: Parents are home with their kids doing home schooling, trying to work, trying to get their job done, trying not to get fired. Young or elderly people are home alone, in a less nice environment than yours and mine. What could happen, psychologically, when people are being forced staying at home for many, many weeks?

MS: I think a lot depends on how strict the lockdown is. I speak frequently with people in China who were confined to their apartments for nearly two months. That is a serious lockdown. And I must say, I was impressed by their capacity to cope with the situation. But people who weren't in good psychological shape suffered from anxiety and depression to a high degree. People react to such tight restrictions in different ways, of course. Some get angry and rebellious. They chafe at what they perceive to be overly strict parental authorities. Today in Western democracies we're seeing governments assume a degree of control over their citizens that we're not used to. We're accustomed to having a lot of personal freedom. Adolescents here, especially, don't react well to strict rules and regulations. We see college students partying wildly on the beaches in Florida, and young people also here in Switzerland staging noisy protests and complaining that their youth is being denied the normal freedoms that are to be expected. Another type of reaction is depression. If you're confined to a small space, an apartment in a city, say, and you're alone, your mood may turn to hopelessness as you entertain dark thoughts about the future.

There is a tendency when you're not active socially for psychic energy to regress. The psychic energy that is normally put into making plans, socializing, traveling, etc., stops dead in its tracks, and the energy flows backward into the unconscious. We know very well what happens when libido regresses. It activates complexes in the unconscious. A lot of fantasies start appearing, many of them a reaction to prevailing feelings of anxiety and anger. The unconscious is highly activated right now in the collective because of this regression of libido. We see all kinds of conspiracy theories afloat about who is to blame for the Pandemic, and these add fuel to the fires of anger. People are on edge, very impatient, imagining enemies amongst them in the streets and abroad. This edgy mood, of course, also affects family life. When schools are closed, what to do with the small children, how to entertain them, how to keep them occupied? This is a dire problem for parents with very young children. The kids can't go out and play as they're used to doing, so parents (typically a mother, but also fathers these days when everyone is working at home) have to become very creative with them. This is exhausting, and it loads great stress into family dynamics. Couples that are a bit unstable to begin with but avoid open conflict well enough by going to work and spending long hours apart are suddenly cooped up together in a tight space for long periods of time, and this can easily flare up into domestic abuse.

At first, I expected to see a huge baby boom coming after the Pandemic subsided, but I didn't take into account enough the element of fear for the future and the splitting energies unleashed by this type of crisis. It now seems that the opposite is the case: The birth rate has dropped dramatically throughout the world in the past year. Eros has been pushed out the door, and Phobos ("fear") and Deimos ("dread") have taken up residence.

SC: You talk about rebellion. You talk about the loss of libido and possible depression. There are other feelings or other emotions: There is anxiety and panic. There is fear, but also solidarity and an enormous or a new solidarity. I have a very straightforward question for you: For those that are not in psychotherapy, for those that don't have a therapist right now, what would you suggest them? Last week I was talking to Verena Kast (see Chapter 1). She said: it's time to be here, to become creative through imaginations, through painting. She also said: If you cannot leave your house because you're in full lockdown, just be creative and imagine what you will do when this is over or what you were doing last year. I sense she suggests so, to bring some hope into this new condition, otherwise, as you said, we have depression and we become negative. What could be your suggestion?

MS: Well, I would agree that this presents an unprecedented opportunity to engage imagination to explore what we call the inner world, to let images appear, to paint them, to draw them, to become creative with them. To do this kind of work, I would counsel patience. It involves the practice of introversion, which many people are unfamiliar with. This means becoming inwardly quiet and attentive to one's thoughts. If they are negative, give them some space and consider them. It they are positive, welcome them into your house. Entertain these thoughts as you would guests, like Philemon and Baucis welcomed Zeus and Hermes when they showed up at their door in the form of wanderers. It's astonishing how beneficial such practices can be and how productive. This is a time to follow the regression into the unconscious and become familiar with the other personalities dwelling there. We call this "active imagination" in Jungian practice. It's what Jung used during a similar period of crisis in Europe when he created his Liber Novus, the famous "Red Book."

You ask about finding hope during a time like this. The best quality of hope comes from inner sources. It is a light in the darkness. Hope has to spring up from within the individual. When it does, they turn a corner. They begin to imagine new paths of development for themselves, new types of activity that they would not have had time to consider while normally active and busy in their lives. As a therapist, I find that hope comes to a client when a dream presents images of a new future and its possibilities. The dream of a young child is a classic example. Maybe as therapists we can also inspire some hope just by being ourselves with people and showing them that we're coping with this situation that we all find ourselves in. Hope is offered, of course, by religious traditions and their teachings. People find spiritual practices to be a resource, and in this current time of crisis they might deepen their religious life through meditation or through reading the sacred texts and scriptures and through prayer.

SC: Last week, the French president said: "We are at war." The South African president said something like: "Every citizen, male or female, is a soldier right now." First of all, I would like to ask you, do you buy this? Are we at war? Secondly, if we are at war, we are at war with a virus that is something invisible. But war – I am European, you are North American, we know very well that war is the *summa*, the greatest destructive thing. And after war both winners or losers have to face reconstruction. This time, if we claim we are at war, there will be no reconstruction. Buildings, bridges, infrastructures, etc., will not have to be rebuilt, but there will be a lot to be rebuild. So the first question is: are we at war? Second: what will we have to rebuild?

MS: Political leaders speak to a nation, and when they want to mobilize that nation to take decisive action, they will tell them they're at war with a threatening enemy. A perceived enemy focuses the mind and gets people to pay attention to things they normally would ignore. Recently people were sitting around in restaurants in Zurich, mingling freely with others indoors and outdoors, and even though they knew the coronavirus was around they weren't paying much attention to it. Then suddenly the Swiss government said this is an emergency and instituted restrictions. I don't know how many years it's been in Swiss history since they declared a national emergency, but here that's like declaring that a war is on. A national emergency sounds dramatic, and it certainly gets people's attention. So they start doing collectively what is necessary to overcome the danger that is threatening the whole society. They start thinking in larger than simply individual terms. National leaders have to do that, they use the rhetoric of war. It's a way to mobilize the collective. When you're at war, you put lesser concerns aside. Fretting about small things is suddenly out the window, and you start thinking about something that's really essential, namely life and death.

This is a life and death struggle. Many people are dying from infection by the virus, and many more will die from it in the future. If extreme measures aren't taken, the medical systems will be overwhelmed and collapse. People will be dying in the streets, as we see in some countries, because there are no hospital beds for them. Doctors and nurses are working beyond their capacities and are suffering burnout in record numbers. So it is actually very much like a war situation.

About rebuilding after the war, the economists are saying it's going to take years to recover from the effects of this Pandemic. And another question is, will it be the same afterwards as it was before? The wars of the twentieth century transformed Europe. There was huge destruction, and what came out of it afterwards was quite different from what these nations were like before. Will the world after coronavirus be a better world? Will it be a more consciously balanced world? Maybe this Pandemic can become a wake-up call to start paying attention to what is really important, to what our basic values are, and to the human world as a community. The world is not in good shape and wasn't in good shape before the coronavirus hit.

SC: This lockdown forces us to stop with our frivolous post-modern life and activities. It forces us to take distance from what I like to call *the lust* *society*, an *all you can eat society*, and *the bulimic society*. A society rooted in the *external*. In the p*ersona*. This lockdown is, somehow, forcing us to look inside, even to go inside and into the depth. Some can do this, others cannot.

But let's stick to the concepts of war and – even perhaps – the Great Depression and let's link it to what you said before about big dreams and your patient's dreams. Do you see a possible turn – like the turn after the Great Depression – towards dictatorship? We are coming from years of new populism, right-wing Populism. What is your opinion?

MS: What the political ramifications of this will be is hard to say. The Great Depression of the 1930s coincided with the appearance of the great dictators of Europe. In difficult times like we see today, with the huge discrepancy between the rich and the poor and the middle struggling, people start looking for a saviour. They want immediate solutions to their social and economic problems, and in their mounting anxiety, fed today by social media, they are disinclined to think clearly about ultimate consequences of proposed solutions. And unbelievably, many fall for the most fantastic promises and outlandish theories. Thoughtful people today are very worried about what we see as movements that would undermine trust in democracy. This plays into the hands of the "strong leaders" who want all the power at their disposal. They have no time for debate and free elections. We know that democracy is a very difficult form of government. It's full of conflict, argument, disagreement. And when you're at war and when you're in a crisis, you don't want that. You want everybody heading in one direction.

So, yes, I think there's a real danger that so-called "strong leaders" will appear and convince people to follow them and to change the systems that we're used to that include space for discussion, dialogue, debate, disagreement, voting, all of that. But I do think that people will fight for democracy. Most people realize that in the long run, democracy works better for everyone than tyranny.

SC: The German sociologist Ulrich Beck underlined in his masterpiece *The Risk Society* (1992) the need for *methodological cosmopolitanism*, and – looking at how things stand right now – I sense that methodological cosmopolitanism is really what we have to face. This emergency cannot be taken care of by one nation only. It was a Chinese thing in December 2019 (and we, the Westerners, looked at the Chinese with superiority), then it became an Italian thing at the end of February 2020 and many Europeans countries looked at Italy with superiority, as if we were bringing the plague because of our inaccuracy and approximation. And now it is a European – as well as global – thing. No one excluded! And perhaps, Europe, as concept of Union, is going to survive or die because of this.

Apart from this, Beck claimed that there is no distinction between nature and society. Following Beck, Covid could be seen as nature, and nature is affecting society. Therefore, global risks are affecting society. And this brings us back to war and death. I would like you to go back to the concept of death and ask you: Why are we so afraid of death (after Second World War)? Why have Westerners put aside the concept of death?

MS: In the early 1970s, Ernest Becker published the bestseller, *The Denial of Death*. He reminded us that death is a topic we should not push under the rug. It is a major theme in existentialism from Kierkegaard to Sartre. People have been thinking about death, but recently it's been more like a panic, more emotional, not merely intellectual. I went with my wife to our doctor the other day because she was having some difficulties with an infection, not coronavirus, thankfully, but something else. And he said to us, as an aside, that if you have been infected with the coronavirus and you take Ibuprofen to reduce the fever, you will die. And then he got very excited and dramatically made a cross with his hand. "It will put you in your grave!" he said with almost hysterical intensity. I would say he was possessed at that moment by the numinosity of Death, which was of course all around him in his practice. We sat back in our chairs stunned and with big eyes as we listened to him. Wow! We didn't know ibuprofen could do that to you. The sense of death in the air and much stronger right now than it was before the pandemic struck, no question. The fear of death is archetypal. We're animals. We want to live. Every animal will do whatever it can to survive. It's built into our nature to want desperately to survive. It's an instinct. There is a profound fear of extinction, that we will lose our being, lose our essence. If we die, we will be no more. Of course, some people like the idea and that's why they commit suicide. They want to get out of the vale of tears.

But the realisation of death immediately brings up the question of an afterlife. Death and rebirth are a pair of opposites that invariably come in a package. What happens after death? Until modern times people have pretty much universally believed in life after death in some form. And so as people come into contact with the immediately threatening presence of death, they will start thinking about the afterlife a lot more than usual.

Some years ago, I was on a boat with a group of people and a crew in the Galapagos Islands. There were three groups of people on board: the crew members, who were Ecuadorian; a group of Italian tourists; and a group of American tourists. There were about 20 of us in total. At some point on the cruise, I got the idea – I don't know why – to take a poll. I would ask each person as occasion permitted: do you believe in life after death, yes or no? If yes, is that life personal or is it more general, like becoming part of a larger whole? The crew members, who were all, I assume, Catholics and raised traditionally, said they believe in life after death and that it's personal. Their individual souls will survive in the afterlife. All said that, except for the captain. He said, no he did not believe in any form of afterlife. The Italian tourists all said "No, absolutely not, there is no life after death." I found out they were all anti-clerical and thought the Church was a fraud and the Pope was a joke. They resented the church and for this reason expressed a negative view. As for the Americans, they said "Yes, there is an afterlife but it is not personal." Later I had the opportunity to sit in conversation with one of the Italian women, and I asked her to explain her answer to me because I was so surprised that the Italians, whom I had assumed to be good Catholics, all said no to a belief in an afterlife. And she said, "Well, I said no because of my husband. He's really anti-religious. He's an atheist, but I'm not so sure." And then she told me a very moving story that contradicted her negative answer. After her mother died, she told me, she was sitting in her room by herself thinking about her, and suddenly she felt her presence in the room and something surprising and mysterious happened that convinced her that her mother was really there, that the spirit of her mother was in the room with her. And she added, "I think maybe there is something after life, but I can't say it publicly."

I think people have experiences that they don't want to talk about because they feel sort of embarrassed because it's so against the modern Zeitgeist. Many people have told me of their experiences that after somebody's death strange synchronistic events happened. If people pay attention, they start noticing synchronistic events around them that give them some hint that life continues beyond this material world. There is a theory that religions are born out of the experience of death because that's where you experience the soul's reality most strongly. The spirits of the ancestors continue after you see the body being cremated or buried. In many cultures, the people have little areas of the house where they keep a picture of the deceased ancestors and place flowers in respect and honour of them, and one day of the year they have a memorial for them and believe that they return from time to time and are otherwise present to them in the other world.

I think this coronavirus pandemic does bring the topic of death into the conversation, and while people are afraid of it, I would hope they also look at it squarely and think about it. Everybody eventually is going to have to face the question of what it means.

SC: As you know I am Italian. My country is really on its knees. Almost one thousand deaths. It's too much. We Jungians – and I would like to ask this question really with respect for those that lost their life and their families – look at death metaphorically. You wrote a very interesting book, titled *In Midlife* (1983), and you underline that during midlife crisis, something has to die and what has to die is the persona, so that the Self will be able to be. So that we will get in contact with our Self; every crisis, every depression as a transformative push. You said it about wars in Europe before. What are the positive sides of this crisis, of these metaphorical death of our society, as it is right now? I was shocked when I read in the news that dolphins were swimming in the Venice canals[1].

MS: Yes, I saw that …

SC: … nature is coming back. For me Covid-19 is nature telling us: "Hey guys, it's too much. Stop it now!" Especially when world leaders, first of all Trump, are denying climate change, are denying that we are really killing nature and deniers are losers. But it seems nature found a way to stop everything.

MS: I think of the coronavirus pandemic as a part of the more general world crisis that includes climate change and the exhaustion of natural resources. Scientists estimate that we, at the present rate of exploitation of nature, humans will exhaust this planet in 50 or 75 years. That's a very short period of time considering the long history of the human race. There just won't be enough of the essentials to sustain the species in its present numbers. Without a shadow of doubt, there will be, in the near future, all kinds of huge and terrible consequences if we can't gain some perspective from this present crisis and begin to take measures. And that's a big IF. If we can learn from these relatively small crises that we are facing now, maybe there is a chance that humans will be able to offset worse things to come in the future when nature will really show its disregard for human beings. Basically, we have overstepped our boundaries. I believe this was innocent at first, but now it's not. We know better, and it's up to us to take appropriate action. This type of overreach is the story of Faust as told by Goethe two hundred years ago. Faust cannot stop himself from continuing to expand his reach before it consumes him. Hubris is the basic sin, according to the ancient Greeks, and there's going to be a huge price for it, as the Titan, Prometheus, experienced.

What I would hope is that this Pandemic will be a game changer that leads people to reformulate priorities. If we could come to terms with our true state of affairs as a species, blessed with consciousness and some degree of foresight, and consider our proper proportion in the great scheme of things, we could live longer and better attuned to our natural world. This type of reconsideration of how to live well in harmony with ourselves and nature is a slow, step by step, process. Maybe it will begin now on a global scale.

SC: I agree. I hope that change will bring more pluralism, more respect, less top-down approach from some countries to the others and real cosmopolitanism, otherwise we will face total destruction. And to my mind comes Jung's dream of the apocalypse (this dream that nobody really knows about – or almost nobody – because von Franz heard it from Jung). And such dream was so powerful that he was so scared to write about or even to share it openly. Hopefully we will be able to learn from what we are going through. … Thank you, Murray.

MS: Thank you.

Note

1 On March 20th 2020, the CNN (as well as other international media outlets) share the news that "These dolphins took a day trip up Venice's Grand Canal." Online at: https://edition.cnn.com/travel/article/venice-canal-dolphins/index.html   (accessed October 14 2021).

References

Beck, U. (1992). *Risk Society: Towards a New Modernity*. London: Sage
Becker, E. (1997). *The Denial of Death*. New York: Free Press.
Stein, M. (1983). *In Midlife*. Ashville: Chiron

Chapter 3

Illness as Metaphor

Paul Attinello

Attinello considers that, although Covid-19 and HIV/AIDS are very different illnesses associated with different phenomena and psychological patterns, there are deep levels where parallels can be found – e.g. our relationship to illness and death, the way panic or avoidance reveal themselves, and personal, cultural and political evaluations as well. Sontag's books on illness and AIDS are both valuable and problematic, as was her changing relationship to her own cancer and death over several decades. Attinello recognizes that he has come to consider his fear of death very seriously in his work on AIDS, and he did so also in his Jungian training and personal analysis. He realizes that he has also come to a very different relationship with that fear – one that now is not that terrifying, but relatively calming. The interview continues discussing the political and communicative chaos that appeared in the first month of the epidemic, linking it to different cultural and psychological interpretations. Ultimately, the author wishes to return to a basic ground of existential awareness around this crisis, which is also, unavoidably, a space for change.

Stefano Carpani: Doctor Attinello, Dear Paul, good evening and thank you joining me during the current Covid-19 crisis. First, let me ask: how are you?

Paul Attinello: I'm good, actually, I'm doing rather well. I'm almost cheerful, which is a little strange – we might talk about that.

SC: As you mentioned in our previous conversation (Carpani, 2020), being HIV-positive puts you in a risk group nowadays. How do you feel, and how do you feel about that?

PA: I feel physically fine. As I've told you before (Attinello, 2020), I made a mistake with my medications three or four years ago. Since that time, I've been on more toxic medications and have frequently felt mildly ill, though not terribly so these days. I'm fine – really, totally fine. Sixty-three years old, but no problems.

The whole question of what it means to be HIV-positive with Covid is complicated. The UK, of course, only started warning HIV-positive people to be careful very late, and there have been people online asking: does it matter if I'm HIV-positive? What does AIDS have to do with Covid? What does this

DOI: 10.4324/9781003266402-3

mean, what do I do? There are ways that these viruses, these conditions, are completely separate, but also sort of related.

Given my health condition, as I understand it, I was curious. I wanted to talk to my doctor about the situation. I, of course, take medications, as I've done for more than thirty years. They protect the immune system, but with HIV the medications don't completely repress the virus. They can't. So, the virus is present – it multiplies quickly, and it's destroyed quickly. So, there's constantly this sort of battle going on – at least with the older medications that was true, I'm not sure the current ones are quite as bad. Well, that was all they could do, that was what was available at the time. That's why they are saying that, as people with long-term HIV get older, we're about ten years older, physically, than our chronological age.[1]

My doctor's response to all this was: that has not been proven, don't worry about it. So, I do have a sense that – yes, I'm 63, but probably physically a bit more beaten up than that. And certainly, people in the HIV groups here in Newcastle, and people who are HIV-positive online, will be worrying more, or worrying less. Actually, I'm not sure people with HIV are more worried than people who are not, in this crisis. Certainly, the government has classified us, saying: yes, you're like older people, people who have, perhaps, lung problems, that sort of thing. So, it's an interesting thing: we get, as it were, the benefit of that attention.

SC: And in the past few weeks – and you mentioned this, look at the UK: in Cardiff, there was a huge concert by *Stereophonics* (*BBC News*, 2020), a big concert with many people. While almost the entire world is in lockdown – yesterday, in India, one point three billion people went into lockdown. I don't even – my mind is not able to imagine how that could work. I have been very angry, perhaps that is the right word, at the German government, saying: what are you doing? What are you waiting for when you see what has happened in Italy, what is happening in Spain, even France? Macron went into lockdown saying we are at war, but as soon as Merkel spoke the Germans followed. Of course, you have teenagers, you have the rebels, but Germany has a very low rate of increase for either people infected or dead. These situations could help us to talk about social dynamics, how people interact …

PA: In the face of death. Not just how people interact, but how they interact in the face of death. And that big split that you're worried about seems to me to be the difference between a material reality and something that seems to be a symbol or an image.

SC: But even about denial: because you ask, what is going on in the UK? And if I look at denial when thinking of the group you are in, and the question would be, is denial perceived differently, and is it in fact different? If you are HIV-positive, you know that if you get a very bad cold, you could have trouble.

PA: Yes, you know, I don't get extra medical support because of my age, I get it because I'm HIV-positive. I get a free flu jab, as they call it in the UK, a flu shot, every fall. So, I've already gotten that this year. But I think this is about confronting illness, confronting death. And, as far as I can tell, everybody who's HIV-positive has essentially already done that. People I know and people online – there may be complaints and arguments about various things, but any question of: should you be taking care of yourself, getting out of public places, that sort of thing – HIV-positive people have simply decided: okay, no question. I think we had already passed that point, which is really the hard part, because this is about the fear of death, panic around death, which is absolutely at the core here. There are these two enormous strands – actually, there are probably about ten enormous strands, you're also talking politics in this context. But two things that I always think about around AIDS, two things that are always in the background, are: one, the inability to really grapple with ideas of death, especially for modern people living with relatively good health care, with no deadly, rapidly proceeding pandemic since the Spanish flu, which was in 1918–1920. And then the second thing will be: do people have a visceral sense that something is happening, or are they just being told about it.

So: real and symbolic. Because that is confusing people all over the world – it is the entire problem of 'I don't believe it until I see it,' which has been complicated by the incredibly messy politics of the last thirty or forty years, especially in English-speaking countries. We, in the larger English-speaking nations, now have some of the worst governments I think we've ever had, so trust levels are minimal, chaos levels are high – the state of not believing what you're told is very common.

I've been surprised that the English are being relatively well-behaved, at least the ones I'm seeing in the north, but there are disturbing stories. It's not just that people are still going to a rock concert in Wales, the event that everyone has been talking about, those are minor stories. But there are other events you would think of as insane, but they're so localized, maybe they're inexplicable. For instance, two or three times in the last few days there have been news reports that someone has destroyed three ambulances in a Midlands town, and then someone else does the same to delivery wagons for hospital goods in another town. Why would anyone do that? Now, that's insane. That behaviour is not merely: I'm going to ignore this (Covid), and it should not be my problem. That state of mind is more like – it's very hard to tell because it's so strange, but it feels as though it represents something more like: *bring on the end of the world.*

SC: Let me go into a direction that would perhaps not make me popular. I want to use an author we both like. You know Susan Sontag – this is the Italian version of *Illness as Metaphor* (Sontag, 1978). She starts at the very beginning, saying that: illness – she talks about cancer, then she talks about HIV, maybe we should talk about Covid-19 – illness brings up punishment fantasies, fantasies around a certain situation. She also says, and I look at this when thinking of the HIV-positive community:

> Nothing is more punitive than to give a disease a meaning – that meaning being invariably a moralistic one.
>
> (Sontag, 1978, p. 58)

You as a gay man, as an HIV-positive man, you went through this shit, excuse my language. In the past, punishment was God's punishment. We are in a society after Nietzsche: God is dead. If we were Freudian, we wouldn't like religion much because it's an illusion. But, as Jung says, let's look at spirituality. What is the meaning, what is the symbolism of what is going on right now? And I think Sontag gave us the answer. She says:

> A disease of the lungs is, metaphorically, a disease of the soul. Cancer, as a disease that can strike anywhere, is a disease of the body. Far from revealing anything spiritual, it reveals that the body is, all too woefully, just the body.
>
> (Sontag, 1978, p. 18)

Tuberculosis was so much linked to Romanticism, Baudelaire and all those guys in Paris, Violetta from *La Traviata* … tuberculosis is a sickness of the soul, because it's metaphorically linked to the lungs, those sicknesses affecting the lungs are a sickness of the soul.

PA: There are about four tricky directions here. Number 1, when Sontag is saying these things in the 1980s and 90s – she will first have cancer in the 1980s, which is when she writes *Illness as Metaphor*, and in it she is defending herself brilliantly against metaphorical reflections of her cancer, against people saying: why do you have it?

She'll write *AIDS as Metaphor* (Sontag, 1989) later, when she has recovered from cancer for the first time – she'll end up having it three times, but she feels very strong at this point (Roiphe, 2016). Strength will be very important for her in relation to her cancer, and she'll see the same even more insidious, nastier projections of sin and darkness and mistake and error onto people with AIDS, because it's sex and it's drugs and you're all terrible people, that kind of thing. Brilliant, brilliant, brilliant argument. Here's the interesting problem, and you will also know this as an analyst. In cultural theory, which I've taught and written about for decades, and which Sontag is practicing here, there is a long tradition that comes from Adorno and the Frankfurt school which says: I will argue with this cultural position and I will present very clear arguments about the underlying interpretations, in order to show you that you're being foolish so that you will be more clear-headed and won't be so mystified by these cultural mistakes.

Of course, as Jungian analysts, we would say, quite differently: any symbol that comes up matters. Some of them are more reasonable or less reasonable than others, but they do matter, you do consider them. So, you take them on board. That would certainly be the methodological explanation of why Sontag makes this claim – she's defending herself, she's saying: I have cancer, it's merely a disease, it doesn't mean anything. Then later, for her friends, she'll similarly say: AIDS is merely a disease, it doesn't mean anything.

And to this day, the clinical psychologists here – I live in Newcastle upon Tyne, and one of my HIV-positive groups works with the clinical psychologists at the city's Royal Victoria Infirmary, and they are brilliant. A lot of what the clinical psychologists do here is to tell people that the fact that they have AIDS or are HIV-positive doesn't mean anything. It's a really, really important defense. But I would say that behind that, at a less rational level, it *does* have meaning. It shows up in our dreams, it shows up in our imagination – you can't magic that away. I would of course reassure anybody who has HIV: it is not their fault, it doesn't mean anything. But at the same time, in a real depth psychology, which assumes that the ego is not in charge, and that our work goes far past the materials that our egos intend to control, we would have to say: do you *imagine* that this is your fault?

SC: Let me respond to that. I follow you. Perhaps, if we were following Giegerich, we would say that there is nothing to understand (Giegerich, 2010). I should accept it, the end of meaning is actually to stop trying to understand, is my guess. But if we look at Jung's *unus mundus* point of view, I follow your meaning, and I give you another proposal following, again, Sontag. She says that tuberculosis was presented as the prototype of passive death, often as a sort of suicide, as in romanticism …

PA: Of course: it will be languishing on the couch, it will be the poet dying, the opera singer fading away dramatically and erotically. It'll be beautiful, it'll be sensual, it'll be …

SC: So, punishment … and those who were HIV-positive, who were living in a 'lustful' world.

PA: Which is where the 'innocent victims' come up. You remember, that was a nasty little phrase that became a big problem – and then nobody said that phrase anymore. But the idea, of course, hangs around as a shadow behind AIDS. And obviously – I am tussling with you about this a bit – if you had an analysand who had HIV/AIDS, there would be a point when you would say: do you feel guilty for having this? And you'd go *through* it, because you can't assume, you can't simply say, well, you shouldn't feel guilty, and expect that it all stops there. That's a cultural discussion, it's not quite enough for analysis.

SC: The moralistic punishment – you *are* wrong: you behave wrongly, not according to the rules, to the norms. And then you must be punished, of course. Let's look at this:

> TB was represented as the prototypical passive death. Often it was a kind of suicide.
>
> (Sontag, 1978, p. 24)

Let's swap tuberculosis with Covid. Covid-19 could be represented as the prototypical passive death. Because if we say that this sickness takes over the lungs, then you cannot breathe. If it is a sickness of the soul – how is that suicidal? I don't think that people who get Covid-19 are consciously suicidal, but society is suicidal because we haven't realized that we really have to do something about it.

PA: Okay, here's another side, though. All three of these illnesses are different. Tuberculosis was mysterious, obscure, you couldn't tell how it happened. Different symptoms would show up, it was slow, and the body would become feverish and languishing. So, you would get a lot of projections onto that, it was a very sort of magical illness. One of the reasons people go from tuberculosis to AIDS is that they are both illnesses that have a kind of glamour. Does that make sense where, for instance, cholera doesn't have any glamour at all? It's interesting that in *Death in Venice* people are dying of cholera, and Aschenbach will die of cholera at the end. It's not really an exotic or interesting illness, it's just grotesque (Mann, 1998).

Then AIDS will have all of its complex cultural background, it'll be associated with drugs at a time when drugs are fascinating and terrible, and with gay sex at a time when people are not dealing with that well. It'll be associated with sex, period, at a point where Western urban cultures are trying to be less oppressed and oppressive about sex, but they are not doing a very good job of it. They're still struggling with the meanings and projections throughout the 1980s. So, it will be just like a complex. "See, my complex was right, sex is bad and gay men are terrible!" So that's rather simplistic.

Covid-19 is, of course, closest to a cold or a flu. Unlike tuberculosis and Covid, AIDS is really strange because it is a meta-disease – you don't actually die of it, you die of other things.

Covid-19 is close to cold or flu, which are very familiar, everybody knows them. I get the feeling I don't know if I can judge this, perhaps a doctor could say it more clearly. But wouldn't you say that a cold and flu are the most everyday illnesses there are? Stefano, you have two children, you have a family. You absolutely expect that this will happen all the time – until it doesn't. You deal with it, you tell your children, you know: use a handkerchief, don't rub your nose on your sleeve, why are you coughing? I remember my own father telling me I shouldn't cough so much, go get a handkerchief. This is a familiar homey, everyday illness transformed into something kind of awful. With Covid, the lungs get too congested: that's the part we find frightening, isn't it? It goes beyond the normal, but it is related to something very familiar. So, at that level, these diseases are all completely different. Does that make sense?

So, the level where they do intersect, the level where they are similar, at least for me, is the terror of death and, of course, the entire complex of illness, fear … (pardon me, I'm coughing, that is interesting).

So, for instance, the part that scares me – this is really interesting. As I said before, I'm relatively cheerful these days. Since it's now, what, the 25 March, 2020, and as you know, because you saw these things back in early March, weeks ago we were already getting messages from Jungian colleagues in northern Italy, therapists and doctors, and they were very serious. They said, take this seriously, which for me at least – I think you were closer to this, you probably knew it a few days before I did …

SC: I was in Italy when the outbreak was there, I was in contact with Jungian colleagues with whom we created a support group for medical doctors, nurses and all the hospital staff, to give them psychological support. And I openly suggested that people stay home in our forums and even privately.

PA: You've been there, yes. And you know that we got messages from our colleagues Monica Luci and Antonio Lanfranchi and others, around the beginning of the month when you were already engaged in this professionally.

I think the last day I was out in the town, about a week ago, I got a phone call from Antonio, a colleague of ours who's a doctor and an analyst who studied with us, and he said, do you have a mask? No, what should I – should I buy a mask? And he told me which mask to buy, he told me: this matters. He's a cardiologist, he's a doctor, so when he tells me, I listen. You knew these things a little in advance of me. But for me, sometime between the 5 and 8 March, I began to take seriously what our colleagues and friends were telling us. So, from then I did start to just avoid contact with people, and I did go into lockdown about a week earlier than the university here. But resistance has been high, you know this.

SC: Absolutely.

PA: And some of it is: I don't believe it until I see it. And of course, some of it is: people have said, here's this virus, which is the flu or cold – people do get very alert around the word virus ever since the 80s, when it developed into a cultural complex around AIDS. But they also think: oh, this is like the flu; and then we say, well, it's fairly serious; and then they say, oh, should we *do* something? There's that very dark conversation that not many people have had, but our colleagues have told us: that this death is not a good one.

SC: It's not a good one. And we should thank all those medical doctors who are on the front lines. The advice that is coming to us directly, not just through the news, is that this is a really terrible disease.

PA: This is hard; this is hard. And I think that what I was leading to before, when you were asking about me and my health … I haven't been terribly worried. At an abstract level – well, it's not an abstract level, the terror of death is very important, and I think, for me, this is a core issue. Not many people can quite get near that level, but that's really the core of this. For me, it doesn't scare me that much. I kept thinking: I've been here – fine, if I'm gone in a month, I'd better update my will, and I don't know who's going to take all my books somewhere – but the situation doesn't shatter me, which is very interesting.

SC: But this is because you have integrity, and you went into self-lockdown.

PA: No, I think it's because I've been doing death for so long.

SC: And that's why you have integrity, as John Beebe would say (Beebe, 1992).

PA: Okay, well, I think it's been a hard lesson.

SC: It is a very hard lesson.

PA: But just to finish that – there was a part that still worried me a bit, and in the last two days I've realized that I'm not so worried … I don't know if I should be.

Here's an unpleasant subject. In the last year, I've been teaching my course on AIDS and culture at Newcastle University. And my students in that class this year tend to be introverts, smart but quiet, they're all sort of on different planets. And several times this year, much more than ever before, I kept *apologizing* to them, saying, I'm not sure I want to show you this video, or talk to you about this material, it's too dark. Interestingly, when we met this week online, they were completely ready for me to talk about Covid-19 in comparison to AIDS, because they've been thinking about it. It was like: oh, yeah, we get it. That may seem a bit peripheral, but you can see how all of this is almost overly entangled.

The thing that has worried me is – I'm not good at the suffering of the body. That sounds so abstract, it's not the suffering of the body, it's really: *I feel terrible*, and the experience is really blunt, it's really here. And you know how that changes time: when you feel sick, time is just stuck. You don't get to go to imagination, you don't get to go anywhere, you're just stuck in the body and the suffering. And I kept thinking: if this happens to me, how terrible would it be? And you never know until it's happening.

This is always a question around, for instance, Tibetan Buddhists who meditate on death. I honestly think some of those who meditate on death are really ready for it – and some of them aren't. And you won't know until you get there. Our culture is not very good at this, but over the last couple of days I've been feeling – this may be a delusion of mine – that even if I get ill and it's really painful and I die, I'm not sure it would reach a point where I think: this is so awful, I wish I never lived, or this is so awful, I just … well, I'm not sure, but it feels as though I would think: ah, this is miserable – but okay, I've had a good life.[2]

SC: Let me go back to the symbolism. Now, again, following Sontag, we look at Novalis who said, between 1799 and 1800, that perfect health is interesting only scientifically. What is really interesting is sickness because sickness, Novalis says, belongs to individualization. For us as Jungians, individualization – individuation – is very important. Our own personal individuation, but also the world, the mundus individuation. And to this I link something else: Stendhal's *Armance*, when the anxious mother is reassured when the medical doctors say to her, your daughter is not really suffering from tuberculosis, she suffers from black bile, melancholy and dissatisfaction, which is usual among young people of her age and condition (Stendhal, 1975). My thesis is about individualization so, the sociological becoming of someone in a post-gender, post-nationality, post-religious society, a liquid society where we lack Jung's individuation, really becoming ourselves. And in fact, Sontag asks the question: are tuberculosis and melancholy synonyms? Also, Paul, what is suicidal in the world right now? Perhaps our chronic melancholy, never satisfied. I've been thinking these days: if Bauman said we live in an epoch that is about liquidity, so, from one job to another, from one partner you go to another, everything is liquid (Bauman, 2000). So, you don't go through the headache of a problem, because as soon as you have a problem, like Calvino said, you go to another city that has no such problem, but the same entertainments (Calvino, 1979). Aren't we now living in what one could call an all-you-can-eat society, all-you-can-eat restaurants, you can eat everything? They are about bulimia; society is a bulimic society.

PA: In an enormous world, the fact that a bad or toxic thing exists – does that mean that it is the nature of the world? And remember that I spent the 80s and 90s doing far too much Adorno, so I absolutely understand the argument. But I wonder if it's true or if it's merely a partial view. In other words, you can find examples, but are they the totality? I would question that.

SC: There are many who would say, as they said about tuberculosis, maybe even about HIV and that kind of thing, that the sickness is an occasion to finally become good, become better. And this is for me a real delusion or naive point, looking at Covid-19. Oh, the world will be different, so different that – that what?

PA: Okay, in relation to AIDS, what are your definitions of being good? There are probably many definitions, but the two big ones are, first of all: I shall behave better, I won't do drugs and have sex and all that sort of thing. Or secondly, what I think a lot of people have really done is – well – individuation. You become more yourself. You realize that the world doesn't give you everything. You get past childishness. You may know this classic line by Kimberly Bergalis, in the late 80s – a young woman who was infected with HIV by her dentist, and took him to court, where she said: I'm a good person, this shouldn't happen to me. But we realize that's just nonsense, it doesn't mean anything at all.

SC: This is exactly what I wanted to get back to.

PA: And Sontag is saying something similar. She is saying it somewhat defensively – and brilliantly, and assertively. She knows she can win the argument because she really is smarter and more powerful than any of us – it's a bit like reading Giegerich. But then the question is, is what she is saying *always* true? Because Sontag will run into trouble, as I've told you – a lot of trouble, later. So.

SC: Because otherwise one could really get off track and say, those that get sick, or those that die, are only those that want to die. Well, we've got to think. Or with Keith Thomas – the happy man, the happy person doesn't get sick (Thomas 1997). But for me …

PA: But this is just like Louise Hay! An American – she had recovered from cancer, and she told people with AIDS that you can heal yourself from your illness by mantras and saying the right positive things to yourself (Hay, 1988). She was doing this in the late 80s – it didn't work very well.

There is a version of this that goes back to the body-mind duality. What is the phrase – dual-aspect monism. The body and the mind: that whole sense that the body and the mind are one thing, which has two facets – we are confused by this because our sensory organs and some aspects of the brain and perception give us the illusion that this is a brain that is in a body, but really, they are one thing. This is a very important discussion that I take very seriously, being myself a not very physical or energetic person in the world. It's a real lesson for me, it's like: no, you *are* a body, you just are.

Now, of course, psychosomatics, and the entire world of 'I can cure myself' – there is a long history of this. ... I don't know if you have analysands like this, but a fair chunk of the people who see me are in the world of yoga and alternative therapies, a lot of dear friends are associated with that kind of thing. And there are times when they are thinking: if I have the right beliefs, and have no anxieties, my body will be cured. And my response is: well, good luck. And I say good luck because, if this body-mind is one thing, that does *not* tell you that the ego can give directions to the entire mind and the entire body, simply dictating: now I will cure myself. The ego just isn't that big a deal.

SC: And it's a bit of an inflation.

PA: Of course. I'll 'make' myself cured.

SC: I was listening to the BBC yesterday on my way to work and they were talking about the Spanish flu. So exactly one hundred years ago ...

PA: I was reading about the other day ...

SC: The world, Europe, was at war. But the Spanish were not at war, so they were the only people who could count how many people were dying from the flu. And there was someone, an archbishop, who said: don't do social isolation, come to church, pray – and the city where this foolish archbishop said this became the city with the largest number of deaths. So, we have to be reminded that science is very important, and other things are not.

PA: Well, when you say science is very important and other things are not – remember that science is going to follow a fairly logical deductive approach to this illness. And we do have a lot of government instructions that can get a little complex. Now, you know, any scientist is smart enough to know that any studied process is not certain and won't happen in the same way in every case. But when you communicate those complex uncertainties to a public audience, people will then say, oh, so you don't know for certain, they don't hear the details of it. And the other problem is that when we do get logical, rational instructions for what to do to take care of this virus, behind that discourse there will still be chaotic emotions and chaotic reactions. That doesn't mean you act on them. But a lot of people will, and every individual will tend to struggle to decide which set of reactions they take seriously. And sometimes it takes a while ... except we don't have time.

SC: Following up on the concept of individuation for the *unus mundus*, we are in lockdown, and certain countries are in full lockdown. My country, my city, Milan, where I come from, Spain, France, and many, many others, Germany, Switzerland – the UK is not in full lockdown, but …

PA: It's getting there a little more rapidly than I expected.

SC: You know the number of cases in the US, in New York. So, Edmund Burke on the French Revolution – he said, talking to the French people: your current confusion is similar to a paralysis – it's the source of life itself (Burke, 1790). We are in a paralysis. But I look at my patients, they cannot stand still. Instead of a time of modesty, a time of depth, a time of meditation in the way Jung uses the term, people are locked down, engaging in WhatsApping, Skypeing, YouTubeing, yoga lessons, Netflixing, or some may *Netflix and chill* – if you know what I mean – but this is really hyperactivity instead of a time of – perhaps, guys, slow down.

PA: Well, again, I think this can be interpreted in several ways. I mean, this situation is not uncomfortable for me. My life is perhaps too quiet over the last decade. This time has not been very strange for me. For many of my students and friends, it obviously is strange and uncomfortable, especially the extroverts. The first few days, the extroverts were just nuts – irritable, looking for problems, complaining about everything – you could tell who was more extroverted from what they were saying online. But some of my students have been playing music and even recording songs, complaining about being in lockdown, but with a smile, so it's a bit of a joke. I know that people are doing different activities, but they're not terribly – some of them are involved in care of the self, which I think is not such a bad thing, whatever Foucault says. Some of them tend to be creative, some of them tend to be …

SC: Depressed?

PA: No, well, a lot of them seem to be having fun. Now, that's England right at the moment – things haven't really hit us yet. There are people who will complain about being a bit stuck, a bit bored. And by the way, I do have to admit, I have a large flat all to myself, but some of my students whom I've seen online – it does look as though they have basically one small room, which would not please me. But I don't know – they don't look as though they're in bad shape.

SC: Perhaps this is what you said before: the threat is not there. Yes. It's like being at war – when the US was at war, but the war was in Europe, was in Japan, and so was not really a threat. We have to be really serious about this. One day it started in China, and I think the majority said, oh, it's so far away. It's like years ago with SARS. It will never get here. But there's a difference. I don't remember the numbers correctly, but ten years ago when the SARS crisis happened, there were only a few million people flying around the globe. Now there are like ten times as many.

PA: Well, I'm not sure it's that so much as that these illnesses are all different. This one moves fast, that's one of its problems. This one literally moves through a population more quickly – and also it takes a while for symptoms to show up. That's one of the problems – it keeps spreading through a population before anybody gets sick. So, I think that's been more confusing – these problems didn't come up with SARS, every one of these illnesses is a bit different. And as I say, at one end, it's all about the fear of illness and death, which is the same for all these things. At the other end, you'll have different experiences that will change the way people manage the illness, more at the ego level.[3] Does that make sense? So maybe the ego is busy with the details of each illness, though at a deeper level, there's a panic that's further down, further away, but still modifying behaviour in parallel ways. Does that make more sense?

SC: It does. We have a couple of minutes left before we have to end this and maybe we can really try to – we were talking about meaning, and for me, the meaning of what is going on is really the shift, the move, from outside to inside.

PA: Okay.

SC: From an entertainment society, a bulimic society, an all-you-can-eat society into something else, maybe because I'm in my early 40s, so in what Verena Kast, Murray Stein, and others call the midlife passage (crisis), which is really the shift from the persona – from what society taught you or your family taught you, what you got into, perhaps the self – from ego to self, to know more about yourself, so individuation.

Today someone on Facebook posted: pandemic crisis, environmental crisis, work crisis, welfare crisis, human relationship crisis, psychic crisis. And then this person had this sentence from Antonio Gramsci, from the *Prison Note-books* (Gramsci, 1992–2007), and he said: crisis consists in the fact that the old dies and the new can be born. But, in this time, this interregnum, many things happen. And this man made a comment saying, yeah, but how long does the crisis go on? Well, as Verena Kast taught us, crises are short – otherwise they are not crises, because depression is something else. The Great Depression of the 30s. So, let's be very clear: a crisis has a start and has an end. If we keep saying crises are years long, then we become like the Italians, including myself. We find excuses to not face that the new has come.

PA: All right. Well, there is the big, mystical conversation, which I really like, and I really believe, and I really can't prove, which is … I'm not sure I would put something causative in that discussion, that would be like Jung's *AION* (Jung, 1983), right? The English-speaking nations, especially, have screwed themselves up so badly in the last few years, it's unbelievable. The low levels of trust and support – they're just absolutely broken. You get a crisis and all of a sudden – real and symbolic, you can't mix them anymore. You can't say, well, maybe it's okay that the president's crazy, maybe it's okay that the prime minister doesn't care about people at all. Then all of a sudden it is *not* okay, because when you're actually facing real death, physical death, chaotically released among the population, among people – you know: your grand-mother, the guy who lives next door, or *you* – people stop saying, oh, I'm sure everything will be okay. And then, all of a sudden, people say no, they start to insist on real leadership, real government, real social connection, real environmental and economic decisions that make sense. You know, that did happen after World War Two, and it has happened at other points in history.

So, I do feel as though, even for the woman from down the street – my neighbourhood, I live in a lovely little sort of neighbourhood next to a huge park. I'm very lucky, actually. And they'd already set up a system where several people in the neighbourhood are wandering around checking up on people. I'd bought some medical gloves online and they were the wrong size. I messaged the neighbourhood group and said, does anybody want these gloves? She came and picked them up, and she stood in front of my door, we were about ten feet apart. She picked up the gloves and she said: well, I hope that maybe this will cause people to think and suddenly take things seriously, and that will heal the incredible mess that, certainly, the UK and the US and Australia are in ...

I'm thinking very much of the English-speaking nations, because that's where I've lived, and this situation is why they're such a mess at the moment. But, for places all over the world, there seems to be a certain amount of: no, you *must* take this *seriously*. So that is what I look for.

SC: Thank you, Paul, because this example you just gave me makes me realize that, aside from modesty, depth, meditation, care is also fundamental.

PA: I have an image – can I end with it? This was the first thing that came to me, some days ago, and it is how I've felt through all of this time. It is really my relationship, as a person with AIDS, to the current crisis.

And it's just an old man in the forest – robed, this looks like a fairy tale, or something medieval – digging for certain plants, looking for certain special things. And it is as though he hears something, or senses something, and he raises his head, and what he senses is familiar to him. And he sighs. And he packs everything back into his bag, and he goes to his hut to prepare to take care of people.

And that's how it has felt, a sense that this is familiar, that I absolutely know this. And somehow, I'm not terribly worried, but that's merely because I'm feeling: oh, *this* again. So, I guess, as therapists and analysts everywhere, we have to take care of people in the understanding that everything in the situation seems to be new – but it is really incredibly old, this is the oldest stuff that there is.

SC: Thank you, Paul.

Notes

1 This applies only to people who have had HIV for a long time, who took earlier, more toxic medications, or who were without medications for a long time. Those infected more recently who are on newer medications will not generally have this kind of cellular damage.

2 I now realize, some months after this interview, that my father John Salvatore Attinello said something very similar when he was diagnosed with late-stage leukaemia in 2000. I doubt I could have felt such a thing about myself at that time, but in 2020–2021 it seems very clear to me – which makes me grateful to him, as well as to my later studies and analysis.

3 I now think, eighteen months later, having engaged in much discussion and teaching of comparisons between AIDS and Covid, I am more aware of differences in people's reactions to the two diseases – which suggests different interpretations that can be related to our ideas of the nature of archetypes, or of culture, or of emergent aspects of archetypes and culture.

References

Attinello, P. (2020). "C. G. Jung and thinking about HIV/AIDS," in Carpani, S. (ed.) Breakfast at Küsnacht: Conversations on C. G. Jung and Beyond. Asheville, NC: Chiron, pp. 13–34.

Bauman, Z. (2000). *Liquid Modernity*. Cambridge: Polity.

BBC News (2020). Covid: 'Wasn't our call' to cancel Stereophonics Cardiff gigs. *BBC News Wales*, 11 November 2020. Online at: www.bbc.co.uk/news/uk-wales-54976503 (accessed 10 October 2021).

Beebe, J. (1992). *Integrity in Depth*. College Station: Texas A&M.

Burke, E. (1790). *Reflections on the Revolution in France*. London.

Calvino, I. (1979). *Invisible Cities*. London: Picador.

Carpani, S. (2020). *Breakfast at Küsnacht. Conversations on C.G. Jung and Beyond*. Ashville: Chiron

Giegerich, W. (2010). The end of meaning and the birth of man, in Collected English Papers, vol. *IV: The Soul Always Thinks*. New Orleans: Spring, pp. 189–283.

Gramsci, A. (1992–2007). *Prison Notebooks*, vols. *1–3*. New York: Columbia University Press.

Hay, L. (1988). *The AIDS Book: Creating a Positive Approach*. Santa Monica, CA: Hay House.

Jung, C. G. (1983). AION: researches into the phenomenology of the self, vol. *9/2, Collected Works*. New York and Bollingen: Princeton University Press.

Mann, T. (1998). *Death in Venice and Other Stories*. London: Vintage.

Roiphe, K. (2016). *'Susan Sontag,'* in The Violet Hour: Great Writers at the End. New York: Dial Press.

Sontag, S. (1978). Illness as Metaphor. *New York*: Farrar, Straus & Giroux.

Sontag, S. (1989). *AIDS and Its Metaphors*. New York: Farrar, Straus & Giroux.

Stendhal, A. (1975). *Armance*. Paris: Gallimard.

Thomas, K. (1997.) *Religion and the Decline of Magic: Studies in Popular Beliefs in Sixteenth and Seventeenth Century England*. New York: Oxford University Press.

Chapter 4

Compensation

John Beebe

John Beebe touches upon Jung's concept of extraversion and introversion stating that living in a country of constitutional excitement, it was hard for him as an analyst in the USA to proof the existence of introversion. Coronavirus pandemic and the consequent lockdowns are showing that energy is drawn from within, when people is to be alone. Stefano Carpani reports that during time of lockdown he observed people becoming hyperactive, entertaining themselves with Zoom calls and online activities. He wonders if we are missing the opportunity to take a new perspective on the world. Applying Susan Sontag's work Illness as Metaphor, a disease that affect the lungs – as Covid-19 does – stands for an illness of the soul. Could the affluent society perceive the seclusion caused by Coronavirus as compensation at all? Beebe seizes the opportunity to discuss the complexity of metaphors and shares his experience as medical student when he learned how violently the body wards off illnesses – to the extent of dying from it. Here the compensation would demonstrate itself worse than illness itself. Beebe urges committed attention instead of defensive extraversion. For him it is a chance to take better care of oneself and each other.

Stefano Carpani: Doctor Beebe, dear John, it's really nice to see you in good health and safe at home. First, let me ask you, how are you?

John Beebe: Physically, I feel well, and psychologically, like everyone else, I am on alert. I seem to have a space, especially in the middle of the night, to sit with my thoughts for two or three hours and have the luxury of reflection. Those are precious moments, when my psyche will not let me sleep but also does not want me to think in a directed way. They give me the strength I need to take care of the patients I see.

I work at varying times seven days a week. I do this because I have people around the world that I speak to, and I need to adjust my schedule to theirs, which means spreading mine out. This much is easy when patients are met by electronic means from a home office.

SC: How do you feel about these days?

JB: I feel as if we are in the grip of a gigantic compensation. If one goes back to the very beginnings of Jung's work, even before he met Freud,

DOI: 10.4324/9781003266402-4

when he was still imagining himself to be a natural scientist, he was doing research getting people's associations to stimulus words to see if he could map out their complexes in a very scientific way. He noticed that people approached the association testing situation in two different ways.

So, as early as 1904, he developed the idea that there are two types of attitudes that most people take when they are called to associate to a stimulus (whether that is a word association test or a pandemic). One is the extraverted attitude. A woman scheduled to take the word association test could walk into the testing room and notice the beautiful salmon colour that the protocol list of 100 words was printed on. "You must love looking at it when you are scoring it," she would say. In contrast, a typically Swiss man might come into the office and restrict himself to just listening to the stimulus words and, looking straight ahead, attend solely to the interior of his mind to observe the exact moment at which each true association first appeared. Jung came up with the words we use today to express this difference: Extraverted and introverted.

Living in a hypomanic country like America, it has been hard to agree with Jung that there really is such a thing as introversion, so the pandemic has been a revelation that Jung was after all right. You can draw energy from within when you have to be alone.

Yet I find I can rarely be alone without some media going. I think that must be because I am totally fascinated by how other people are coping with this strange time. That it must be a compensation for at least some kinds of extraversion is obvious. The poet Wordsworth in his poem titled *The World Is Too Much With Us,* said so long ago, "getting and spending we lay waste our powers," so it makes sense that from time to time there will be this kind of comeuppance driving us to introvert again.

But a pandemic is such a violent compensation, one that reminds us that Nature, which creates situations, is not a respecter of persons. Our global situation is what I reflect upon in the middle of the night, listening to my ideas and feelings until something like insight emerges. Even when this takes several hours, the effort is not exhausting. I am glad to have made room for some make-up introversion.

That I am a psychiatrist has not helped me get to this, because psychiatry is ambivalent about introversion. More than once in my own fifty years in practice, some of my colleagues have argued people who are habitually introverted are either schizoid or avoidant. Others have said, more softly, that it should raise the index of suspicion of clinicians that a personality disorder might be present when one sees a patient's libido taking an introverted turn. Amid a virus that so often begins with a respiratory attack, it might be time to counter this notion. Imagine, if pulmonary physicians were to say that inspiration, taking a breath in, is pathological, and that expiration, letting a breath out, was not. We would not have enough respirators to make up for that error. So, I cannot endorse the kind of psychiatry that would begrudges us what we do when we shelter at home, and what I myself do to make the most of this time has taken me back to early Jung.

SC: I am reading again Susan Sontag's *Illness as Metaphor* (1978), and you make me think of that because you mentioned lungs. At some point, comparing tuberculosis with cancer, she says that cancer is an illness of the body because you can locate it in the body very specifically. But she says when the lungs get infected, they become ill metaphorically as well. When we mention lung disease, we are talking about an illness, a sickness, of the soul. I link this to what you said about compensation. I have been thinking what is going on? Until lockdown we have been living in what I call *the lust society*, an *all you can eat society, the bulimic society*, and now we are experiencing a compensation of too much entertainment, lust, unnecessary stuff, into modesty, depth, maybe meditation, maybe more care. Or is this an illusion? Is it naïve to hope that the compensation for too much extraversion, hopefully, will help us to look anew at different aspects such as modesty, depth, meditation and care? I say this because I am really puzzled when I see friends, or I hear patients, or I just look outside the window and I see people, that are hyperactive. What is up? All day on Zoom calls, all day doing yoga online, meditation on YouTube, baking bread, coking, exercising indoor. I would say, just as my very first therapist said, switch off all your technology and give yourself a rest. Slow down, go with nature. Is this crisis a cry to go with nature instead of going for technology, money, speed?

JB: I certainly understand what you are saying. But I am going to resist your metaphor for a moment before returning to it. I think we all learned a lot from Susan Sontag. She was a brilliant person, very available to others, and I met several people who knew her personally. So, she was someone that was around from the very beginning of my development. Once someone I knew was on a plane next to her and handed her a journal article of mine and she seemed to like it, I was pleased by that, although I never met her personally. So that was kind of a lovely thing. But the article she liked was an essay called "The Trickster in the Arts," which happily I am going to be sharing with you in a more final form for your book *The New Ancestors* (2022). And why I feel she may have liked what I had to say about the trickster in that paper is that she understood how *tricky* metaphor is. She felt her work, *Illness as Metaphor* was a warning against using illness *naively* as metaphor. That does not mean – we are human – that we cannot draw, and must not draw, messages from what happens to us and begin to imagine. We are naturally metaphoric creatures, we just are.

It was the novelist George Eliot who first warned us that our minds can be trapped by the metaphors they take up. So, what I would say about the reason Susan Sontag was complaining about the romanticism with which tuberculosis was received in fiction as a metaphor for illness in the world soul is that it trapped our thinking further. About this, Sontag was right. My literary tastes were cultivated in my college years as an American studying English literature in the 1950s, by concentrating on Henry James, who loved George Eliot most among the nineteenth century novelists not least because his female characters, like hers, were often survivors. One of them, however – Milly Theale, the title heroine of *The Wings of the Dove* (2008) – was a tuberculosis victim. She is Christian love incarnate, finer and more generous than any healthy person could be, her compassion transfigured along divine lines because she is dying – of tuberculosis. Not even her doctor, Sir Matthew Hope, can save her. All that is left her is to make a special sacrifice of self that will allow friends who cannot love her enough to live. James is too great an ironist not to see that those her generosity leaves behind will feel too guilty to do so.

This is horrible, but the reality of tuberculosis is more horrible, and contemplating it is salutary when the disease is viewed less romantically. When I went to medical school, one of the things I learned early on was that the body in its attempt to ward off the bacillus that causes tuberculosis develops these enormous fibres, fibrotic, strong, inflammatory reactions called tubercles, to save the lungs from the invading bacteria.

People dying of tuberculosis of the lungs can no longer breathe, but not necessarily because of the bacillus, but because the physical compensation of the body against it, walling it off, had also become a barrier against the exchange of carbon dioxide for oxygen. It seemed to me as a medical student that the compensation was worse than the disease itself, and I kept asking my professors, if the body did not ward off the invading bacilli with a tubercle, would the bacilli themselves have cost just as much damage in the long run? How would they have done it? Did the body need to do this to stop that? No one seemed to know.

I still cannot answer the mystery of why compensations must be so violent. All I can say is that I know nature compensates because it lets me see that it does, violating its own essential rule, best formulated by Heraclitus in the 6th century BCE, that "Nature loves to hide." So, when I see a compensation that is kind of obvious, I say how did this happen, what did we do?

And I think that's where Susan Sontag's warning about grasping at metaphors to answer that question guards against the abuse of the victim that can be set in motion by posing it. Coronavirus victims are not getting their comeuppance for their countries' turn, through the logic of globalization, toward excessive extraversion: that is not why they are being forced to die alone, even if our effort not to have that fate has put those of us who have not yet been infected by the virus in virtual lockdown

Many of us are being punished by that compensation on our part. One of the harshest penalties imposed by lockdown, one I have not had to pay, since I can do psychotherapy from a room in my home using a computer, is underemployment. During the pandemic, I first heard about the extent of the impact on unemployed parents whose children's schools were closing, I was thinking about that the kids would be able to go home and work from the computers the way I was doing. But it was reported that it was an even worse disaster for parents to have them at home rather than at school and at risk, because the families at home had been depending on a free school lunch to assure their children got fed. In many households, lunch at school was the only dependable meal these children had been getting every day. So, the question had become, is it even ethical to ask children to stay at home? Even if the lunch is brought there, it only tempts the rest of the hungry household to share it with the child for whom it is designated.

That is the kind of problem I wake up in the middle of the night to spend some time with. And I think this need to confront ourselves with what the coronavirus came not to solve, but to get us to contemplate, has been felt by all of us. That more is wrong than meets the eye is not something you have to be a Jungian analyst to know. To realize it, you just must expand the time you spend quietly paying attention. The best thing about sheltering at home is that it has given us time to do just that.

I cannot be sure, however when I do the work of contemplating that this time seems to require, that I am truly being introverted. Rather, I think my extraversion is no longer defensive, but genuinely engaged with something out there that we all need to know more about to take better care of the others around us and ourselves. When I bring that engaged attention to my work as a psychotherapist, I seem to be more effective. It is what has helped me most to help people hold their lives together while they try to get these dangerous days. I think that is so because I have already met the pandemic in the middle of the night, when I can engage with myself as well.

SC: Thank you, John.

Bibliography

Beebe, J. (2022). The trickster in the arts, in Carpani, S. (Ed.) *Anthology of Contemporary Clinical Classics in Analytical Psychology: The New Ancestors*. London: Routledge.

Eliot, G. (2008). *The Wings of the Dove*. London, Penguin.

Sontag, S. (1978). *Illness as Metaphor*. New York: Farrar, Straus & Giroux.

Wordsworth, W. *The World Is Too Much With Us*. Online at: www.poetryfoundation.org/poems/45564/the-world-is-too-much-with-us

Chapter 5

The Suspension of Time

Davide Favero and Stefano Candellieri

These two three-way dialogues took place, the first one, at the very beginning of the pandemic, which was particularly violent in Italy in spring 2020, and the second one a year later during the second wave in spring 2021. By freely discussing, the authors questioned themselves on what was happening at a psychosocial level, in Italy in particular, and in the Western world in general, focusing not only on the most immediate level of the ongoing traumatic experience. They referred, on the one hand, to illness and death and, on the other hand, to the claustrophobic experiences of the lockdown, but also on the pre-existing social critical issues that the Covid-19 pandemic contributed to make more evident, such as individualism, anomie according to Durkheim, the pervasive spread of digital tools and social-media, the emotional-cognitive dissociation of a human being on the one hand hyper-technological and on the other prey to primitive and pervasive emotional states. The contents of these dialogues will remain highly topical even after the pandemic emergency will be over.

Part I

Stefano Carpani: Dr Candellieri, Dr Favero, Dear Stefano and Davide, you're the founding members of the Turin Psychological Medical Center, which opened in 2003. How are you?[1]

    Stefano Candellieri: I would say, "good and bad." Good because I'm fine, my family is fine, professionally fine because I'm working, I have the opportunity to continue to work and that keeps me intellectually alive. I have my patients to thank for that, who assiduously continue coming to my office in person. The therapeutic journeys we undertake are life journeys, so they're truly also a major support to me as a therapist. Bad, however, as a citizen, because the feeling I run into the most these days is sadness over the many, many deaths we have had in Italy: today we surpassed 12,000 deaths from coronavirus. Sad for the doctors, the nurses, the support staff, who've worked so hard in hospitals and ambulances making enormous sacrifices; sad for them and their families. And I'm sad about the situation we're in, with these deserted, melancholy cities. I've had the opportunity to go out every day to

DOI: 10.4324/9781003266402-5

come to my studio and work, and so every day I cross these lunar landscapes, in these truly deserted cities, with hardly anybody around, and all that undoubtedly provokes great melancholy. People have reacted, there was the singing on the balconies, for example, but it's undoubtedly a sad and melancholy scenario, and there's a nostalgia for the way we used to be up until a few weeks ago. And it's sad for all of us who are stuck in our houses, and especially for the young people who find themselves going through all this without enough support from us, because none of us has gone through an experience like this, it's utterly exceptional. So, to go back to your question, I'm fine, on top of things, I would say, but also quite sad. Not especially worried. I'm essentially optimistic about how things will go, but yes, I'm sad.

Davide Favero: Yes, well, I would second what Stefano just said. I feel the same way. I'd like to add a consideration regarding the lockdown measures which are at the origin of the collective confinement caused by this period we're going through. These measures are experienced by many people, certainly by some patients I treat, but also acquaintances I'm in contact with, as a sort of interval. Therefore, in a way, the collective is waiting for an anomalous period, which has created a discontinuity with respect to the past, to end. This discontinuity, which indisputably exists, in my opinion, can't be understood as an interval. I mean that once the interval ends we can't, the way you can when you're writing an essay, for example, pick up where we left off. We are in the face of a true paradigm shift, which will inevitably lead to a break with the past and that will likely extend far beyond the measures laid out by the lockdown. I make this claim because the discussion of the interval splits the groups of people I see these days, i.e. the ones who experience it as that, as a hiatus, and the ones who can see the paradigm shift and the start of a transformation that will go on in time. I imagine that in the mid- to long term we will eventually resume the majority of our pre-existing habits, but, in any case, it will take a long time. Therefore, the present is a kind of suspended time. And it's important for people to understand that a suspended time must be experienced, must be lived, it's a time when it's also possible to try something new. Yet to their detriment, many people experience this time as a waiting period, a non-time. A time that can't be used in a constructive, creative way. Now, I don't want to digress too much, because the question was about how I'm doing, but to say how I'm doing, adding on to what Stefano said, I can't do without making this preliminary point. I am called to live in a time that is discontinuous with respect to the past, and that will continue to be discontinuous for an unknown amount of time. So I'm trying to winnow all my actions, my thoughts, my feelings, with this factor in mind.

SC: Davide, let me say that I'm with you, because I also have this feeling, this experience, even with my patients. And before we get to talking the suspended time of today (which many are beginning to talk about in Italy), I would like to talk about the emotions of this period. Stefano noted the sadness. Davide brought up the interval, which is not an emotion, but can be linked to emotion. There is nervousness, anxiety, anguish, fear, panic. I would like to use the next few minutes, if you agree, to look one by one at those emotions your patients bring to you, in the hopes that this will help the reader. How can people get through this suspended time and navigate the emotions we're experiencing – even if these are the same emotions we have had for forty-five years, but that now arise or are perceived differently because we've so consumed with the activities that fill up our days.

DF: The primary emotional tenor is of the depressive type. That is, the sadness Stefano talked about earlier, after a few weeks of lockdown, has turned toward the depressive polarity. A symptomatology has begun to appear that includes anhedonia, abulia, apathy, ataraxia. Individuals are unable, despite their initial resolve, to complete the vaguely euphoric goals they set for themselves when lockdown went into effect. Flour and yeast flew off the supermarket shelves: people started baking at home, making cakes, making bread, making things from scratch, which, incidentally, are excellent activities in themselves, but from the psychological perspective, suggest a manic reaction, i.e. a reaction of non-acceptance of the depressive condition that was beginning to emerge; in other words, there's been an attempt to flee a state of suffering by recourse to activity. A recently published Lancet study[2] (2020) clearly delineates two opposing psychological attitudes of people under quarantine. On the one hand there is a so-called "manic-compulsive" attitude, on the other there is an attitude more oriented toward social relations and altruism. So the Lancet study, which is a meta-analysis, a review of other studies on the quarantine, says exactly that: some react to a depressive condition, as quarantine inevitably is, due to the objective loss of certain individual liberties, habits, and so on, and some react manically, risking long term psychological damage, even severe. Yet those who are able to construct or at least invest in the relational-affective dimension, altruism-based and otherwise, have a good chance of coming out unscathed – which is not to say without any degree of suffering but at least having maintained the proper mental hygiene for coping with quarantine. Thus I would recommend people to resist autistic urges, regressive urges, which the present situation nonetheless provokes, in favour of activities focused on others: friends, loved ones, relationality in general. Activity need not be manic. We need a certain kind of activity (relational); this is fundamentally the emotional repertoire we need to stimulate. Not mania or compulsivity, but their opposite. Ideally, letting in a little bit of this dimension of sadness, of the depressive type, without fear, without being afraid of getting crushed by it.

SCa: Yes, I agree. The emotions we've seen recently – not so much in the patients already in therapy, who, so to speak, can collect the fruit of their labour and thus on average are better equipped, as much as in people in general – the emotions we've seen were initially a slightly hysterical reaction, with anxiety, as Davide was saying, immediately followed by a sort of euphoria: "This is my chance to finally read *War and Peace*, to pick up the guitar again, go back to studying, finally get my house organized, etc." Except quickly realizing the infeasibility of these plans. Most people didn't succeed in following through with these plans, and so also felt guilty, inevitably, in my point of view. Because the climate in which we're immersed, an alienating climate, would require disassociation to be particularly creative while stuck in the house with this anguished climate across the nation right outside the door – I'd almost consider it pathological if someone could disassociate to such an extent from what is going on outside. So most people failed to follow through, and as a result felt very frustration. Gradually, then, first came guilt, then frustration, and finally more overtly depressive conditions began to emerge. What I try to do when these therapeutic cases come up, is support the person, pointing out that this a significant transition. As Davide was saying, a euphoric response, when it occurs, is not positive. On the contrary, we must face the sadness. One of the latest posts on our Facebook page ("Gorgoni Psicoanalitiche") talks about Pier Paolo Pasolini's movie titled *The Gospel According to St. Matthew* [Il vangelo secondo Matteo].

During the opening scene, as the Three Kings are arriving, there is a heart wrenching musical score, a spiritual sung by Odetta Holmes entitled "Sometimes I Feel Like a Motherless Child." We quote this song because we see it as particularly apt for representing the moment: we are orphans of a world we've left behind, and we're disoriented and lost. It's good to get in touch with this mental climate and put aside the banners, the anthems, this initial euphoric response. The sooner we get in touch with our sadness, the sooner we become truly creative. To become creative, we must get through this phase. We've yet to reach the time, in my opinion, for creativity.

SC: In my conversation with Verena Kast (see Chapter 1), the world-renowned Jungian psychotherapist and former president of the Jung Institute in Zurich and IAAP, she said, "you have to aim for creativity." But, precisely, the first step is denial, the second step is acceptance of the moment you're in. Another important point, these days – we see this in our patients, friends and perhaps even in ourselves and in social networks – is the theme of addiction. People spend day and night on Netflix, on Tinder, sending and receiving WhatsApps constantly, taking online yoga classes, relaxing with online meditation, you name it. ... What do you think of this fact, or the fact of those who are in total denial: "As soon as this is over I'll have a five-litre gin and tonic." "As soon as this is over," you name it (again!).

SCa: I see it as connected to that "mania" Davide spoke about, that is, to the fact that the initial wave of anxiety was followed by this slightly euphoric response. Let's not forget – to introduce the theme of war, which I would like to circle back to since we're all infected by this metaphor – that soldiers in war used to get drunk before battle: in World War I cognac and grappa flowed like rivers. That cognac becomes Netflix, becomes little games on the telephone, this suggests a climate of battle, a reaction something like the assault troops had in WWI: drink, get intoxicated, and jump into combat. It's certainly a physiological phase, but one that must be abandoned as quickly as possible in order to get in touch with that same void, this alienating climate we're living in, the profound sadness I mentioned before. The sooner we get in touch with it, the sooner we can become creative.

SC: Also because if you go into battle drunk, it ends badly. You're not lucid enough to handle combat. Pope Francis said, "Let's not call it war, let's call it a storm." I wonder if this is a more apt metaphor for this moment. The president of France has too talked about Covid as a war, where every citizen is a soldier. But, perhaps, since it is a war against unknowns, against a virus, against something invisible, we need to change our words too ...

DF: As I brought up before and Stefano reiterated, I believe it is the euphoric responses that, at least initially, avoid confrontation with the depressive mode, which is a mandatory phase to go through in order to "digest" everything that's going on. They are also an expression of this temporal suspension which some people still don't read as necessarily "continuous" time. What I mean is that, acknowledging the break with the past that has been created, the present is a "continuous" time that will keep going for quite a while. This implies that for some people, the most addicted, the ones holding their breath waiting for the bad times to end in the hopes that they can go back to the life they had before, it becomes complicated, and so I think that there is conceptual orientation that should be modified as early as possible. We must try to help, not only our own patients, but also with interesting initiatives like your interviews, try to spread the message as widely as possible that the world after a pandemic is transformed just as it is after a war – albeit in different ways. Therefore, to continue with the analogy, undoubtedly the world goes on and a war becomes a historical fact that is described and circumscribed, or rather, compartmentalized: similarly, in twenty years the pandemic will be an "objectivized" story, but it is not yet so at this moment.

We are now living in pandemic time, just as people in the past lived in wartime. This similarity serves not to forecast a theme that we should address later, but to say that pandemic time is a specific kind of time. I had the fortune of being raised by two grandparents, so people who were quite elderly, in fact I skipped a generation; my grandfather was born in 1904, so he lived through the Spanish Flu, World War I and World War II. When he would tell us stories from his past, whether about the pandemic, war, or anything else, he would prefaced his story by saying: "In the time of ... " "the war" or "the pandemic" precisely to indicate that it was a different time compared to the time right before a war breaks out or a pandemic hits. So I insist on this point because it's absolutely fundamental that people abandon the illusion of a brief transitoriness, of an unusual and abnormal period. Unfortunately, just today I read that a second wave is starting in Hong Kong and a second lockdown, after they had practically eliminated contagion in their first wave. It's useless to say that all epidemics, and pandemics even more so, return, there's no way to quash them on the first try, at first contact. So we have them for a long time. The psyche needs to adapt to this time. The psyche has no hope of coping without putting itself out there.

SC: Fear and uncertainty are also common emotions these days. "Fear" because it's been many years, if not decades, since something like this has happened. The "uncertainty" is about how long it will last and when we will return to our normal "life" and what the aftermath will be like. What do you think?

SCa: I want to step back just for a second, because in reality there's another emotion – if we want a more complete list of what we're dealing with in this period – is anger. Here in Turin there have been instances of people inside their houses going to the window and railing against people out on the street jogging – and this before the prohibition against going outside to run – or who looked askance at people walking down the street. So another emotion that's going around is anger, and, in this regard, I'd like to go back, quickly, to the theme of the extremely abused war metaphor, because it's a problem I feel strongly about. Maybe "storm" is a better image than "war," but as a doctor I'd simply like to speak in terms of a "health crisis." Lately I keep thinking of Wilfred Bion (2018), a famously provocative spirit, who said "When there are a lot of individuals here, there are also a lot of thoughts without a thinker, and these thoughts-with-out-a-thinker are floating around somewhere. I suggest that they are looking for a thinker." Bion introduced this notion, which I find extraordinary, of thoughts that circulate from mind to mind and have a life of their own, of a thinker who believes they have "copyright" over their thoughts but that can in fact be unknowingly "colonized" by thoughts circulating in society. Cultural semiotics uses the concept of the "meme," introduced by Richard Dawkins in the 1970s. A "meme" is a minimal unit of significance, we could say an elementary idea, that self-propagates like a virus and that seeks nothing but its own survival. "War," in my view, is one of these elementary ideas, one of these memes, that can penetrate our minds as a metaphor to represent the Covid-19 pandemic only to cast off the idea of the epidemic and take an autonomous direction, ultimately leading to increased aggression. In the end, in other words, we risk finding ourselves at war against another person (a passer-by, a neighbour) and not against the virus. That's why war is a metaphor that, in my opinion, should be discarded as quickly as possible, and we should stop saying "doctors in the trenches," etc. Anger must absolutely be metabolized, worked out, and put behind us, so we can find ourselves with the feelings you were discussing – disorientation, emptiness, the sadness we'll have to carry inside for a while, maybe for a long while, certainly for weeks and months. Only after that, I reiterate, will the time come for us to be creative and vital.

DF: Yes, the war discourse is also a springboard to other ideas, because, in the meantime, the similarity is apt for a host of reasons, banally because of the limitation of individual freedoms, because of a situation of objective peril that people are experiencing, because of the evacuation of individual responsibility in favour of the larger role of institutions. Certain analogies hold up, but we can't run the risk of talking about a health crisis by calling it a war, it seems absolutely essential to specify this phase. Moreover, to complicate the issue, in war there is a physical or objective enemy; in World War I, which was trench warfare, there were specific fronts where the enemy forces were located, people knew, gave them a name, knew who they were fighting against, where and when, they gave a specific name to what was happening around them. Even in World War II, air raids were announced in advance by sirens alerting people to imminent danger, which was visible at its origin. Whereas now in this health crisis, the enemy is invisible. Because, sure, we've seen images of Covid-19 under the electron microscope, but that's not representable in the individual psyche nor in the collective psyche. This is an enemy that we are fighting which is for all intents and purposes invisible, that anyone could potentially transmit. And therefore everyone is potentially an enemy, a fact that creates a psychological storm in each of us, even in the people who think they're immune. In reality no one is immune and I'm not referring to immunity from the virus but immunity from this impossible mental representation, because let's not forget that the deepest and most terrible anxiety is so-called "nameless" anxiety, whereas an anxiety with a shape easily becomes a fear, which is more manageable: in the face of an anxiety with a name you shift into fear, the two terms are almost indistinguishable when you know why you're anxious. But in this case the enemy is really boundless, with hazy boundaries and therefore really very powerful. Stefano and I have had a symmetrical approach to patient management in these weeks, Stefano has continued seeing over 80% of people in his office, was able to go on like that and the other 20% remotely, whereas I see 15–20% of people in my office and all the others on Skype. Well, lots of young people I treat and who with "reason" might feel pretty safe because of course the virus affects everyone but we know that worse effects are correlated with age, and in fact I see many young people who are terrified, anxious, and don't leave the house for this very reason. Because they aren't able to come up with a mental representation of the element they have to protect themselves from, defend themselves from. So this anxiety also needs room for expression. It will take time and as Stefano pointed out before, people who are already in psychotherapy, especially psychoanalysis, are automatically better protected because they've developed a habit of working that allows them to dream, and to dream not only at night but when they're awake, therefore to represent, to imagine, in other words, to have representations that are effective in handling such a dramatic situation.

SC: I'd like to move to the concept of suspended time. However, I would like to make a preface first. In my opinion, after Bauman's "liquid society" (2000), the last few years have been characterized by what I term *bulimic society, all-you-can-eat society*. You go to a restaurant, pay 9.99 euros, and eat as much as you want. Or you go to a chain store and buy a T-shirt for one euro, and just not use it or throw it away. We live in the society of *hyper-entertainment* and the superfluous. Is the Covid the antithesis to all this or am I a deluded naïf? Can we look at the post-Covid moment as something new, as a more modest era? Will we move from extroversion to introversion, to meditation, to taking care of ourselves and others differently?

And so, talking about suspended time, will this time be a space for reflection, for learning the art of patience, without being a time that's really scary. What are your thoughts on this?

SCa: Picking up on Davide's comments, it's truly a frightening space, also because it's a space that must be explored from scratch. We're not used to this space, except perhaps those of us who are older. I was born in 1963 and as a little boy I lived through austerity, the years of terrorism and the so-called "strategy of tension," but the current situation is completely different from all that and so, just as we don't have antibodies against this new virus, nor do we have "psychic antibodies" against it; we don't have the tools, we have to create them. One theme, which I'll just mention very briefly, is that we're going to need lots of culture, culture is the most abandoned sector right now. We're going to need poets who can "dream" what we're going through, artists, filmmakers, painters, and so on. We're going to need a collective effort to dream this new experience we're going through, just as, in individual therapy, dreams have an enormous function in working through trauma. We'll need a lot of culture. If we have, at the same time as reanimation in intensive therapy, a sort of "social reanimation" that helps us to dream, to imagine, to explore, to build up "antibodies" against this new unknown space, then we'll be able to emerge enriched by this experience. Otherwise, the risk is grave regression, not only social and economic but also political.

DF: Of course. I completely agree with what Stefano said. I wouldn't expect otherwise, having collaborated for so long. So our thinking is aligned as well. I would add, though, to what he said, and returning to your prompt, that this globalized-late-capitalist society, as it was prior to the paradigm shift triggered by an infinitely small (and this is an extraordinary paradox), not to say, atomic disaster, but it was the invisible that managed to bring the turbocharged machine of this advanced capitalism to a halt. History teaches us that probably, over the mid- to long term, capitalism will reorganize and exploit the situation, its methods becoming even more efficient and its products even more effective. But this time we have an interesting opportunity because this machine running at an unsustainable speed did stop for a bit. And that never happened, except in analogous situations like pandemics, like wars. But it's the first time that it has stopped in globalized society. The speed of capitalism was slower in the past. It's an extraordinary opportunity for collectivity. And we're already seeing phenomena from a collective point of view. To pick out a simple example, a shift of the dimension of the superego from the individual to the institutional, the social. I mean, today it is the state telling you – and it's not a nation, a mayor, a president, but administrators who govern billions of people – "Stay home, you can't work. Or if you must, work less, work remotely, slow down." It's a completely new message. This message, however, produces a shift in the superego, this exempting the individual of responsibility towards production, makes it so that the individual can experiment, be liberated, albeit temporarily, from that unconscious conditioning that has consumed them since birth, and that induces people to produce without thinking about the why, the how much. That's why the present is an absolutely fertile moment, as if the virus enabled a tilling of the soil and now it's up to us to plant the seeds for something truly worthwhile to grow. We have this big opportunity. But it won't be simple, because, I repeat, over the centuries capitalism has always proved able to overcome any setback. But we have great luck, too: just when we were despairing and were almost convinced and resigned we'd have to live with the excessive powers of finance shaping governments' political and economic decisions. So there is hope …

SC: It's as if this invisible virus has managed to stop the alienation Marx talked about and Chaplin so elegantly mocked. I'll conclude our conversation by thanking you and returning to your words: the moment for creativity will come, but this is a moment for sadness, for the awareness that we are going through a difficult time, as every crisis begins and ends; your idea of the hiatus, Davide, and that this will be done when we start dreaming again, as Stefano said, thinking of social and cultural revival in our country, and that Europe, hoping it remains united, can enter a new phase. Thank you very much, I wish you well, because we need it.

SC and DF: Thank you! Best wishes to you as well!

Part II

SC: Dear Davide and Stefano. We spoke a year ago when we had just gone into the first lockdown. We are now one year into the pandemic and into another lockdown. Before talking about this past year, I would like to dedicate, if possible, this conversation of ours to a dear friend of yours and our colleague, Dr. Simonetta Putti, who passed away earlier this year. You were both at the IAAP conference in Avignone where you presented a paper, I met her there. What is your memory of Simonetta?[3]

DF: To be extremely concise, I would say that I remember Simonetta as a very frank colleague, not one to mince words, so to speak, that is, a direct person who would get right to the point of an issue, without shying away from subjects that could be a little disturbing. She didn't use anaesthetic and I always appreciated that a lot. Moreover, her talents as a psychoanalyst, both in terms of her level of culture and the compassion she devoted to her patients, were extraordinary. Truly a great loss.

SCa: I second what Davide has said. For me, it's a huge void. Over the past year we discussed everything that was going on, and perhaps we can bring up some of those points here tonight. Simonetta and I wrote each other since we couldn't see each other in person, she was in Rome and we're in Turin, and we both commented on the things that went on in this long pandemic year, trying to reach beyond the manifest surface of things, trying to get past the pictures of army trucks transporting coffins and the ill in intensive care, past the virologists' commentary, and understand what was happening in the social fabric. As an interlocutor, from not only the psychoanalytic but also the intellectual point of view, Simonetta leaves a huge void, besides, of course, from the affective point of view. A very beloved person, and as Davide said, very candid. It's truly an enormous loss.

SC: I didn't know her as well as you did. I went to see her in her studio in Rome to record an interview with her, and she wanted to talk about the concept of the limit. Aren't the last twelve months about the concept of limit and boundaries? What has happened in those twelve months?

SCa: I can start, in memory of Simonetta … Well, I won't hide that – and those who know me are aware – but I've been highly critical of the way the pandemic was handled in Italy, the country I obviously know best … but in these months I've tried to go beyond political-organizational management of the pandemic in the strict sense. I'll make my point by referencing the epilogue of Tolstoy's *War and Peace*. These last pages of the novel, which readers often skip, contain a significant historical reflection, in which Tolstoy poses both a full stop and a few interrogatives that he leaves unanswered, interrogatives that in my view were later taken up by the great twentieth century thinkers, the great psychoanalysts and sociologists, for example. The "full stop" Tolstoy poses is the conviction is that heads of state – at that time kings, emperors, generals – are not in fact the true architects of history. This reflection is articulated over several pages and leads to a question: if it wasn't, for example, Napoleon who ordered the Russian campaign, then what led to the mass migration of millions of people, what led to the millions of deaths? We ask the same question about World War I, the Shoah, World War II. From Tolstoy's point of view, heads of state are certainly partly responsible, but somehow they ride a tiger which today, over a century after Tolstoy, we could call the collective unconscious. So momentarily shelving the various Napoleon I or III or our own Premiers, our reflection must focus on the social fabric, or rather psycho-social fabric, and that brings me back to this last pandemic year. Beyond the mistakes that were made, beyond the initial disorganization with something that nobody expected … . Here I must make an aside: for many reasons it's kind of funny that we didn't expect it, because there were three pandemics in the twentieth century alone: the terrible Spanish flu in 1918–1919, the Asian flu in 1958, and the 1968 one known as the Hong Kong flu. Back to what I was saying, beyond how the pandemic has been managed, what we have seen is a very long lockdown which people have been fairly cooperative with, and one can't help but wonder why. A first, easy answer is the obvious one: people are dying of Covid-19, going to the emergency room and causing overcrowding in the hospitals, and as a result, lockdown is simply a necessity. I don't dispute this view, but it seems insufficient.

It seems to me that our society was "ready" for this long lockdown. For a few years now David and I have been reflecting on certain aspects we've been seeing emerge more and more not just in our psychotherapeutic practices but also at the social level. In 2014, for example, we wrote a piece on "autistic barriers" not only in psychotherapeutic work but also as an aspect of society, and on that subject, I'd like to mention, in passing, the phenomenon of Hikikomori, which is increasing noticeably. In this same period, we've reflected – to add something else to the mix – on what we could call a very regressive and primitive collective unconscious, and we wrote a paper on the phenomenon of "Santa Muerte," a very widespread cult in Latin America. I'll come to my point. My impression is that the Covid-19 pandemic was a kind of "perfect storm" that brought out something that was already boiling under the surface: a very strong tendency in our society to withdraw into the self, what we call in psychoanalytic slang "autistic shutdown." The technological means we have at our disposal have facilitated this progression enormously, or perhaps it would be more accurate to call it a regression. On the other hand, our society, in my opinion, has some strongly primitive aspects at the level of mass psychology. We have this, as McLuhan (1994, p. 18) called it, "digital idiot"[4] – which we all are to some extent – a hypertechnological and hyperconscious man behind which hides the psyche of a primitive, a caveman. These two dimensions, the autistic and the primitive, already very present, in my opinion, in our society, have exploded because of the pandemic. So on the one hand we have a dramatic order to remain homebound, over the course of this long lockdown, using the tools we have available to us, from cell phones to computers, and on the other we have a collective psyche that is profoundly suggestible to what's going on, primed to act like a barbarian horde – I'm thinking of the online "shitstorms" in this period, the extreme polarization like everyone taking sides as pro- or anti-vaccine. Basically there's a proliferation of this human type who is on the one hand hypertechnological and hyperrational and on the other "hyperbarbaric," who in my opinion was "precipitated," as in a chemical reaction, and violently brought forth by the pandemic. This is one of my early reflections that I shared privately with Simonetta in recent months.

DF: Stefano mentioned Napoleon, as cited by Tolstoy, which reminds me that in just a few days, on May 5, 2021, it will be the bicentenary of Napoleon's death. In 1804 he produced the famous edict of Saint-Cloud, an edict which declared that the dead were to be buried outside the city walls. It was an edict motivated primarily by political and sanitary reasons – the same reasons motivating health policy decisions given to us today – an edict that shook up the populace's habits quite a bit. Why am I mentioning Napoleon and the edict of Saint-Cloud? Because even then our Foscolo and Pindemonte, inspired by pre-romantic English graveyard poetry, reacted vehemently against this edict because at the time there was a kind of closeness, friendship, with death; not to say that people longed to die, but that death was considered as inherent to life. And living and dying weren't so separate or distinct. They were two temporally diverse conditions in a single symbol, as we trained Jungians would call it. Well, it seems to me that in this pandemic year our repression of death has become even more pronounced, the displacement of death to a distant land, or even, we have become more distanced from the experience of suffering, in an unprecedented way, unlike anything that has happened in the past. We were willing to trade part of our freedom to chase a little safety, which, moreover, is deceptive, because safety, as we know, is by no means given with certainty. We could respect every possible guideline for preventing Covid-19 contagion and be infected nonetheless. So we are seeing a sort of, as the philosopher Han says, algophobia in this age, or fear of pain. Aries, the French historian, has discussed how death was domesticated in the past, because the dying person was surrounded by family, there existed a certain ritual in passing into the afterlife. Friends and family gathered, then at a certain point the dying person turned toward the wall, turning their back on the present, which might also include children. It was the possibility of staying close to the dead, keeping vigil over the dead, touching the dead. This all waned a bit over time ... maybe Stefano would like to continue on this subject?

SCa: Yes, I'll take up your thoughts and return to one of the images I mentioned earlier, one of the most shocking images of this long pandemic year, repeatedly shown by the mass media: the image of intubated intensive care patients, which along with the coffins on the military trucks, has strongly impressed itself on us, our feelings, our thoughts. This year I found myself reflecting on these images, on what they had touched inside us, and I'll address this point by taking a small step back from it, because one of the readings that has often come to mind is Roland Barthes' famous *Mythologies* (2013), an extraordinary book, and particularly extraordinary is the last chapter in which Barthes reflects on "mythical thought" in our modern society. Part of his reflection centres on a photograph from the front page of a newspaper. The newspaper was *Paris Match* and the photograph was of a young black soldier saluting the French flag with a blue sky in the background. Barthes' reflection is easy enough to explain. It starts with the consideration that this photo, which could have ended up in this young soldier's family photo album, instead winds up at a newspaper office and is published in a very prominent position on the cover: at this point it is no longer the same photo and in semiotic terms it becomes the signifier of a second semiotic system. Put simply, this photo becomes representative of another value system, and doesn't end up as a memory in a family album, but goes on to embody something that from Roland Barthes' point of view we could call French imperialism, France's destiny as a "great empire." Barthes' reflection here, which I recommend reading, is very sophisticated. He doesn't say: "This photo is a symbol of French imperialism," but rather, "This photo is French imperialism," which thereby transforms it into a concrete reality, which is not symbolically represented but "is" that soldier. And Barthes' reflection focuses on this second order system, which we could call a rhetoric of power, a political rhetoric: in essence a system that is "embodied" in that image. Barthes, incidentally, also hints at a possibly psychoanalytic point of view, but since the fifties when he wrote that text, many of the fruitful developments that have taken place in psychoanalysis in recent decades had not yet happened. The fact remains, from Barthes' point of view, that the image of the soldier at the centre of his discussion can also somehow be considered the equivalent of a dream image. Even in a dream we may encounter concrete objects, such as a house, that really exist, but that are no longer objects in reality, and by representing it, embody something else, another "second order system," in this case our unconscious, of which the dream object is not simply a symbol: if I dream that I am alone and lost in a big airport, that image "is" my loneliness, "is" my disorientation. I say this in passing but also to skip a step and get to an important point: somehow, when we look at a photo in a newspaper, we're dreaming. This is Roland Barthes' point. We're seeing something else even subtler and more invisible. And so my question is: what did we see, or rather "dream," looking at the coffin picture all these months? What did we see looking at a picture of an intubated person in ICU? We saw "facts," some will say. Sure, but we also saw something else. Those pictures represented something inside us. To follow Barthes, those photos also represented a rhetoric of power, they also represented a particular message, at most in a positive, perhaps psycho-pedagogical sense, like images of disease on cigarette packs: "Watch out or this could be you." But that's not what interests me. I wonder, rather, at the level of the collective unconscious, what we saw looking at those pictures. One answer I give myself, which is certainly provisional as I don't think any of us has the answer in our pocket, is that looking at those photos we "saw" several things. First of all, we saw death in the way we experience it today, as something monstrous and terribly scandalous, and here I want to connect back to Davide's reflection. There's another anniversary coming up: in 1822 Alessandro Manzoni's *Adelchi* (2019) was published, with the famous chorus about Ermengarda's death, a death described in such a vital way that I don't think another poet could do the same today. Today, for us, death is more scandalous than ever. And this is another topic that I discussed often with Simonetta: the monstrosity of death today. So looking at those pictures, in my opinion, what we saw first of all is the modern idea of death. Something awful and completely disconnected from life, of which death is actually part.

Then I think we saw other things as well. I think we also saw, provisionally I mean, something punitive, certainly in part evoked by the rhetoric of power I spoke of earlier. We saw those who don't behave properly or who are the victims of others who don't behave properly being punished. This is what happens to libertines, in modern terms. Yet, to go a little further, we saw something else too: I think perhaps we saw our society in the mirror. I think, in fact, that our society is in intensive care, precisely because of the type of humanity that has taken shape, where social relations are suffering enormously. I have the impression that in that photo we saw, as if in a dream, ourselves. We are a society very much in crisis and in my opinion Covid-19 has simply brought this profound crisis to the surface. We're all hooked up to machines. Maybe even the money we receive from the European Union eventually risks becoming a kind of life support. When we spoke a year ago, my idea was that culture should be the real reanimating force, but instead the terrible thing in this past year, the last six months in Italy in particular, is that culture has been wiped out: theatres, events, cinema, all activity that could broadly be called cultural. And so to me it really seems like those pictures showed us our mirror image, which is that of a society profoundly in crisis, in intensive care.

SC: True, a society profoundly in crisis! I want to challenge you: Barthes was a giant, but he wrote what he wrote in *Mythologies* in 1957. The world was very different because it was less technological than today. The cover of a newspaper or a magazine, or a news article was the only piece of information or picture of a day (or the whole week). Everything was contained in that picture and information. Today we receive numerous images a day. For example, of all the pictures and images we've recently seen on TV, the image of the military trucks transporting coffins from Bergamo to the crematoria outside Lombardy, had a huge impact on me, stayed

with me until now, and I feel it will stay with me much longer. Such an image – I would propose – encompasses everything. It encompasses everything and will stay with me for a long time because it has a powerful and highly symbolic meaning. Indispensable! Going back to Barthes, my provocation is: can we keep this image (or other images) in us long enough for it to have an effect?In Italy, former Prime Minister Conte,[5] who did what he could and I believe did his best, considering our system, was replaced by Professor Mario Draghi.[6] And Draghi chose General Figliuolo as head of the task force to implement vaccinations and handle the emergency. This is a very important symbol, is it not? In a nutshell, can we stay with an image long enough for it to lead to transformation, or do we get rid of it and our memories along with it?

DF: But one thing must be said: at the international level the strategies for managing the situation didn't seem so dissimilar to me, even if a few different things were tried – I'm thinking of the strictness in China, the laissez faire climate in Sweden, the contradictions in England. ... In the end, the results, at the level of epidemiological data, at least from what you read, don't seem to have been all that different. So the first reflection I'd like to make is that the political management of this pandemic has been homogenous at the transnational level, I don't see one country significantly more at fault or more virtuous than another. And the fact that it has been transnational leads me to another reflection, which is that in some way the crisis should have been thought through. In my opinion, any theorization of the crisis has been conspicuously absent. We must acknowledge that politics has to respond to crisis situations very quickly, they don't have the time at their disposal that, for example, science may have, or generally speaking, culture, which base their logic on careful research into primary sources, materials, selecting the most appropriate methodology and thus generating an elaborate and complete analysis. Decisions have to be made quickly in politics because in any case immediate solutions need to be provided. So what has been missing is a theorization of this crisis. But not so that anyone could have known in advance that Covid-19 was coming, no one could have imagined Covid-19 or what sort of real-world consequences it would cause, but in general, epidemiology studies pandemic situations, and they have always existed, as Stefano reminded us, from the plague as in Alessandro Manzoni or even before smallpox, up to the flu of the last century, the so-called short century. Well, if we know that pandemics exist, there must necessarily exist forms of responsibility in which politics assumes the onus of governance in preparing a crisis management strategy a priori, and above all, in constructing thinking around pandemic crises.

SC: Let me interrupt you here, because I want to share something with you. A few days ago I was talking to a colleague (also a Medical Doctor), who says to me, "How come, a year after the pandemic, with all the information we have (I have about 20 articles here to read) do they talk so disparately?" This question is important: why, with all the information we have, does everything look so disparate? Another question is: one year after the pandemic, why has it not been possible to understand who is really in danger? Why is it that the elderly ninety-year-old lady doesn't get sick, or if she does she has very mild symptoms, although she has hypertension, she has this, she has that, but then the young man under thirty gets sick and dies? There is total confusion.

Surely, we've gone from fear of contagion to the fear of death, but as long as contagion and death don't affect us, they don't exist. The only certainty, in my opinion, is the difficulty in verbalizing and recognizing emotions. It is no coincidence that in this year we find the vulnerable: crying, anxiety, irritability, nervousness; the children: hyperactivity, attention deficit, they seem possessed, they can't keep still.

I like what you said, Davide, about management, theory, even more than management, because there was a void. Which is not an inner void, but really a political, strategic void.

SCa: May I make a comment "off the record"? As a doctor, I couldn't say ...

SC: This is really important: "as a medical doctor, I don't know what to say." In the past twelve months everything and the opposite of everything has been said. One example: a year ago, as soon as lockdown started, Salvini said "let's open everything." He wanted to save the economy and was utterly ignorant about what was going on as it happens for populist leaders.

I sense that what happened last year was only about nature and Covid-19 is nature, and nature always takes its course. Nature knows. Nature knows what's best, but when that happens, human beings intervene with technology, with medicine ...

SCa: I confess that in this year I've followed all the health regulations, in the studio I have always followed all the hygienic recommendations, masks, etc. However, personally, I have never been afraid of Covid-19, I think that nature takes its course, that we must certainly equip ourselves as best we can, but we can only do so if we think that the pandemic is a health emergency and not a war. Something that happened right from the start, however – and, to follow Tolstoy, I don't believe that the responsibility lies only with politicians, I think it was something that came from all of us – was to experience it as a war. If it becomes a war, in my opinion, it simply confuses matters, because it's no longer a health emergency and therefore is no longer rationally managed as such. I will make an aside on a fact that strikes me greatly: my medical association in Turin publishes an updated list of colleagues who have died in this pandemic year called "The fallen of Covid-19." Personally, I don't agree at all. These colleagues, to whom we express every gratitude died on the job, died in service, they didn't "fall." This is to say the power of this image of war, which in my opinion has also kept us from having a generally better equipped policy, precisely because the pandemic was not handled as a health crisis. I would add to this: why was it experienced as a war? I go back to what I was saying before: there is the buried shadow of a very primitive man within us. We are hyper-modern but fundamentally tribal. And so war is embedded in our minds. This has led us to make bad decisions, to the point of having an Alpine General in charge of the emergency, a general whom, based on my experience as a medical officer in the Alpine Corps, I must confess I like much more than Arcuri and consider more capable, I say so openly. But I see him in line with this image of war that is so widespread. I would place the image of war within a broader social context, which is my real concern, much more so than Covid-19, which is this society, which is at once hyper-modern and deeply primitive, and therefore extremely confused: in this perspective, not in a clinical sense, it is a schizophrenic society, dominated by chaos. If you'll allow me a joke, Stefano: influenza seems to have disappeared in these past months but in compensation we have a lot of "influencers," a word that curiously has the same etymology, and it all makes me reflect on this chaotic society where there's no longer authentic culture in circulation, but fragments of ground up, homogenized information, distributed in a totally uncritical way. Influencers, a particularly apt term now, since they're a kind of viral superspreader, superspreaders of cultural garbage, to put it a bit harshly, of ground-up, chaotic information, which bounces around like the memes we mentioned last year, from head to head, in this great collective chaos. It's very difficult, clearly, in such chaos, to coordinate management of a health emergency such as this pandemic was and continues to be.

SC: Also because, if you'll allow me, the noble level of politics, within professions, in places where decisions are made, where that theory, that strategy that Davide was talking about, is reduced to bar-room squabble. In one of his fundamental texts, Dr Wolfgang Giegerich (2010) emphasizes the difference, paraphrasing Berkley, between having opinions and thinking. In my opinion, Davide, this is what you mean as well. Theory is the difference between arguing, bar-room talk, opinions that are always clichéd, a paper you read as I did to prepare for our conversation, but with interesting insights, and understanding why, and actually thinking.

DF: Think how in "classical" culture, doxa and episteme were opposing terms. Doxa, opinion, and episteme, knowledge, after which epistemology is the discipline that studies knowledge. Thus, of course, what you're saying is absolutely true. But I'd like to linger on another aspect. All this later had repercussions we've observed in our daily work with patients. This sacrifice of freedom for the benefit of presumed safety. ... We've seen patients giving up living fully, the same as happened to the Epicurean sage. I remember in this regard a beautiful image in Lucretius, which Blumenberg cites in his *Shipwreck with Spectator* (1996). He recounts that in the second book of *On the Nature of Things* (2001) Lucretius describes a boat in trouble, tossed about by the waves, which risks sinking, and he takes solace in the fact that his feet are on solid ground. Not because he sadistically delights in the misfortune of others, but because he himself is in a condition of safety. This metaphor has been systematically reprised throughout the history of Western thought and interpreted in various ways. But one interpretation that seems to me fundamental is the one that states that if you want to keep your feet on the ground, you don't set sail, you give up travel, you renounce that very crossing which is the true horizon that gives meaning to existence. It's not so much the destination but the journey, as we all know. So we've seen some patients give up planning to some degree. Romolo Rossi (2004) used to say that a euphoric plan, by giving you intermediary or even distant goals, helps bring a little brio to existence. Well, now our patients are really all a bit spent. They're waiting. Last year, when the three of us met, we talked about that suspended time, and we were already pointing out that we were going to need to interpret it, that time, to not let time continue on its own but live it, and again today I reiterate this same need, which is absolutely fundamental!

Because in times of war, going back to what Stefano was saying, what happens is not what's happening now. If we go back and read Elsa Morante's *History* (2000), where she masterfully describes what life was like for those who were not directly involved in the war effort, but in everyday life, in urban areas subject to air raids. Well, people went on living, they went on doing everything they possibly could, of course within the limits set by the danger of bombings, thus heading to shelter when it was time. But in the shelters, there were people making love, there were children playing, all this in the presence of others because they had no alternative. Yet life, rhizomatically, in the shelter, went on all the same, what a beautiful image that is! Whereas what I've observed in the lives of many is precisely this abdication of the journey.

SC: We had talked about suspended time. I have to admit, I had never liked it much, and after our conversation – thanks to a chat with Susan Rowland (see Chapter 6) – I started reflecting on the suspension of certainties. For me, to ponder this, Covid as the suspension of certainties, is rather more interesting. Today, the only certainty we have is that we don't know how long this will last, a bit like a war, but we are not in a war. There is a void. What is the emptiness that your patients experience? In my opinion, it is the opposite, it is the antithesis, the enantiodromia of desire. But not that desire we felt until last year, the desire or "The Necessity of the Superfluous." That's it, desiring itself is something generative, a way of putting something into the world, bringing it forward, making it grow and then leaving it to its own path. In my opinion, the void in which we find ourselves is precisely the lack of desire. Or aborted desire.

SCa: I agree, we live in a society where desire is a desire for the superfluous, a sterile desire. But the humanity that made it out of the Spanish Flu and World War I – fifteen to twenty million died in World War I alone and fifty to a hundred million died of the Spanish flu – had perhaps a contradictory desire for thought, the kind of thought we were talking about earlier. That world saw the movement of one of my great loves, T.S. Eliot, the poet of "The Waste Land," composed immediately after those terrible experiences. It was a world that was hungry for culture and thought. Nobody would publish Eliot today. I confess that on the individual level I am very optimistic, and by individual I also mean my patients. Yet I am very pessimistic in social terms. Because I feel a lack of authentic culture, although we have a large number of "experts," a plethora of experts.

I do not want to discuss here, except in passing, Ortega y Gasset's critique of the figure of the expert (1994), whom he calls a "learned ignoramus," the sort of ignoramus who, being experts in one field, assume they're experts on everything. And to Ortega y Gasset, experts – which I also found in Tolstoy – are very dangerous. We have a plethora of experts and influencers who make up this perpetual culture grinder. Meanwhile that we actually need – although I don't see it on the horizon – is thought, culture. As we said last year, we need poets, musicians, theatre people, artists who represent what is happening to us on the collective level. We do this in psychotherapy rooms. In this regard, this subject always reminds me of a passage from a beautiful book, *We've Had a Hundred Years of Psychotherapy – And the World's Getting Worse*, in which Hillman (1993) proposes the consulting room as a "cell of revolution," a place where the "big bang" of thought can take place. So, we psychoanalysts do it in our consulting rooms, but I don't see at the collective level, at the social level, intellectuals, or poets, who are able to set thought in motion as we do in our therapy rooms. A motto I've always liked from '68 in France was the reversal of "we want actions, not words," so it was: "we want words, not actions." I've always found this beautiful, despite the violence of that period. I would like true, authentic, considered words, not those of the people like Scanzi or Tosa here in Italy. I would like words that convey thought. I don't see anyone on the horizon who can do this at a social level. We, of course, will continue to do so in those revolutionary cells that are our psychoanalysis rooms.

SC: I agree. We Jungians, unlike those claiming that "God is dead" (Nietzsche, *The Gay Science*, 1974) or that "Religion is an illusion" (Freud, *The Future of an Illusion*, 2008), following Jung, look not at religion but at spirituality. We look at spirituality without religion.

Last week, in *El Pais*, Pablo d'Ors[7] (who is a priest and a writer) stated that the pandemic conveys two messages: one ethical and one mystical. The ethical message of Covid-19 tells you that we can't continue living the way we've been living until now: producing and consuming unchecked, traveling constantly, and wanting to live and experience everything. The mystical message of the Covid-19 says that we must – circling back to you, Stefano – a sense of humility, silence, contemplation and meditation (which are Jungian themes).

But let me be frank: I'm becoming pessimistic, and I don't think what we said last year is correct (moving from extraversion to introversion). I was naïve! I believe that the crisis we are in (spiritual and cultural) is so deep, that, with Covid-19, nature wants a total reset.

DF: You've touched on some big topics. I'll add another, which is love, which is eros, and which has shifted enormously. This whole affair has been, if you'll allow me the term, highly anti-erotic, and so we also need to go back to falling in love. I remember in Piedmont′ dialect you say, or at least we did when I was young, that when you liked someone you'd say "*ti prendevi un'imbarcata* (you've embarked)." And that meant you had a crush, etc. This slang reminds me of the French *embarqué* and Pascal's famous phrase, "Vous êtes embarqué," (1950)[8] which says that we're already on that boat sailing through the waves, we can't think about not being in it, we can't delude ourselves into thinking we can stay out of all this, so to me it's absolutely essential we add this other dimension. Rediscover desire, rediscover that deep drive that makes it possible for us to enter into authentic relation with the other. We're already doing this at our studio, in our rooms, where we constantly dream with our patients, in our discussions. And dreaming serves precisely this, to generate a perspective. Jung teaches this well. Our dreams are perspectives, but then those perspectives must be faced in some way. They must be inhabited, we have to find a home in a perspective.

SC: The concept of Eros is so important and you mentioned making love in bunkers, in shelters, going back to making love, creating, falling in love, not necessarily with a person, simply ... falling in love. Even, perhaps, falling in love without the butterflies in the stomach, a sign of teenage love, because the butterflies in the stomach instead of love are about a projection (hopes and expectations) of love. Therefore, it is not love. Jung said that eros is fundamental, because if eros is missing, there is no relationship. Jung said: "a couple," husband and wife, whoever, can sleep in the same bed for fifty years, but if eros is missing, everything is missing. You've mentioned many times, Davide, the concept of sailing, embarking ... Ulysses, the great navigator. On this, I often propose to my patients – following a lecturer at C.G. Jung Institute in Zurich (and I apologize for not remembering her name), who said that it's one thing for Ulysses to listen to the Sirens' (Homer, Odyssey, Book 12.153) song while he's tied up and can't jump into the water, and it's another thing to invite the mermaids onboard and strike up a conversation with them ...

DF: What you're saying leads me to the fact that today, even in our sectorial discipline, psychology, positive psychologies for the most part, those that aim for overall well-being, and therefore try to ward off pain. But let's remember that only the simultaneous presence of pain, anyway, only the tragedy of existence, the tragic, is what truly gives life depth. We can't do without it. And so we can only truly meet Eros when we'll be able to meet at the same time in this other dimension from which we're all escaping. In social terms, speaking of mass flight from pain, let me remind you of the opiate crisis that kills as many people in the United States as Covid-19; there are big prescribers of these painkillers that obviously cause dependency and can later attract people to turn to the black market to fight addiction, as happens to heroin addicts. Prince died of it, Tom Petty died of it ...

SC: We're back to Simonetta Putti and the sense of limit/boundaries.

DF: Exactly.

SC: You mentioned Hillman earlier. You have to mention the great master, in my opinion, of psychoanalysis, because we are Jungians but we are also Freudians, with distinctions. I think we're coming back, since in '29–'30 it will be the centenary of the publication of Freud's *Civilization and Its Discontents*. A necessary discontent of civilization, which we would like to remedy instead. I thank you, I greet you and I wish you well!

SCa and DF: Our pleasure. Thank you!

Notes

1 The first part of this interview was recorded in Spring 2020, during the first lockdown.
2 The psychological impact of quarantine and how to reduce it: rapid review of the evidence. Online at: www.thelancet.com/journals/lancet/article/PIIS0140-6736(20)30460-8/fulltext.
3 The second part of this interview was recorded in Spring 2021, during the second lockdown.
4 "Our conventional response to all media, namely that it is how they are used that counts, is the numb stance of the technological idiot. For the 'content' of a medium is like the juicy piece of meat carried by the burglar to distract the watchdog of the mind."
5 Giuseppe Conte is an Italian jurist and politician who served as Prime Minister of Italy from June 2018 to February 2021.
6 Mario Draghi is an Italian economist, banker, academic, and civil servant who is the current Prime Minister of Italy since 13 February 2021. He previously served as President of the European Central Bank (ECB) from 2011 until 2019. Draghi was also Chair of the Financial Stability Board from 2009 to 2011 and Governor of the Bank of Italy from 2006 to 2011.

7 "La búsqueda espiritual de nuestro tiempo," online at: https://elpais.com/opinion/2021-04-02/la-busqueda-espiritual-de-nuestro-tiempo.html.
8 Pensées, fragment 397.

References

Barthes, R. (2013). *Mythologies*. New York: Hill and Wang.
Bauman, Z. (2000). *Liquid Society*. Cambridge: Polity Press.
Bion, W. (2018). *The Italian Seminars*. London and New York: Routledge.
Blumenberg, H. (1996). *Shipwreck with Spectator: Paradigm of a Metaphor for Existence (Studies in Contemporary German Social Thought)*. Boston: The MIT Press.
Brooks, S. K., Webster, R. K., Smith, L. E., Woodland, L., Wesseley S., Greenberg, N., and Rubin, G. J. (2020, 14–20 March). The psychological impact of quarantine and how to reduce it: rapid review of the evidence. *Lancet 395 (10227)*: 912–920.
Dawkins, R. (2016). *The Selfish Gene*. Oxford: Oxford University Press.
Freud, S. (2008). *The Future of an Illusion*. London: Penguin.
Giegerich, W. (2010). *The Collected English Papers*, vol. *4: The Soul Always Thinks*. New Orleans: Spring Journal Books.
Hillman, J. (1993). *We've Had a Hundred Years of Psychotherapy. And the World's Getting Worse*. New York: Harper One.
Homer (2006). *Odyssey*. London: Penguin.
Lucretius (2001). *On the Nature of Things*. Indianapolis: Hackett.
Manzoni, A. (2019) *Adelchi*. Milano: BUR Rizzoli.
McLuhan, M. (1994). *Understanding Media. The Extensions of Man*. Cambridge: The MIT Press.
Morante, E., (2000). *History*. Steerforth: Steerforth Press.
Nietzsche, F. (1974). *The Gay Science*. London: Vintage Penguin Random House.
Ortega y Gasset, J. (1994). *The Revolt of the Masses*. New York: Norton & Company.
Pascal, B. (1950). *Pensées*. London: Routledge.
Rossi, R. (2004, December). *"Seneca o Nerone? Philosophe, cura te ipsum." Journal of Psychopathology 10 (4)*.

Chapter 6

Psychosocial perspectives and Covid-19

Andrew Samuels

Does the coronavirus create a momentum that leads to change? This is the crucial question Andrew Samuels approaches in his talk. The Jungian analyst pleads for people working in the psychologic field to reach out into the world and exchange knowledge with professionals in the field of social matters and politics. Psychology can help transformation during a crisis like Covid-19. As an example for this psychosocial approach Samuels names Accogliere le ferrite di chi cura, an initiative that Stefano Carpani and Monica Luci – among others – took to provide free psychological support to Covid-frontline health workers in Italy. Unusual concepts that adjust therapy to an outer event are necessary because going back to normal is not possible anymore. He laments the words "We are all in this together" that came up shortly after the lockdown as it something that does not reflect the real situation. Millions of refugees were not in the same position as those that can lock themselves into beach houses or cottages. To him change in a world of climate crisis and economic inequality is not easy. And that is where he sees therapists come in insisting on change and facing the struggle together with progressive forces.

Stefano Carpani: Professor Samuels, Dear Andrew, good evening. Let me say that it's very, very nice to see you, though, of course, through video. How are you?

Andrew Samuels: I had a bad experience. I came into contact for a prolonged period of time with somebody who later that night got the virus. And then I had the unpleasant experience of counting the days because you have to get to fourteen days without symptoms unless one has it without symptoms. You know there are two groups of people who count the days: one is prisoners – and the other is people waiting for an infection to manifest in them. The experience left me with great energy and energy to think about the future, energy to think about possibilities. But not energy, by the way, to get all excited about how wonderful this virus is. Isn't it great that "dolphins swim in the Grand Canal in Venice" (they never did!), and look at all that poetry and all those rural images and all that happiness? To me, this is something I find so difficult. Maybe it's my personality, but I can't get

DOI: 10.4324/9781003266402-6

involved in all this optimism and positivistic I can think and I can see a future and I can hope, but I cannot join in this Panglossian access for those people watching this. Dr. Pangloss was the tutor of Voltaire's Candide when he saw the colossal Lisbon earthquake, refused to accept it was a bad thing, and said "everything is for the best in the best of all possible worlds." So to me, one of the main enemies of a satisfactory reconstruction is sentimentalism. That's how I am personally, but I hope we don't just stick to me in my personal situation.

SC: Going beyond sentimentalism. Does the coronavirus crisis tell us something about the limits of psychology?

AS: I'm really glad you asked this. I mean, I am an enthusiast for psychology in relation to social and political problems. I spent my career developing ways that can be operationalized. But I'm also a skeptic. I have a tragic vision about psychology and politics. There are really serious limits. What I like to see is alliances between the psychological communities and other people who are politically active, who have radical and progressive views, who have a commitment to change and transformation. So psychology on its own? Well, I hate it. But an approach to our current crisis without psychology at all. Well, forget it. We therapists have to find other people to relate to. If I may say something a little flippant, we have to find people to play with. We are playing too much with one another. Swapping theories, swapping quotes, swapping references. Come on, this esotericism, this group introversion must stop. They have to reach out. And actually you and the guys you are with in Italy who are who were the first in Europe to set up a project of a collaboration between therapists and frontline medical people, health people, doctors, nurses, paramedics. This is also an alliance, a partnership. This is psychosocial. This is something in action done by analysts like yourself and others. I'm deeply, moved and impressed because it is not just psychology.

SC: You are referring to "Accogliere le ferrite di chi cura" (*Reaching out to the wounds of health professionals*) – of which I am among the initiators with Maria Giovanna Bianchi, Roberto Grande, Alessandra di Montezemolo, Antonio Lanfranchi, Monica Luci, Chiara Tozzi, and Eva Pattis Zoja – an online free of charge psychological support for doctors, nurses and other health professionals engaged in a frontline battle to treat Covid-19 patients in Italy. In March 2020 we grouped and decided to offer free of charge online psychological support to those in *the front line*. By the end of our initiative (early 2021) we could count on free-of-charge counselling from 150 colleagues (psychologist, psychoanalyst, psychotherapist). I think this is amazing. It is such a generative thing, and we need this in Italy (and beyond).

AS: This experience of your project in Italy shows us that therapy has to change. First of all, the psychoanalytic shibboleths and rituals have to be interrogated even more. Second, the role of the client or the patient, whatever you want to call them, this becomes more and more important compared to the role of the therapist or the analyst. Later in our discussion. I'm going to say we cannot go back to the normal. We cannot go back to business as usual. But that applies to psychotherapy, too.

SC: Another important point is that what's going on around the world concerns racism. Every crisis is a cosmopolitan crisis. We are all vulnerable as well as we are all responsible, as German sociologist Ulrich Beck underlined in his most important book titled *Risk Society* (1992) and later in his post-humous book titled *Metamorphosis of the World* (2017). But what specifically does the coronavirus tell us about racism?

AS: Well, I make a simple response and then a slightly more complicated response because I'm supposed to be a professor and therefore be complicated. The simple response is that people of a progressive inclination have to stand up against the racism, especially in connection with China. And I remember when people started talking about the Chinese virus in London, this together with some friends, we started to eat only in Chinese restaurants. Crazy, but anyway, that's what we did. I don't have much original stuff to say about this, but in the end, the attempt to deflect blame and indeed anxiety onto the other onto another group is a very well tested way that authoritarian leaders function and we need to speak against it. The virus is a good example of risk. What Ulrich Beck said about risk was that you can't control it. Governments cannot control it, technology cannot control it. Having a powerful religious faith cannot control it. Beck was talking at one point about what we call in England mad cow disease, some kind of brain disorder that comes from cows, cattle. This idea that risk means that governments will fail to control things has always been inspirational to me as I work out my ideas about a good enough leader, the one who knows that they will fail and whose job is to become a master or mistress of failure. You cannot control modern and post-modern societies. Maybe you can never control any societies. There's a kind of organic madness that moves in societies.

SC: I agree. People construct a compensatory opposite from what Beck (2017) says when they adopt a "we are all in this together" cosmopolitanism, but we are not all in this together.

AS: Let me focus on the viral therapy situation because I've been writing so much about it. I hear from Western analysts that all their practices are online. Mine is and probably yours is too. What happens is what happens if you don't have a practice that can move online? If you don't have a car to drive to your second home in the country, let alone having such a home? Everybody is telling stories about how they're working in their basement and how interesting it is to see inside other people's houses on the screen and other people's pussycats walk across the computer. It is not like that if you are working in Africa. My friend and colleague in Cape Town, Sally Schwartz has written beautifully about this. What if you're working with refugees? There are 8.7 million refugees in the world, Mainly, they won't get therapy anyway, but they are not all in it together with bourgeois people in Hampstead, Manhattan, San Francisco, Berlin, all of whom post about how they've moved to their second houses, houses in the mountains, houses on the beach, houses, I don't know, cottages, houses, what-ever. This is so insensitive. "I am quietly recuperating with my family in my wife's parents' second home on the coast in X." Horrible.

SC: Immoral, not only horrible! Especially when they brag about having moved to their second houses where they can relax playing …

AS: … piano. And then the local people are saying "get the hell out, go away." This casual inequality is intolerable. And this is what I mean when I say therapy has to change. We really have to address who we are, what our social location is and how that will change. Have therapists and analysts got the same practices we always had? No. The practices will decline in quantity, the shrieks of financial anxiety and panic will get louder and louder and louder.

SC: You mentioned this before. What do you mean that the future means no return to normality?

AS: People say "when we get back to normal." OK, everyone understands what that means. Jung had a great line about normality. He said, show me a normal person and I'll cure him for you. And Christopher Bollas writes about the normative personality or personality as someone is just too normal to adapt. Anyway, we cannot get back to normality in terms of the climate crisis. We cannot get back to normality in terms of international relations, economic inequality, whether it's on the international or national or even communal level. We cannot go back to that. Personally, I don't talk the language of how we are all going to be in solidarity with one another, and work together, and there will be an end of individualism, and Ubuntu will suddenly come in and change the West. Come on. It's just not going to be like that if we want to avoid. The vicissitudes of normality, we will have to struggle. This is not going to happen easily, the powerful will return unless the less powerful do something about it. And here there is a role for therapists, along with other radical and progressive forces, to say absolutely, clearly no return to normality, but there will be a struggle. There will be a huge political struggle. And I'm often talking with people I know in the climate crisis, world extinction, rebellion and so on. And they get this. There is a potential for transformation, but it's up to us.

SC: I want to refer to the end of a movie called "Mediterraneo" by Gabriele Salvatores, who won the Oscar for best foreign movie in the early nineties. It was about soldiers sent to Greece to fight in WW2. They were sent to fight a war they never fought. And at the end of the war, they were so happy, excited to go back home to Italy. And they used to say, we have to go home because it's a new time. We have to rebuild Italy. We can create a new Italy. Then the last scene is forty years after the same men are around seventy years old. So something must have gone wrong. And they look at each other in the same island where they spent the war and they say, well, we went back. We wanted to rebuild Italy, but we were not allowed …

AS: Yes, yes, this is right. You look, you win the war and you lose the peace. After the First World War in Britain, the idea was to create a land fit for heroes. It didn't happen. Look at the 1920s. Look at the Great Depression which affected the whole world. You know, we talk a lot now about the 1918 Spanish flu (also a racist gibe). After the pandemic let us hope there is going to be a terrible economic reckoning. Patterns of employment and unemployment will change. The dignity of work, if it existed before, is surely gone in today's gig economy. And if the dignity of work goes, then fraternity and sorority go too and organized labour collapses in the face of neoliberal power.

SC: This a big threat. I see many people saying "yeah, but I'm working from home, but it's business as usual." Well, I think this had to do with their anxiety, even angst and panic, and that it is NOT going to be business as usual for a long time. But let me ask you one last question concerning the risks of the situation we are in: is there any hope?

AS: Before we can talk about hope, we have to talk about obstacles to it, obstacles within ourselves as individuals, within our culture, within our societies. We are facing what feels like an apocalypse. The hard thing for me to say is that a lot of people may unconsciously feel a pull or attraction towards apocalypse. Why? I think the masochistic tendency in the human psyche – which Freud saw as primary – has a lot to do with this. Our masochistic tendencies search for reasons to be punished, and when you are faced with something like this pandemic (or the climate crisis) there is this attraction. I call it *apocalypticism*. Apocalypticism is an invented word, but it is clear that it is an obstacle to any kind of hope. That's the first thing I want to say with regard to hope. You know, I've written a lot about this, there are different categories of hope. The first category of hope is illustrated in the Monty Python film "The Life of Brian." You know, the one about Jesus. It's a kind of comedy about a guy called Brian who obviously represents Jesus and it's incredibly satirical. So at the end of this film, Brian/Jesus and many, many other people are up on crosses and they start to sing. "Always look on the bright side of life." That's shallow hope and it works for a while. I can't mock or dismiss anyone who wants to look on the bright side of life, but that's not hope, as I want to talk about it in the last few minutes of our conversation.

For me hope springs from taking risks. The narrative I'm always talking about and thinking about in these terrible days is the story of Jan Palach, the young Czech guy who put gasoline on himself and lit a match as a protest against the Russian invasion of Czechoslovakia in 1968–9. You may have seen the pictures of it. Of course, self-immolation has a long history; it's a martyrdom. But this was political. And I think there's many other examples of how hope and risk go together. As when paramedics in Gaza run towards the fence and get shot as they run to do their job, dressed in their uniforms. They are taking a huge risk and out of such behaviour comes an authentic hope. Sometimes people take a huge risk in communicating across the divide, enemies talking to one another, people who have perhaps on both sides of a conflict. This happened in Northern Ireland. It's a huge risk to talk to the killer of your child or your brother. Hope needs to be based on risk and I think, in our generation right now, the possibility of constructing a genuine hope on the basis of risk exists, but who is going to do it? The younger people are going to do it! Not baby boomers like me. By the way, the etymology of "risk" from Latin means "running towards danger." Not walking, but running.

As well as being scared, I found that I didn't really care when I was facing the possibility that I would get this virus. It made me think it is going to be OK if I die, and I wrote this in several places. Everyone was very surprised because it's not my normal style to try to write in this kind of way. Maybe I'm being sentimental even though I don't want to be sentimental. So, who is going to be responsible for rebuilding the countries of the world? I can't imagine how the United States can rebuild when the both the presidential candidates are in their 70s. Where are the younger people? Is the idea that we elect older people because they are safe, they have a reliable demeanour or something like this, or is it just normal to do it?

SC: Time of risk and time of courage …

AS: Courage! Yes! Winston Churchill, whom I don't usually quote, said "courage is the virtue that guarantees all the other virtues." Martin Luther King wrote this: "Courage is an inner resolution to go forward despite obstacles; Cowardice is submissive surrender to circumstances. Courage breeds creativity'"

SC: Courage and creativity is what we need. And perhaps it is what my generation needs to learn. My generation needs to learn from our parents, from you, those in your age group. My parents are more or less your age. And also, it's our time to become generative, to have the courage to put something new into the world, to let it grow and to let it go. Otherwise, there will be a big mess. Thank you, Andrew.

AS: Thank you. That was a very, very interesting conversation. And I felt my heart rate go up in the conversation, which for me is a good sign, because for me to be bored is the worst.

SC: Yeah. And hopefully many people will read it and ponder on it, reflect – and take action. Thank you.

AS: Let's see.

Bibliography

Beck, U. (1992). *Risk Society: Towards a New Modernity.* London: Sage Publications.
Beck, U. (2017). *The Metamorphosis of the World.* Cambridge: Polity Press.

Chapter 7

The Suspension of Certainties

Susan Rowland

According to Susan Rowland the unconscious is overwhelming us in the form of coronavirus and climate change. What is remarkable is that Jung already dealt with transdisciplinarity from a contemporary perspective, through art and knowledge, as he provided the language to explain psychic images. For Rowland, who herself bases her work and research on arts, creativity is at the heart of who we are, and being creative is only possible when we have no certainties of any kind. The coronavirus, she states, functions as an invasion of the unknown psyche into our collective world that questions everything we knew. However, giving up on certainties we are able to change and adapt. Susan Rowland and Stefano Carpani look at the meaning of technology in a time of coronavirus. Many of us turned inward but in the sense of entertainment by Netflix and Co., while there are other uses of technology, think of the British physicist Stephen Hawking, who was trapped in his own body due to ALS disease, but used technology to turn outward and to communicate his findings in science. Rowland speaks out for a new view on technology and the possibility to see in this situation a chance for individuation.

Stefano Carpani: Doctor Rowland, dear Susan, how are you?

Susan Rowland: I am well, I am sheltering in place as most of the world is and generally feeling anxious and stressed like everybody else.

SC: This was actually my second question. How do you feel about the whole coronavirus emergency?

SR: Well, I've obviously been thinking about it a good deal. I teach Jungian related material to graduate students, so it's something we've been discussing. One thing I find very helpful is the very simple notion that the unconscious is that which overwhelms us. And I find that a useful starting place with people who are not educated in Jung, because it is my job to too often educate them from the beginning that makes a kind of sense as to why depth psychology, Jungian psychology is important. The unconscious is that which overwhelms us, which suggests that the coronavirus is the unconscious. And I think that's a useful, even correct way of looking at it, because we are material and spiritual beings. The coronavirus has a material and spiritual dimension. So there's that.

DOI: 10.4324/9781003266402-7

And thinking of it like that sees I think puts us in the picture. It's not the coronavirus is something out there. It's actually part of our reality that we're dealing with. And in terms of what Jungians believe about the unconscious and the psyche, we can start to see possibilities of for the future in the immense suffering and destruction that we're facing. The other thing that I find it useful from a kind of imaginative point of view is alchemy. So I've been discussing it with my students in our chemical terms as a kind of alchemy of the collective, a transformation of the collective with us in a very dark Nigredo state where we're forced to get to the *prima materia*, the core stuff of our existence and what matters to us as human beings, as individuals. But more securely, we're being forced to get to the essence of ourselves as families, communities, nations and collectives.

SC: Talking about alchemy, we cannot avoid the question who was Jung or who was, who is your own Jung?

SR: Well, I've never been able to get away from Jung the person as such a kind of useful perspective and as somebody who is a Jungian but not a clinician, that's an interesting position to be in. But my research for thirty-five years has been into Jungian psychology, Jungian writing and then in the context of the arts and in the context of gender. I've published a lot on Jung's writings. And here I have a very distinctive position because my view is not Jung the person matters, so much as Jung the text. And I'm not interested in questions like what did Jung really mean by this? Because although that's a very normal way to approach Jung's writings, and I'm not saying it's wrong, it's not a necessary way of approaching Jung's writings because it is buying into a very cultural notion of an author and the idea of an author of a piece of writing as the God of the text.

The author owns the meanings of the text, and we can get to the ultimate meaning of the text if only we could get into the mind of the author. This is a very common approach. It is an OK idea, but it's a very cultural idea. It was invented more or less about the time of the of Romanticism and Jung himself has an interesting relationship to romanticism. And what we see when we kind of put this idea of the author as god next to Jungian psychology is that the idea of the author is the privileging of the ego. It is the notion that there is a single fixed meaning to a word, to a sentence, to a whole piece of writing. This fixed meaning stems for the fantasy of single coherent author intention.

And that's OK. But it really isn't Jungian because Jung is all about not privileging the ego. What I find fascinating is that there is quite a lot of evidence, if you read Jung carefully, that this is an attitude he actually understood and was writing from. So, for example, he says of his own theorizing, nobody drew the conclusion that if we take the unconscious seriously, then all our knowledge must be incomplete and moreover, to a degree that we cannot determine. Now, that's a really radical statement. This is Jung in the Collected Works. It comes in his essay on his psychology saying that there is no *one* kind of truth here. There is no absolute truth because we don't know all the stuff. Therefore his writing is fascinating to me because he writes from a kind of honouring of mystery and unknowing and the possibilities that meanings will continue to be generated over time. Around his own work, his book, *AION* (Jung, 1979), for example, is a demonstration of symbolic systems ending with his own theory as a symbolic system that will change, that will be superseded. To me Jung is a modernist, he's an arts-based researcher, he's a performative writer, he's a trickster writer. And he's a comic writer. Comedy is really important to Jung's writings. Freud is in essence tragic. Jung is in essence comic both in the sense of there are jokes and they matter, but also in the sense of divine comedy and the way comedy is about death and rebirth, death and rebirth of meaning is included there.

SC: It is interesting to talk about death and rebirth at the time of coronavirus. But I want to stick to your attitude towards translation. There are people like Dr Giegerich[1] who say an author has to be read in the original language, otherwise you cannot really grasp the essence. What is your take on this?

SR: First of all, I respect that. I have been critical in my publications of Giegerich. I have been critical of Professor Sonu Shamdasani, but my criticism says what these scholars are doing is perfectly legitimate. My criticism is of their attitude that what they're saying is the only perspective. I think multiplicity is at the essence of Jung, and multiplicities are the essence of the kinds of scholarly work that I do.

And if we take what you've just said about Giegerich, if you want to get to the essence of an author. Yes, fine. If you want to treat Jung as an author, as someone who is able to control the meanings of the words he uses, then fine. Clearly, it's important that most of these words were first written in German, and I respect that. But first of all, I think treating anyone as an author-god is not Jungian because Jung was all about dethroning the ego and dethroning fixed meanings.

So it's a cultural fantasy to treat Jung as an author, a cultural fantasy that is very much tied to certain trends in Western modernity of the last few hundred years. Here, let us accept that translation is a fantasy. Languages are not mirror images of each other. They do not translate, you know, not in the way we imagine translation. Now, of course, translation occurs. I read translations. My work is looking at Jung in English translation., I can understand people who say that is not really getting to Jung because most of these texts were originally written in German. But it's still that is all part of this fantasy ethos that is ego privileging in Western modernity. The fantasy of translation privileges, the ego at a number of different levels.

One of them is the fantasy that things can be translated and another of them is the fantasy that the author authorizes. Think about it. In English, we talk about the authorized version of the Bible. People, Christian communities have continually tried to produce their version of the Bible and they argue and fight one another and historically have killed one on another because of their translation of the Bible.

If you stop having a fantasy or fixed meanings, then it is possible to reimagine a relationship between different perspectives on a text that is not one of conquest and annihilation. So with translation, on the one hand, I get that people are making a very conventional, I would say, but reasonable and widely held objection to somebody working with an English translation of Jung and claiming to be a Jungian, but I still say that my work is profoundly Jungian because it destroys the ego and looks for the way in which the texts themselves are fluid and playful and multiple, that they have many voices in them.

The unevenness of Jung's writing is because he allows different archetypes to come into the writing. Now, this may sound weird, but it isn't weird because it's saying Jung is a kind of novelist more than he is a traditional scientist. We have a lot of conventional expectations about what science is like and that the division between science and the arts. Again, one of the great schisms of modernity has meant that this is privileging of the ego has become a sort of dogma that has restricted and poisoned a lot of our knowledge as well as our social being.

SC: You have your own approach to Jung, and I would dare to say "a reformed approach to Jung." What is Jung's relevance today?

SR: Well, I think Jung's relevance today is enormous because I think this notion that the unconscious is that which overwhelms us is, again, a central Jungian perspective that remains a viable starting point as we face the pandemic and climate change. And it is a kind of practical way of dealing with those overwhelming things that we are facing as a species, not even as a culture, but as a species. So the coronavirus and the other overwhelming thing is, of course, the climate emergency. Both of these are the unconscious and very real and immediate ways. Jungian psychology is a way of facing that without being overwhelmed and made, simply paralyzed by kind of fear and terror. That's a big point, but obviously extremely important.

There are two things about Jungian academia that I think are very exciting and very new. One is that Jung anticipated the Transdisciplinarity of Basarab Nicolescu (2008) which I've been working on and writing about for the last couple of years. And Transdisciplinarity is a way of bringing all the academic disciplines together in a way that has a social, ethical and religious vision that is about the whole planet working ethically together, while respecting and making room for each other's differences.

Jung really does anticipate that if you kind of dig into some of his attitudes to knowledge, for example, now as part of that, there is a new way of doing research called arts-based research. And it's out there. It's in the social sciences mainly. And it's new because it's not art as a result of research, it's not art about research, it's not art illustrating research, it is making art as a way of making knowledge. And it's new that the academy is doing this. It started in the late 1990s. Arts-based researchers are really interested in the image, the psychic image and intuition.

They don't have a very good language for exploring the psychic image. Jung provides the language for exploring the image, intuition as well. In fact, Jung's full functions are really quite helpful here. So sensation and thinking and feeling and the whole kind of ethical way in which the psyche would work. Another way of putting this Stefano, is that Jungian arts-based research is doing psychotherapy with the world.

What you do as a clinician with a client, the way you kind of work together in a kind of temenos and create something. Well, that's what psychological arts-based research does. Jungian arts-based research materializes the psychic image. Also I must stress when I say arts-based research, I'm using arts, plural. It's not limited to painting. My own arts-based research practice is fiction writing, but any artistic mode is enhanced by being research because it takes art out of its box that it's been put into by modernity. Moreover, art as research is enhanced by a Jungian perspective. Because that way we can kind of negotiate the role of the psyche and the role of the psyche going out into the world. Because arts-based research has something for Jungians in that it has art, which is a system, has a heritage, it has a cultural location. It has ideas and philosophies already with it. So by doing arts-based research, Jungians can get their Jungian work into the world in a way that communicates with it. That is so much more difficult to do when you're writing as a clinician and trying to explain why what you do with patients is so important.

SC: Can you say a little bit more about how you engage with patients with your arts-based research? How do you work with them? I can imagine active imagination as we are taught in training, sand-play and even poetry. What is your take? Can you share something more?

SR: Well, it comes down to the image and Jung says the image is the is the kind of emanation from the unconscious. It's our sense of something from the unconscious and yeah that can go into active imagination and then materialized in art. So the image generates the writing of a poem or the image generates a painting, the image generates music. I actually have a dissertation student, PhD student, who talked to film directors about the psychic image. It was a very real conversation to them that the psychic image inside of them led them to produce certain types of work. Whereas you might talk about dreams with patient. That too is arts-based research is taking that psychic material and making it visible and communicable through the medium of analysis. After all, isn't analysis art?

SC: Analysis as art. Interesting! I intentionally avoid to add anything, hoping our readers will be able to think about this and find their own conclusion.

One of my clinical supervisors – Giegerich in fact – years ago suggested me (when I was working with a patient who claimed she was writing a letter to her father for many, many years, although she was not able to finish this sentence) to tell her to keep writing, without having in mind to hand in the letter. It didn't work (so far). This patient is still dealing with the task of writing. What would you suggest her?

SR: I think I should say that arts-based research is not the same as art psychotherapy. They are distinct because obviously art therapy privileges the therapy. That is the important thing, whereas arts-based research is about making art and it won't necessarily make the artist feel better to do it. There is a different pull towards the art and the art is something that goes out into the world. It is not tied to the person of the artist.

It's very interesting. You use that example. I had a student I was teaching who had unfinished business with her mother, and who doesn't have unfinished business with their mothers? And she was a playwright and she wanted to write a play about this and she did, but it wasn't working. She, too, got stuck. And we looked at alchemy. And then having been absorbed in this notion of art-based research and Jungian psychology, she sat down and said, OK, her mother was dead. OK, Mom, you know, come and help me with this. And they did a dialogue. Then the parent came alive. Some people would say her spirit came back from the dead. Some people would say her archetype was activated. However you want to put it, what I love about Jung is that you don't have to buy into one particular reality, that dialogue happened and has gone on and produced the play, which I saw performed. It was fabulous and incredibly funny, I would say, to that patient. On the one hand, why don't you change the media? Why don't you paint a picture or why don't you dance? That would be me, imagining myself in a therapeutic work role. If that person was interested in writing as their art form, their creative practice, I would say it's time to talk to him, your father. It's time to summon him and bring him back.

SC: This leads me to the concept of certainties. At the beginning of this conversation you said that *coronavirus is the unconscious,* that it could be linked to the unconscious. These days, especially in Italy, where I come from, or in Spain, where my wife is from, or any other country, we – as few have authors have underlined – are going through *a suspension of time.* Could we say that night time, sleeping, dreaming, dreams are actually a *suspension of certainties*? A *suspension of the ego*? And you said, coronavirus could be linked to the ego, and from this we could say that certainties could be linked to the ego and coronavirus. Why do we need uncertainties? Why do we need to sleep at night?

SR: Well …

SC: Why is the world suspended right now?

SR: Because we cannot live in certainties. Certainties are not what human beings are. This the certainties or the assumptions that we've taken to be certain about our lives and all our society, we've lived them mostly unconsciously, they mostly just been there. And you can go about your business and you don't think about how all the assumptions that are structuring that. And it seems to be human nature that we need to grow to develop it beyond certainties.

I think this ultimately comes to why do we have to die? Because that is, you know, that is putting a limit to our time. And by putting a limit to our time, it allows us to make certain kinds of meanings that we wouldn't have if we just felt we were going to go on forever. So I would say, and I feel is this is a very kind of Jungian position, that humans are not healthy or alive if they have too much certainty. Also, humans are rather dangerous, if they have too much certainty. They don't agree. And if they're certain about the things that other people don't agree on the community kind of breaks down as in the United States where I've lived for ten years. But you can tell from my accent, I'm not indigenously American. In the United States, there's been a kind of paralysis in the politics because there have been two sides, both full of certainties and an inability to change, adapt, appreciate the other position. And all of that is being challenged by the virus.

The virus is a kind of invasion of the disruptive, unknown psyche into our collective world and challenging all sorts of basic assumptions, including the assumptions that we are individuals. We're all being asked to stay at home in order to save lives that we can't see and can't know and be certain about. And yet also that life might be our own. So we're being asked to act as part of a collective in a very urgent way. And that's what that's wiping away a certainty that I think perhaps particularly in the United States, but also in the European world, we've had this sense of ourselves as individuals, as a single being, as autonomous. We can make choices. We can do all these things with our lives. Well, we can't do most of those things now. And it's essential. So I think it's about being alive. I think it's about being happy. I think it's about the human nature that we need. And it was absolutely right. We are beings that seek meaning. And you can't if you are too full of certainties, then you are dead because the meanings that you are you have them unconsciously. They aren't real. And you are kind of empty because you're not interacting with meaning and you're not creating meaning. Put another way, creativity is at the heart of who we are. We have to be creating in a very broad sense in order to go on living.

SC: ... And too many certainties, perhaps, bring stagnation, which is the opposite of creativity.

I want to share a dream with you a patient brought to a session today. The dream is the following:

First part of the dream: I am dancing with Stephen Hawking.

Second part of the dream: I am trying to figure out how to teach yoga to Stephen Hawking, who is someone unable to feel and to breathe.

I was very much touched by this dream, not only because Stephen Hawking was a B.A. student at Trinity Hall (Cambridge) where I also studied. And I couldn't stop thinking that both Hawking and I were in our 20s and in perfect health when at Trinity Hall. Then Hawking went studying for his Master and PhD degrees, and he "lost" his healthy body. He became "trapped" in a body that didn't support his genius mind. After listening to this dream, I started thinking of us now, locked in a body, in the house, in a box, and I also pondered about *the impossibility of creativity*. Today in lockdown so many people get addicted to Netflix, Zoom, WhatsApp, Tinder, baking bread or vigorexia, beyond their usual addictions. And I find it poetical that this patient dreamt of dancing with Hawking and even trying to figure out how to teach him yoga, although he has respiratory problems (coronavirus is about this, right?) and he doesn't feel. Derived from this: We really have problems with feeling nowadays. With the feeling function. What comes to your mind?

SR: *The Enchantments of Technology* (2005) – it's a book by Lee Bailey from a Jungian point of view about technology and arguing really just what you've said, that there's been this radical split, ultimately this notion of us being subjects and everything out there being objects which happened to Stephen Hawking in a sense that he had this fabulous mind and his body was an object really that he couldn't connect with. And as you said, we are in our houses and we think of out there as an object that we're not connected with and that could include the house itself. And you're right. Addiction is a way of avoiding that problem. But it's only a way of imagining ourselves in the world with this split. I mean, Stephen Hawking is an incredible example and an incredible hero. He still needed his body. The body was, you know, it was still that which was keeping him alive. There was still that connection between the mind and the body. However, difficult it might be for us to imagine it and technology which we've split off from. And the obvious example here is the American obsession with guns and this notion that, you know, guns don't kill people, people don't do. So it's all right to have a gun. Well, if I pick up a gun, I change, you know? And so we have this on consciousness of how we are psychically invested in technology. And this book by Lee Bailey, it's very good on this. It was published in 2005 before social media, before we found out after 2016 that basically social media had invaded people's psyches and elections had been manipulated through this. So we are part of this technology, but we have this terrible unconsciousness of it. We're not conscious of the way social media manipulated us then and is manipulating us now. So I think that what one of the things you may be pointing to is we are called upon to try to get out of our own consciousness around technology ...

SC: What I tried to underline is that until two weeks ago or a month ago, we lived in the absolute external world, the extroverted world. Now we are for forced to stay indoors and to leave the certainties of the extroverted world (that became suspended with the lockdown), what I call *the entertainment society, the bulimic society* or the *all you can eat society* and yet – as Stephen Hawking, who went inward and found resources he was unaware of, before his body dumped him – we might find resources we were unaware of a month ago.

SR: Yes, I totally agree with that. But I don't think that's the whole story because he went inward and he went outward.

SC: That's right. Thank you for adding this.

SR: What if he had cared less about the world? No, he would not have done his work and he certainly would not have communicated it to the world. So it's not just about going inward. It is about going outward too. And we need to find ways of loving one another through technology. We need to find ways of loving one another at this time of isolation. And in a way, you could say all the anxiety that there is a kind of very pragmatic, concrete thing here. And that is, you know, the world everybody every country in the world is trying to get ventilators and, you know, and companies who make calls, making ventilators and etc. So there's all that kind of anxiety and that understanding that this is this will save lives. But also people are finding ways to help one another via this technology that we're using now. So there are signs of fertility in the darkness, but it's it is a very dark time and. What I think is a very important myth of our situation with technology is it's Frankenstein. The Frankenstein is our mistakes with technology, because Frankenstein was created out of fear and could not be loved. It was a technology that could not be loved.

And similarly, we created nuclear weapons out of great fear and an inability to love. So I think we're kind. I think what people are starting to discover is they could find ways of expressing and living their love for each other. And I mean this in all kinds of ways into including helping people in their communities that they will that there is a chance that they can get beyond addictive and deadly technology that you've pointed to in the bingeing on Netflix. There is a chance that people are starting to individuate that technology. I'm not saying that problems with technology will be over in six months' time. But I think our relationship to it is being forced to change because this is the only way we can be with our friends and other members of our family and also take part, do our work, be with our colleagues, be with our students.

Stephen Hawking went on because he loved the world, because he wanted to contribute and he was spiritually excited by what he could contribute, and that spirit enabled him to survive far far longer than most people with his illness. He was a kind of medical marvel. And it must've been because his spirit infused his body and vice versa.

SC: Thank you, Susan, it was a pleasure to be here with you today (also thanks to the help of technology!)

SR: Thank you Stefano. It's been lovely and I really appreciate what you're doing and I'm very honoured to be part of this series. Thank you.

Note

1 Private conversation 2016.

References

Bailey, L. W. (2005) *The Enchantments of Technology*. Urbana and Chicago: University of Illinois Press.

Jung, C. G. (1979). AION: Researches into the Phenomenology of Self: Aion: Researches Into the Phenomenology of the Self *(CW 11)*. Princeton: Princeton University Press.

Nicolescu, B. (2008). *Transdisciplinarity: Theory and Practice*. London: Routledge.

Rowland, S. and Weishaus, J. (2021). *Jungian Arts-Based Research and "The Nuclear Enchantment of New Mexico"*. London: Routledge.

Chapter 8

Fraternitè

Ursula Brasch

Ursual Brasch focuses her talk on breath and breathing, emphasizing its being crucial for every living creature. In the context of the Covid-19 pandemic it gains even more meaning. The symbolism of breathing refers to a connection between the outer and the inner world, between the body and its environment, which is deeply disturbed in the pandemic. The question is if this effect on life will be like a wake-up call, a point in time when real changes happen. She uses the atomic catastrophe of Chernobyl as an example for a slow change that occurred over the course of thirty years. In Germany it led to the strengthening of the Green party and the exit from nuclear energy. She applies Erich Fromm's theory of the father and mother complex to show how our behaviour prevents us from real change. People cry out for father state for protection as well as a softer force – the mother – to cure their anxieties. This creates a dependence and prevents from development. As many feel restricted in their actions due to lockdown, she suggests to think of freedom rather not as the freedom to travel but taking care of oneself and beloved ones.

Stefano Carpani: Dear Mrs Brasch, dear Ursula, thank you for giving me the opportunity to talk to you again. The last time I was in your praxis, close to the Black Forest, now I am in lockdown in Berlin, you"re in lockdown in the Black Forest. My first question for you is: How are you?

Ursula Brasch: Thank you, Stefano, I am fine. I can find positive things to say about the lockdown. I am not forced to travel so much, a lot of things that have been left behind can now be worked on. It is also good to have time and space for all these things.

SC: How do you feel?

UB: I can say that I feel recovered and well-centred and I enjoy to be so close with my family. It was a very new experience and a very good one for everybody.

SC: Germany is in partial lockdown. The north of Germany, where I live in Berlin, has been little affected. How is the situation in your area?

UB: Our area was quite more affected, but here in our surroundings, there is nobody ill, nobody was in contact with the virus, so life was calm and people were taking care of each other. Of course, you could see this, but since

DOI: 10.4324/9781003266402-8

the weather was so wonderful everybody was outside going for works, taking the distance, but with the kind of friendliness and tolerance, also really taking care of each other, which was a good life to have in the last two-three weeks, beside everything else, of course. Our immediate life here was very calm and good.

SC: When you and I were talking a couple of days ago about this interview, you touched two points: *Atmen* and the soul. What are those things? Perhaps you may use a language that anyone watching here can understand.

UB: Ok, I will try to put it in easy words. What I was thinking was, of course, that this is very Jungian, that you ask yourself what is the symbol of this whole situation? Can we understand the global situation psychologically with the help of this symbol? Because it immediately started that virologists, people from natural sciences, gave explanations, and this drew the whole understanding of the virus in a specific direction. It is, like you said, about anxiety, about the virus, about anxiety of apocalyptic fantasies. Of course, it is a pandemic and, of course, it is a problem that many people are dying from, but there are many aspects to understand as well, I think. One of them is to see this from what the virus is doing in a symbolic way. So, what is the virus doing? The virus is attacking the breath, the lungs, and in German the word for breath is *Aten*. Taking a breath is the first thing we do when we arrive in this world and it is also the last thing we do. So, the *Aten*, the breath, is connecting us with the world beyond our body limits. The breath is within our lungs, but with the breath we are connected with the world, and without it we cannot participate in it. It is impossible. The German word *Aten* is coming from the Sanskrit *atman* and the meaning of it is "the breath of life." It is more connected with the undestroyable essence of life. This is also the essence of mind and the meaning of it is the soul. So, it is the question about how we are related with ourselves but also with the world, about how we are related with the soul, both our soul and the soul of the world. And it is interesting enough because, as far as I know, what I have understood is, that the virus is not attacking the nucleus of the cell, it is destroying this little, alveoli in the lungs. Again, it is not attacking the cell, its core, it is attacking the way that we are related to the world, how we are in a relationship. This seems to be so interesting to me. We and our relationship with the world. And I do not have to repeat myself in saying that this is the discussion: "Friday for Future," in politics, the crisis of democracy, the economic consequences of globalism, all these things. This was already a problem before the pandemic.

SC: I find very interesting these lungs, soul, issues or links that were mentioned by Susan Sontag in *Metaphor as Illness* (1978), and I have underlined them in a couple of interviews. But this is also a matter of – when you talk about breathing – the lungs, the air, a movement from the outside in to help us oxygenate ourselves. An exchange between the outside and the inside: We and the world. I always say that this is a crisis about the suspension of our certainties and the movement of our external world and the inner world. What can you say about this, Ursula?

UB: Well, I want to refer to it again in a very symbolical way, through images. Because after what you have said as well, it is the question (with all these crises happening, this is always the question): "what is the challenge for our consciousness?" We are talking about the relatedness, our relationship with the world and about the relationship with ourselves. Everybody knows, the virus started in China. Since the Jungians see fairy tales as an expression of the collective unconscious, I remember a Chinese fairy tale, that is quite parallel to a German fairy tale. It is about the relationship between a protagonist, a so-called hero, and the world. If you allow, I want to talk about this fairy tale in order to explain what the archetypal background could be.

SC: Of course!

UB: It is also to answer your question: "how is this related with our experience of the world inside and outside of us." So, in the German fairy tale, the devil has three golden hair. And, to summarize it in short, in this fairy tale a young man is falling in love with the daughter of the king and he wants to marry her and after many detours and experiences he had to go through, he finally marries her. I do not want to go into too much detail, but one of the most important plots of the fairy tale is, that the king says: "Well, I cannot give you my daughter because you did some strategies to arrive where you arrived. Before I give you my daughter, you have to go to the devil and there you have to take three golden hair from him." And the hero says ok and he goes. On his way, he has these famous challenges. These challenges are interesting, because they concern the everyday life of people living in a village. In one of those challenges, it's about a dried-up well. The second time, a tree doesn't carry fruit anymore, and the third time there is a man driving a ferryboat, he always has to cross the river back and forth, and he can never stop. Finally, the hero arrives in hell and he takes the three golden hairs of the devil and with these three golden hairs he can solve also the three challenges and finally he can marry the princess. So, in general we can say this German fairy tale is about going to the devil, going beyond limits and solving at least the father complex. And while he is solving his father complex, he is also solving collective questions. Now, in the Chinese fairy tale, which is quite parallel to the German one, the protagonist has a similar problem with his later mother-in-law: he wants to marry a girl and the mother-in-law says no. It is not so easy to marry her daughter. To do so, he has to go to Buddha, and he has to take three golden hair from him. And the same things happen. The protagonist is going beyond the limits of the world and on his journey, he also faces three collective challenges. There is one challenge related to a big chicken. Interestingly, this chicken is sitting on a tree. This chicken sings so beautifully in the night, that all the people that live in this village have to get up and work in the night and sleep during the day. So, you see the normal rhythm of day and night that is disturbed, because the bird is singing so beautifully. So, because of something very beautiful, the natural balance is not in order. This is the first connection where I thought: "Ok, this is very much connected with what happened before the corona crisis," that we were, let us say, kind of suffering from so many nice things we always could do and which needed our effort, our energy. Some beautiful things like travelling, meeting people, spending time in big public events, visiting concerts and museums, using modern shopping malls and so on. We could do this without limits, whenever we wanted, wherever we wanted. All the possibilities of modern life, which on the other hand, started to destroy our natural balance, messing our natural rhythm. This is one collective challenge to solve. The second task is also very interesting, because it is about two phoenix birds who are always eating the harvest of another village. The harvest was rice, and it was a wonderful, big grain rice. Since these phoenixes were always eating the rice, the people were starting to starve. Something very collective, the richness of the western world on the back of the poverty of the rest of the world. So, you see something very interesting and collective. And finally, he also comes to a place where it is about a ferryman asking him something. In the end, he comes to Buddha, he takes three golden hairs, he solves the challenges. The interesting aspect here is, and I like this very much, he also gets presents, he brings them back to his little village, where he comes from and one of the gift is the rice, which is of a very strong and effective variety, but he is only allowed to eat one bowl of that rice a day, not more than that. Something bad will happen to someone who eats more than one. Another gift is the chicken. He got a code and when saying this to the chicken it is giving golden eggs, but again not too much, please. The advice every time is not to overdo it. And to use the gifts only when he really needs them.

He brings these presents back to his mother-in-law. Now she has to say yes to the marriage. He marries the daughter, and he is then kind of a rich man but, since the mother-in-law is very greedy, she is doing some tricks to lure him out of the house. She takes the rice and the chicken eggs, and she eats to much so that she destroys the rice, then she destroys the eggs and then she explodes and dies. Then, he buries her, and after one year an orange tree blooms on her grave with nice orange fruit. Two things are interesting here.

In this fairy tale it is about overcoming the mother complex. It is about being greedy and is about that something so precious and important like the rice and the chicken eggs are not for your individual benefit but for the collective. The orange tree as well is something collective for everybody. When connecting this with the symbol of the virus and what is actually happening, I come to the question "what is the personal and collective challenge?" According to the fairy tale the challenge would be to go over the limit, in order to find something important outside of our personal limits. With our breath, with the *atman*, we can go over the limits and try to connect in order to find something new, that we can integrate in our lives in a new meaning of progress. And the question is: "what is the solution here? What is the progress here?"

SC: And the answer is?

UB: The answer I found is something I read from Erich Fromm. He wrote this fifty years ago! He talks about the sibling complex, saying that we have to overcome the mother complex and the father complex. He means as long as we are attached to the father and to the mother in a wrong way, we suppress ourselves. Actually now, the father complex is, what happens now: everybody is crying for the State. The State, as the father, has to solve all the problems well enough. It looks like as if in Germany this really works, and the state is very supportive, but it does not release you from finding your own ideas, developments, to overcome the crisis. On the other hand people develop anxieties, they need to be protected, they want that somebody takes care of them. This is the realm of the mother.

When you depend on this, when you do not mature and take the chance to develop, you will be stuck in the call for "I need to be provided, I need to be protected," and you start to depend on these people that seem to provide you with everything you need. The solution Fromm offers is the sibling complex: it is to find the relationship with your brothers and sisters. Because there you can have both, you can have the feeling of family, the feeling of connection, the feeling of equality, without depending on and not suppressing. Not in a hierarchy. You are all peers. You are free.

This you see in the fairy tale as well, the protagonists bring back the solutions for the collective problems, and then they establish a new relationship. It is a relationship between the protagonist and the woman. For me, the whole question is how we can arrive to overcome this dependency we have on the political and economic structures in order to be more related to each other, not in a linguistic way, but in a way where we can share and have a good community.

SC: You mentioned Erich Fromm. Erich Fromm said in *Escape from Freedom* (1941), when you think of the mother complex and the father complex, that when we are not able to sustain the responsibility coming from freedom, we give back these responsibilities to the authoritarian figures, to the authoritarian father. And this led to wars such as WWII. Many commentators and many state presidents use the concept of "war," the Pope uses the concept of "tempest," and before asking you if you are happy with the metaphor of war, I want to ask you another question: What is going to happen in two weeks, in a month, in six months? Are we really able to hope for development, for change, or are we too naïve? Because I personally have hopes of a better world, a modest world, a world of caring, but twelve years ago we had a financial crisis brought by the bankruptcy of Lehman Brothers, and nothing improved from then. Seventy-five years ago, after the end of WWII, Primo Levi said that nothing was going to be the same after Auschwitz, or, how can there be life after Auschwitz? Well, the world on one hand is improving technologically, but also is going its way. German Sociologist Ulrich Beck said that the world is out of joint (2017). Shakespeare and Hungarian philosopher Agnes Heller (2000) suggested that *time is out of joint*. So, are we naïve? Can we hope? Are we at war?

UB: We are not in war and, as I said to you before, I do not like these war terminologies. This is a terminology working with anxiety. If we are naïve or not is not important because there is a constant change. It will change. The question is whether we can influence it or not, and since I am a psychoanalyst, I would think that with a new consciousness we can influence things in a good way, there I am very positive. Let me give you another example that was much more important for me when I discovered it. In 1987, there was Chernobyl, and to say something very personal, the catastrophe of Chernobyl was much more affecting and difficult for me than this crisis now. I will tell you why. I was a young woman, I just had a baby, a boy, and I was pregnant with a second one. At that time nobody knew or could say what was going to happen. And, of course, it was very concentrated in Europe, but with this nuclear accident pregnant women and children were in more danger than the others. So, I remember very clearly sitting in my apartment with my little boy, pregnant and being strongly afraid. Fortunately, the media were not so strong at that time, but on the other hand, at that time, there was real isolation. There was no internet, everybody was in a lockdown in a very strong separation from each other, in real isolation. I remember it strongly. It was about always asking the doctors if this could impact the children, and nobody could answer this. So, as a pregnant woman I was in fear thinking about what would happen to my babies. And all of us know how strongly this influences the development of our babies. Personally, that was a much deeper crisis than this one. But one of the consequences of the crisis was that after thirty years we have reduced the nuclear centres in Europe, and at least we are close to the French border, now, after more than thirty years, they have closed a nuclear centre in France which is directly at the German border, and which was all the time, in the last years, risking a nuclear accident. Small one, but it was. So, for me, it took some time, but something changed. It was also the development of the Green Party in Germany. So, on a political, on an economical, and on a social level, something happened. On one hand, I say: "Well, I am optimistic, this will change something!" On the other hand, there is the psyche, and in the psyche there still is a very strong movement, always to regression, to going back to the father and to the mother complex, going back to crying to the authorities, and to give over the authority to the so-called strong persons who are offering a solution, and, of course, these political people like to use the terminology of the "hero" and of the "war" because, of course, if they find a solution later on they can use it, but the price we pay is that we stay immature, not being part of all the necessary changes that have to come.

SC: You are an expert on I-Ching. What does the I-Ching have to say, or what comes to your mind when you link the I-Ching with the coronavirus crisis?

UB: Of course, I did. I was asking the I-Ching, and the hexagram that appeared was, "43," "breaking through," and when I got it, I remembered that Helmut Wilhelm, the son of Richard Wilhelm wrote about exagram "43," "breaking through," that this hexagram requires totally clear, very conscious, actions on something unexpected that suddenly breaks through in normal life. So, breaking through is a kind of psychotic situation and the commentary of the hexagram is clearly speaking about something happening unexpectedly. All the conscious means, individually and also in group, are required to overcome this very critical situation. Here in Germany it seems to be better, compared with Spain or Italy and many other countries, where we have much more great personal catastrophes. So, the I-Ching is talking about a collective disaster. The collective and the individual must be reacted on it with strict, clear and well means.

SC: Now that you have mentioned Spain, I want to ask you another question. You know that I am Italian, that my wife is Spanish and that two of our daughters were born there, the third one was born in Berlin, so we are a very European family. The more I think about this crisis, the more I think that it is now the time of grief. In Milan, there are more civilian deaths than during the Second World War. In the past few weeks, when the lockdown started, many people got a bit manic: cooking bread, cooking amazing lunches and dinners, yoga, meditations, Netflix and whatever. Now we do not know what to cook anymore, now we do not know which new book to read, and, believe me, we are lucky here in Germany: We are in a partial lockdown, my parents are locked in the flat and they have been living like this for the past two months, and it is getting out of control. But it is also about death. What is grief? What is depression because of grief? What could be the next step? What can we say to those listening to us that are in deep sorrow?

UB: we need the connecting feeling of love. This is for me also expressed in the relatedness we can have when we have brothers and sisters. It is about looking for each other and showing that even if we do not share one room with each other, in our soul and in our feelings we are there, and we are there with love. Let me give you an example: under normal circumstances, when one of your daughters is going to Spain and you are staying in Berlin, your daughter will never have the feeling that you will not love her anymore, just because she is being away from you. That is because she is connected to you in this love. So, for me, this is important to share with each other, and it has nothing to do with outer circumstances, whether there is a political change, an economical change, or the virus. Let us send these signs every day. The mother of my partner lives in Italy, she is more than ninety years old and, for two weeks, she has been staying all alone in her apartment. The only support we can give is to send her reassuring signs, and to make her feel very close to us, and that we are really taking emotionally care. But, Stefano, to be honest, this is not all. In this pandemic the symptom is a problem with breathing. Our breath is not only connecting us with the world, it is also taking something from the world, because we are processing this in our lungs. So, the question is: what is really giving me this kind of safety, emotional safety, what does really matter in my life, beyond travelling and beyond shopping, and so on? What is it, that gives me a very good feeling in staying at home, seeing in which way I am connected with my family? Of course, many families came into crisis, because the consequences of the lock down made obvious from what they were escaping, so, again, the question is: What is really important for me? What do I have to correct to come to an effective balance? What do I have to finish? What do I have to reflect again? What do I have to discuss with me or the others? The inner process is to reconnect with my wellness, it is facing my anxieties, not to project them, but to face them. This crisis is requiring and showing us all these things.

SC: I wonder whether this is a time for a renewed *Liberté, égalité,* and as you said, *fraternité?*

UB: Yes, it is. It is really about honestly asking oneself: "What is this for me? What does *liberté* mean for me? What does freedom in berlin mean to me?" And you see, is it the freedom to travel to Spain, or is it the freedom how I manage my family life, how I manage those things in my life that are really important? There, I can make decisions.

SC: In a recent conversation with Susan Rowland (see Chapter 6), I mentioned a dream of a patient of mine. She dreamt Stephen Hawking, who was a genius but his body somehow dropped him, and yet he grew inside. Today, thinking of freedom or maybe even liberation, I'm thinking of Nelson Mandela, who was trying to transform his country to end apartheid. He was imprisoned because of his actions and he resisted almost thirty years in a very small cell, smaller than this room I am in now. But he was free inside. This was his strength. So, those that are complaining because they need a haircut, a massage, new nails.... This is really the time to reflect on what we have become.

UB: Yes, it is. Of course, when we think about Nelson Mandela, it is unbelievable what he did, what he managed to survive. I do not know who can do this, but I was also thinking about that with a patient, yesterday, when we were discussing about a German folk song. This folk song was written during the German revolution. There was a revolution in 1848, which lead later on to the reform of Bismarck and too many other developments in Germany. This song starts with: "Our thoughts are free, and you can imprison me and put me in jail, but my thoughts are free and I can think what I want." This is something which is very important in this situation. We have to start to find our own answers according to what we feel inside, and not depending on Netflix, or on what somebody is saying about something. It is, again, about restarting a creativity of my own thoughts and also on my own feelings, that I can have independently from where I am or under which circumstances I am. Maybe this is something that happened to Nelson Mandela, I do not know.

SC: Thank you very much, Ursula!

UB: Thank you for this interview! Thank you for asking to so many people, and collecting so many important opinions, and show them to everybody. Thank you, Stefano!

References

Beck, U. (2017). *The Metamorphosis of the World*. Cambridge: Polity Press.
Fromm, E. (1941). *Escape from Freedom*. New York: Holt Paperbacks.
Heller, A. (2000). *The Time Is Out of Joint. Shakespeare as Philosopher of History*. Lanham: Rowman & Littlefield Publishers.
Sontag, S. (1978) *Illness as Metaphor*. New York: Farrar, Straus & Giroux.

Chapter 9

Nightmares

Renate Daniel

Dreams are the dominating theme of the talk with Renate Daniel. We all dream, every night. But sometimes people just don't recall their dreams. Psychiatrist and Jungian Analyst Renate Daniel makes understand that whether people remember dreams depends on the intensity of emotions within that dream: the more emotions – no matter if good or bad – the less forgettable the dream. At the same time Daniel takes to account the strive of humankind to overcome nature. Sleep as a state of unconsciousness gives up this moment of control. Renate Daniel links this circumstance to the Coronavirus that lets us face death – a part of nature humankind fears deeply. She shares her observation that we would live in a society that is too concerned about the physical death. To that extend that by isolating during the pandemic some people sacrifice the health of the soul – the need to be in nature, to be active or social. Covid-19 – like giving up control in a dream – shows the limits of humankind's power to overcome nature. Even technology as the most powerful weapon to do so, reaches its limit here according to Daniel. In the last part of the talk, Renate Daniel dives deep into the meaning of nightmares. The experience of a nightmare is a soul in distress, as she puts it. It sometimes can be that intense that a physical reaction occurs. But, according to the Jungian, nightmares can disappear when its meaning is depicted. Or: An uninterpreted dream is a letter that has not been read yet.

Stefano Carpani: Doctor Daniel, dear Renate, you are a psychiatrist and a Jungian psychoanalyst. You are the director of programs at the C.G. Jung Institute Zürich. How are you and how has the coronavirus time been for you and the Institute?

Renate Daniel: Well, I had a lot of work, but I was happy to reschedule our program to a video conference programme, and I'm happy that students like it. Also, we all are longing for the time when we can meet face to face again.

SC: This must have been a gigantic amount of work for you.

RD: Yes, it was a lot of work, but I'm happy that we made it and that it worked.

SC: Before looking into the pandemic and your work on nightmares, I would like to ask you few of my usual questions when interviewing Jungians: who is Carl Gustav Jung or who is your own Carl Gustav Jung?

DOI: 10.4324/9781003266402-9

RD: He is the famous psychiatrist from Switzerland. And let's say my Carl Gustav Jung is the psychiatrist who described a concept of the psyche that helps me a lot to understand my clients. But also, my own person, my friends, my colleagues, it helps me to understand the psyche itself and the life as we are living it. And so it's helpful for my work, but for my private life too; for me, his concepts are really very helpful. I benefited a lot from his work.

SC: What is his relevance today in the twenty-first century?

RD: It's a little bit tricky because in the world of science, even in psychology and psychoanalysis, he is not. Jung is usually not quoted in modern books. You read a lot of famous analysts, but he's not mentioned very often. But there are other countries in the world like South America or the United States or in Asia and in Russia, where they read Jung and benefit a lot from his work, but perhaps in the centre of Europe he is not very much appreciated. And today in Switzerland or Germany most psychiatrists or psychotherapists do the training to become behavioural psychotherapists. There is not so much interest in his work, but I profit a lot from his concepts and always use it.

SC: Why is his work not appreciated anymore? I was a student of literature and philosophy in my 20s and of course we read Jung and Freud, but within the Department of Humanistic, not psychology.

RD: There's perhaps one important fact, namely that today's scientific approach wants to bring psychology closer to natural science. And Jung was interested in religion, in the question of meaning, in the mystery of life, and the mystery of psyche. And concerning these questions it's very difficult to give answers and to make research. When you are interested in the mystery of life – this is not very close to natural science. And that's perhaps one aspect. And you know when the Red Book was published, people asked themselves, if he did suffer from a psychosis or something like that. And so perhaps there are many prejudices about his personality.

SC: Now that you mention the Red Book: What is your opinion about it? There are many who love it, those like Sonu Shamdasani for example, and others, like Wolfgang Giegerich who says it shouldn't have been published. What is your opinion about it?

RD: That's a different question. Should it be published? That was the decision of the family. And, of course, it was his own inner process where he found how to work with his images, how to work with his anxiety and all the material that came up to his conscious mind. And that's why it is so important. He made the process himself and he did not only ask others for support or to find answers about the psyche and about psychological questions, but he found it on his own. And that's why, when we are trained as Jungian psychologists, let's say, we are obliged to do self-experience. So, we get to know ourselves. And that's very important when we want to work with others. And in the Red Book we see how his process worked. But we all have our unique own process.

SC: You recently published a book titled Psyche und Soma (2020). In your previous book *Taking the Fear Out of the Night* (2017) you underlined that "some neurobiologists come to the conclusion that we dream primarily in order to solve the problems or develop new ideas." Beyond the neuroscientific findings, you underline that "strategic learning can happen through dreams and that dreams contribute to health." Can you say more about these two quotes, perhaps starting defining what dreams are?

RD: What are dreams? Well, to summarize it, you know, we have experiences when we are awake. Yeah, and there are furthermore experiences at night, while we are sleeping – after we lose control. And in the morning when we wake up, we remember, there was a kind of story, while we were sleeping, and this story was a kind of inner experience. And that's what we call a dream. So, there is a life when we are awake and there is a life at night time. And due to modern research with devices like the EEG one can ask a test person to sleep in the laboratory in order to be awakened, let's say, every 90 minutes or every 30 minutes in order to tell one's dreams. Due to this research we know that everybody is a dreamer. The problem is that in daily life it's difficult to remember dreams. For sure we are all dreaming and it seems that all mammals are dreaming. So, there must be a benefit or it must have a meaning. And already in antiquity, and even in the Bible, there are descriptions of dreams and people were interested in their messages. So, you see, that first of all, dreams are a very old phenomenon and people always paid attention to dreams. And in former times people were convinced that dreams are important or can be important.

SC: You underline that according to the Talmud a dream which is not interpreted is like a letter that has not been read or perhaps was even neglected. That means dream interpretation is attempting to find an answer for our unconscious images and cultivating a dialogue between the unconscious and the conscious. You also say dream interpretation is a dialogue with one's soul. Why? Often people don't look at dreams seriously. Why are we afraid to look at the content of the dreams? Why do we forget dreams so easily?

RD: I can't give you an answer why we tend to forget dreams. But we see the more emotions there are in a dream – for example negative emotions like anxiety, which is why we call it a nightmare – the less you can forget it. When there are not that many emotions in a dream, then it's easier to forget it. And this reminds us, or is similar to the situation when we are awake: because the more intense your emotions are, the less you will forget your experience, an encounter or whatever. And when something is not very important and not many emotions are attached to it, then you will forget it. The more intense the emotions are, the easier it is, to remember the event or situation. If there is a very positive or a very negative emotion in a dream, then you will usually not forget the dream. Furthermore, it seems easier to remember dreams when you are in a crisis, in puberty or in psychotherapy.

SC: You make a difference between what are called big dreams and let's say daily dreams. What is the difference?

RD: Well, be aware, that to all your questions, the answer cannot be that precise. There are vaguenesses and uncertainties, besides the knowledge there is a lot of not-knowing. Back to your question: there can be dreams that are important for humankind. So, when we read in the Bible that the pharaoh had a dream, it was a very important dream because he's responsible for his people. And his decisions may have an impact on the whole people. But everybody can have big dreams. They are usually not talking about father and mother or the external world. They are not interested in your, let's say, your personal environment or your individual problem. But there are symbols, let's say a church or a stone or a large tree, which point to the question of life, perhaps meaning or the mystery of life. That's what Jung called archetypal dreams, because they talk about question which belong to all of us, which are important for all of us. For example the question: Why do we live? Or what is the meaning of life? What is it for?

SC: In your book you also underline that the moment from being awake to the state of sleep is important. You write and I quote: "We can only go to sleep when we let go, when we allow our ego to plunge into the unknown." And you add that this requires the ego to relinquish control. Is this a problem for our society?

RD: Well, let's say the history of humankind is to overcome nature. We would not have a flat, we wouldn't have medicine, we wouldn't have all the technical devices if we had allowed nature to do its job. We want to protect ourselves against the power of nature. We want to live longer. We want to be secure. And this fight against the forces of nature is something that belongs to humankind. We cannot avoid to overcome nature. But we are also a part of nature. And our instincts and our instinctual life is one aspect of nature. For example, we need to sleep. Without sleep we cannot stay in a healthy state. When you are in distress or when you have many problems and when you are pondering about your problems, then the ego is very awake which makes it difficult to fall asleep. But we need to sleep, we want to sleep, but even if we want to sleep, it is out of control for the ego. The ego cannot decide to sleep. On one hand we are able to control, this means we are disciplined beings in some aspects. But for me, it's, let's say, a healthy state if we are able to control what is possible and bear all that what we can't control or shouldn't control. It's about to find a balance between control and no control.

SC: Contextualizing what you just said within the spectrum of the coronavirus pandemic ... is coronavirus about this? Rebalancing, control what we can't control, wake and sleep?

RD: At least, let's say coronavirus faced us with death. We are threatened by death. We don't want to die and death is an aspect of nature, which is Mother Earth. Nature tries to be in balance, and this balance includes animals, plants and human beings. They are born and they have to die and this is necessary for the health of the whole. And now humankind is facing death and this, of course, this causes panic. Due to this danger we stayed at home, and as a side effect Mother Nature got healthier. For Mother Nature, for some animals and plants the lockdown was very positive. They could recover. Yeah, and of course, it was positive for our individual human life, too, because social distancing was the measure to reduce the risk of infection, disease and death.

SC: You said Jung actually made it a pillar of his theory that our life could be divided in stages. Actually, two major stages. The first one, the natural aim, which goes up to 35, 40 years of life. And then the second one, which is the cultural aim. That is when we become aware that we are mortal and why we are so afraid of death and why the coronavirus really, as you underlined, brought up this panic of death. What is your personal idea – not looking at Jung because I know you have many ideas?

RD: This question is too big for this interview. There are many aspects why we are afraid of death. I would need more hours to reflect on that. I guess it is something innate. We don't want to die. And as you mentioned, it was Jung's idea that we have to find our answer concerning death. We do now leave the realm of dreams. Coronavirus showed us that we tend to focus on the physical death. And isolate ourselves and protect ourselves. On one hand, it's necessary and positive, but from a Jungian perspective we are interested in the shadow, which means possible negative aspects. When you stay at home and isolate yourself you can avoid physical death. But something is perhaps dying inside, in your soul, this is a kind of side effect. You cannot hug persons, you don't meet persons, you cannot engage in life. So, while you are protecting from physical death you have to sacrifice something. Not everybody, but some people, understand that they sacrifice fundamental pillars of life when they are no longer able to be active in the way they need to be active. And this can be that you want to work or that you want to go out in nature or that you want to be active in a way you are no longer allowed to do. And so perhaps some have had the feeling that they are condemned to wait for death because they cannot see their grandchildren or see their beloved ones. The needs of the soul are very important during the pandemic and sometimes the dreams can help you to understand what you can sacrifice and what not. You have to keep in mind that health is not only physical health, but includes the health of your soul or your psyche. And the health of your soul has an immense effect on your immune system and therefore on your physical health.

SC: Before we go back to dreams, to nightmares actually, I would like to ask you to share what you told me recently in clinical supervision about death and how you want to die.

RD: To be honest, I want to be awake when I die. Because this experience will be a unique, which means a one-time experience. And I prefer to be awake in order not to miss what happens. I am curious and interested what will happen, Therefore I don't want to sleep or be sedated by psychopharmaceutical medication or painkillers. That's my wish.

SC: Is it possible to imagine that one day we will die? Can one be ready to die, to go? These are important questions.

RD: To be honest I would like to grow old and my role models in my childhood were the sisters of my grandfather, they were in their 90s when they died. So, when I was a child, I was convinced everybody dies, especially women in my family, when they are in their 90s. So as a child it was an unquestioned fact for me, that I will be in my 90s when I have to die. This aspect is alive in me, the hope that I can die in my 90s. But during the corona crisis, when I saw all that, I thought, well, when I have to die tomorrow, it's ok too. This helps me to feel free and to live how I want to live and to be aware what my soul needs and what makes sense for me. But this is something very individual. It is the question what is important in one's life, what can be sacrificed and what not.

SC: For me coronavirus is also about technology, how a nation, how a public health system can cope with such an emergency through technology. Technology in the past decades helped to generate life, to extend life and avoid death. When I compare the pandemic of the coronavirus with the Spanish flu, there was little technology. But nowadays, if I get sick, I will get a ventilator or the needed care (at least in the West). The whole issue about technology is very important. Technology nowadays can extend life or even create it.

RD: Coronavirus confronted us with limitations, and one limitation is the physical death, but there are many other limitations: will there be a bed in the emergency department, will a ventilator be available? Will there be enough nurses and physicians to help me? We have to face our limits and this is very difficult in an epoch when there is an advertising: "Accept no limits." And no limitations – that's a wish but not reality. There are limits in every epoch and these limits are sometimes bitter, tragical or sad. Others feel angry that we have to accept limits. This is something very emotional. Limitations can reinforce emotions.

SC: Let's look at nightmares now. What are nightmares? What makes a dream a nightmare? You explain it beautifully in the book.

RD: Ok, when you wake up in the morning or during night, usually a nightmare is a psychosomatic experience because on the one hand there are these images of the dream. And on the other hand, you have a physical reaction. You are sweating. Perhaps your heart is racing. There are very intense emotions, anxiety and fear. Your whole personality is involved. You have images, thoughts, emotions and physical reaction. A holistic, a psychosomatic experience. That's a nightmare.

SC: Can nightmares be transgenerational or transpersonal?

RD: Yes, I have examples for both things you mentioned. There was a 14- or 15-year-old girl, living in the United States, suffering from anxiety, panic attacks and one nightmare especially came very often. Here she dreamt that she was imprisoned in a concentration camp. Due to her symptoms she met a psychiatrist. During therapy they found out that one part of the family, they were Jewish people, and on the other hand she had an uncle who was a Nazi. And as soon as these circumstances were revealed, the nightmare stopped, and she had no longer any panic attack. So, she dreamt about something that was connected to her ancestors. My conclusion of this and other examples is that the soul is longing for the truth or longing to witness the reality, which should not be forgotten. Very often, as soon as you know the secrets of the family, the nightmares stop. The uncovering of such secrets can be a healing factor. And I know more examples of this kind.

SC: This is an amazing example. Thank you! You mentioned a couple of times *the mystery of life*. Why this kind of nightmares? Why did this young woman or this girl dreams this? Is this a kind of family requirement? Is this a kind of sensibility towards the family? How do you explain that?

RD: I don't know if it's only individual. Perhaps this is one aspect. As I mentioned before, when I give you an answer, this is only one aspect as all these issues are very complex. There are always many aspects, some of them we know, others not. I believe – I have to emphasize I do not know but believe – that dark aspects in the family or even in the society, for example the Nazi situation, need to be seen and to be witnessed and that we have to know that dark aspects belong to life. And it seems that the soul yet is not only interested in joy and fun but wants to see the very dark aspects or shadow aspects that really happened in life. I don't know if this girl I mentioned had siblings and if they also dreamt about this, this would be interesting to see. If one is the only family member who gets such information via dream, the question occurs: is she your chosen? Why? Are these issues important for her, for her soul and for her life? So, we need more research on that. Right now, we have only these single cases where we can see that.

SC: In the introduction of your book you give three examples and under-line that people found individual responses to the nightmares which worked for each of them personally. And you mention that nightmares disappear as soon as their message has been depicted. Can you say more? You said some-thing already, but can you give us other examples?

RD: This seems to be a rule that understanding the message calms you down. This is what I can see. This is my experience. Do you want to have another example?

SC: Yes. That would be great.

RD: What example comes to my mind? As I mentioned, this Hungarian director, Benedek Fliegauf, he mentioned whenever he wakes up from a night-mare, he knows that he needs to make a new film. A new movie. Then he calms down. And he found out spontaneously that he has this task. He has to do something. I give you another example of a woman who was in a concentration camp. She was imprisoned in Ravensbrück, where many prisoners were the subject of medical experiments. These tests were conducted by physicians. And during her time in the concentration camp, this woman did not have a single nightmare. But from the first night on in freedom, she suffered from nightmares and she didn't dare to talk to anybody. But she wrote a diary. And as soon as she had written down everything, all the nightmares and all the cruel experiences she had in the concentration camp, she had no more nightmares. So, she found her answer. She didn't dare to disclose the nightmares to a human being, but she wrote a diary. And then she calmed down. And there were only few circum-stances in her later life when the nightmares came back and she understood that she had to reduce her workload to calm down. This always worked. So even without psychotherapy, if you watch yourself, if you are really in connection with your nightmares and your soul, you will find an answer, your individual answer. What do I have to do to calm down? Because the nightmare indicates that your soul is in a kind of distress. You are facing something terrible, but you can cope with and find your very personal answer.

SC: In your book you write, "writing or drawing objectifies the nightmare experience and make it visible to the outside world." Then you also write "the act of illustrating our dream images frequently as a calming effect on our emotions." What would you suggest to those that actually cannot find this calming effect, those that keep having the same nightmares night after night?

RD: Of course, this is usually helpful. This is something that works very often, but it doesn't work in every single case. To say it in general, I try to find out what is the situation in the dream and what about the dream ego, what is the dream ego facing and are there any resources? Are there any helpers or what could be a helpful attitude in this specific situation? What would be a helpful strategy? Is there anything in the dream that is connected with the outer life when we are awake? This means I try to find a bridge between the unconscious and the conscious world. I try to find out, if there is a message that the dreamer can understand. But of course, this is an experiment. I don't know. I cannot say that this approach works 100 percent. I try to play with these images, associations and emotions that belong to the nightmare. And as far as I see, this works very often.

SC: I remember you describe the example of a boy who was having nightmares and I think he is dreaming of monsters. Can we look at that example?

RD: Yes, it was a five- or six-year-old boy and he dreamt of monsters. He was sent to therapy because he woke up at night and went to see his mother. And that's why she couldn't sleep, too. He then painted the monsters and spontaneously he had the idea to put a spider in front of the monsters. He painted himself and then between him and the monsters, there he put a spider. And isn't it interesting that out of his soul emerged a potential solution? This proves that dreams are not a fixed product or something that is set or petrified. You can play with the dream or you can work with it. So, you can continue the dream process, you can take this "product" in the unconscious or from the unconscious, and make something out of it. Because what did the boy do? Of course, he didn't accept the image as a kind of stone, but worked on it, played with it and thereby added the spider. And doing so his soul calmed down because the spider protected him and the monsters had to face the spider. While he immersed in this process, he had less nightmares. But he forced his mother to write all of them down. He was interested in having a dream diary and to record his dreams. And so, this five-year-old boy found his own way to calm himself down.

SC: That's amazing. Before we conclude, I would like to ask you: can you tell us something about your new book and what you are working on right now?

RD: Well, already the topic of nightmare, as it were, touches psychosomatic issues. Since I studied medicine, I have always been interested in the relationship between psyche and soma. This is a very difficult question. Until today it's a kind of mystery. If I make a psychological process or if I develop my personality, this has always an impact on the body because we are physical beings. And that's perhaps why I was so shocked at the beginning of the pandemic. Working on the new book, in reading the latest research and through experience with myself and my clients I understood on even a deeper level that psyche and soma are very deeply connected. For example, when you are in panic or full of anxiety, then your immune system will not work that good. That's what we know today, that's proven. The psyche has a big impact on our physical health. This means, if you suffer mentally, if you are stressed, the risk of getting seriously ill with the virus will increase, but if you are mentally stable, the risk of getting seriously ill will decrease, because the immune system is more robust. And this may be astonishing, but it is a fact. And as psychotherapists or analysts are working on the psychological aspects, they should be more aware of the impact of their work on the client's body. It is a pity that not many scientists or virologists don't know about this research or are not interested in it. It seems not to be a very widespread knowledge. But it's very important to know that psychotherapy affects the body. And when you are working as a physician, of course, this has an impact on the psyche. And that's what they have to know to, for example, during a cancer treatment. The medication and all the other treatment have an impact not only on the body but also on the psyche. So, all physicians and psychotherapists should know more about this connection between psyche and soma. And you will find out that everybody has a more or less unconscious world view concerning the question about the relationship between psyche and soma. The new book has the intention, that we become more aware of our own world view concerning this topic and that we are better informed about available insights, to which, by the way, Jung has already made an important contribution.

SC: Thank you very much for your time, and I hope to see you very soon again in Zurich.

RD: Thank you, too.

References

Daniel, R. (2017). *Taking the Fear Out of the Night: Coping with Nightmares.* Einsiedeln: Diamon Verlag.
Daniel, R. (2020). *The Self: Quest for Meaning in a Changing World.* Einsiedeln: Diamon Verlag.

Part 2

Chapter 1

How I Was Affected by Covid-19 in My Practice

Misser Berg

The first part of this paper describes what happened in the author's clinic when she had to close it down due to the Coronavirus restrictions. Berg describes the reactions among her patients and the process until and after the restrictions were lifted. The second part of the chapter contains the author's reflections on her reactions and the gradual change in her attitude towards online work from a rather one-sided focus on the benefits of online work to a more balanced position. In this process she recognizes that she received good help from reading papers by esteemed colleagues. She looks into her own mild depression and finds an interesting and most helpful description in Jan Wiener's expression with reference to the Argentinian psychoanalyst José Bleger of what happens when 'the setting begins to weep.' In the conclusion, Berg describes how she is now back to the 'old normal,' albeit somehow changed.

The History

By the end of February 2020, the coronavirus began to spread in Denmark. At the beginning the health-authorities were very calm – in hindsight much too calm. They thought that it was unlikely that the infection would spread seriously in Denmark, because they controlled all persons who came from China and North of Italy, but too late they found out that much more infection came from Austria. We followed the news from North Italy and the insecurity and anxiety increased. The infection began to spread in Denmark, and people in my clinic reacted in very different ways. As we now know, at that time nobody really knew what it was.

One of my patients, a man around 50 with a severe psychiatric diagnosis, whom I had been seeing once a week in my clinic for over seven years, declared that he would try to get infected as quickly as possible to get it over with. I told him that if this were his intention, he could not see me face-to-face in my clinic, because being over 70 I did not myself want to be infected (we knew from Italy that older people got more sick than younger). My patient looked at me with surprise; he was so used to be invisible and without any influence on others, and he had obviously not been consciously aware of the fact that he could damage me. This became the first turning point in our relation caused by the coronavirus. Later, after I had moved

DOI: 10.4324/9781003266402-10

my clinic online, it turned out that being online actually supported him in being much more structured (he used the telephone, because his phone could not access Skype or Zoom). Not having to look me into the eyes enabled him to focus better on himself and the analysis. He is probably the patient for whom going online during the pandemic has had the most positive influence, and since then we both prefer meeting online, and he seldom comes to see me physically.

On March 11 our prime minister, Mette Frederiksen, locked down the country. I also then locked down my clinic (some of my colleagues continued to work face-to-face, but my clinic, being in a garden-shed, is too small for keeping the required space). From then on, I worked by Zoom, Skype or telephone. At that time, I already worked online with several patients and supervisees, so it was not new to me, but still it was a big difference to sit in front of the screen all day and only seeing peoples' heads.

When I contacted all my patients and supervisees and informed them, that until further they had to see me online, another of my male patients declared that he nevertheless wanted to see me face-to-face and that he would turn up at my place at the already scheduled time. I told him that this was not possible, and he then decided to wait until I opened my clinic again. After some weeks, however, he found out that he needed to see me, but he was very much against Skype or Zoom, so we had to try Teams. For some reason Teams and I do not work well together, so at the end, when we had struggled to make it function, he agreed to work on Skype. At the beginning, he was very resistant but gradually he became more relaxed at our online meetings. As soon as I opened again, however, he was back face-to-face which was a relief for both of us.

Another male patient wanted to take a break, but after some time he asked me to talk with him on the phone. At first, he did not want to use Skype or Zoom, but after having tried Zoom with some colleagues at work, he found out that it was OK also to use it for his analysis.

For some reasons, it was the men who were the most resistant to go online in my clinic. I do not know if it is just a coincidence, but also a male supervisee took a long break before he agreed to work on Skype.

All my female patients agreed to continue online. Some of them expressed sadness that they lost travelling up to me; I live around 30 minutes by train north of Copenhagen and many of my patients have over the years expressed how important the lonely train trip through beautiful landscapes have been for them as a preparation for and digestion of their analytical work. Others expressed that they were satisfied with being able to stay at home because of the risk of going out.

Two of my female patients who both on beforehand suffered from heavy anxiety, became terrible anxious when the virus broke out and both have not yet come back to see me face-to-face, but continue their sessions online. They both had to have extra sessions at the beginning to calm them down, and as anxiety makes everything much more concrete and blocks the symbolic function (which already was rather impaired) we spent hours after hours to talk about symptoms and about how to best secure the food that was brought by the online service so it would not infect them etc. One of them, who lives alone, has not seen a person face-to-face for over a year. Now she is fortunately vaccinated and has begun to come out of her house for shopping, but she is still too anxious to see me face-to-face.

My lock-down lasted from March 11 until June 2020 and again from January until June 2021. Between June 2020 and January 2021 my clinic was open, and I had to take extra precautions by ventilating the room, cleaning the door handles, securing that the distance between the chairs was two meters, providing hand sanitizer etc. The use of hand sanitizer created a little ritual: At the beginning I asked my patients to use the hand sanitizer, but after a short while, instead of telling them to do so, and also because some of them did not want to touch the bottle with hand sanitizer, I simply took the bottle and poured the sanitizer on their hands. It happened spontaneously and was a procedure that felt natural at the time, but I must say that I was not happy with either method, and I am glad that it is now over.

I was fully vaccinated in May 2021 and my clinic has been open since June. As most of my patients are also now vaccinated, things are more or less back to normal with those of my patients who come to see me face-to-face. As mentioned above, two of my female patients have not yet dared to come to see me, and others have now become more inclined to ask for an online session when they are busy and can save time by not taking the trip up to see me face-to-face.

Reflections

Already before the pandemic I was occupied with the advantages of online analysis and supervision. I had given online lectures, seminars, and supervision for groups and individuals in places like Kazakhstan and China etc. It was very clear, that online media enabled much more contact with remote groups than before when analysts, supervisors, and teachers had to travel to places far away.

Also in my clinic, online analysis made sessions possible which before had to be postponed. One of my patients could continue her analysis online during a very difficult pregnancy and subsequently during the maternity leave. This was important to lessen the level of anxiety and stress during pregnancy and right after birth. Fortunately, both mother and baby are completely healthy.

In our Danish Training we have candidates from all Nordic countries, and online supervision made a much better frequency possible than before when it had to take place when the candidates were in Copenhagen once a month, eight times a year.

I discussed the benefits of the online media with more reluctant colleagues from the Danish psychoanalytic and psychotherapeutic field and gave several lectures on the subject. My knowledge at that time was very much inspired by John Merchant's excellent article *The Use of Skype in Analysis and Training: A Research and Literature Review* (Merchant 2016) and Alessandra Lemma's inspiring book *The Digital Age on the Couch* (Lemma 2017).

As I already had good experience with using the online media, and as I was a happy advocate for working online, it took me some time to feel and to realise the other side. At first this was not conscious, and instead I gradually found myself being slightly depressed. As the lockdown period in 2020 was less than 3 months and as I at the same time was busy with changing several requirements in the IAAP Education Committee to enable higher amount of online analysis etc. I did not give room enough to what could lie behind my mild depression. But during the spring 2021 where my clinic was closed for more than 5 months, I had to look more closely into the challenges and disadvantages of online work, and actually, it was when hearing Jungian colleagues reporting on how they had changed from being strongly against online media to now embrace the format, that I realised that my perception had taken the opposite direction.

Challenges and Disadvantages

Alessandra Lemma mentions how 'Skype slippage' for both patients and analysts gradually loosen the boundaries. (Lemma 2017, p. 105). My pregnant patient who week after week was lying in her bed, green in her head, while holding her mobile in her hand is an example of this. During my lockdown I did not work from my clinic in the garden-shed because there the Wi-Fi connection is not good enough, so instead I worked from my office inside the house. Here my patients can see what is behind me, and sometimes I have not been as conscious about what I change in my office as I am in my clinic. At a time, I had the grandchildren's teddy-bears and a big red plastic goat standing on the bookshelf behind me. I gave the goat to a little girl, and the next time I saw one of my supervisees, she said: Oh no! Where has it gone? I am also generally more relaxed regarding my appearance, for instance I take off my shoes when I feel like it. Sometimes I also drink a cup of tea or coffee which I would never do in my clinic.

Also, there can be challenges for the patients to find a secure space for the online meeting. Suddenly during a session with one of my female patients her boyfriend showed up. They lived in a single-room apartment with living room incl. sofa bed, and kitchen in one, and he went in the background and made coffee for himself. This clearly destroyed the confidential space and was a clear obstacle for the analysis.

One well-known challenge is when the Wi-Fi connection is bad (I myself have had to invest in a much stronger connection). Occasionally, the technical problems can be used constructively (Merchant 2016, p. 319–320). But mostly I get terribly tired and also irritated when working with patients with bad connections.

However, I think that for me the biggest challenge has been the absence of physical meetings. Although a lot of what is behind you and the patient is visible when you are online, only the top of the bodies can be seen on the screen. Marilyn Mathew describes what was lost during lockdown:

In person, we could be aware of the way someone smelt, walked or shifted position; tapped their feet or clenched their fists. Meeting in three dimensions was a fundamental way in which I got to know, understand and 'feel into' the people I worked with.

(Mathew 2021, p. 465)

Already, in his article from 2016, John Merchant had stated that genuine analytic processes can occur online (see Merchant 2021, p. 488). This understanding is very much in line with my own experience: most of my patients have worked well in the online analysis and I do not think that this would have been different if we had not gone online. But still I got this mild depression during the two lockdowns.

Jan Wiener in a recent paper (Wiener 2021 p. 793–812) writes about when 'the setting begins to weep' She refers to the Argentinian psychoanalyst José Bleger who talks about the analytic setting (session times, fees, holidays, the room etc.) which allows processes to go on within it. The "setting itself can function like an invisible phantom limb, in that we only become aware of it when it is disrupted.... Patients project into this normally mute setting, early primitive symbiotic feelings connected with the mother" (ibid., p. 801). The setting remains mute until it is disrupted and then it may begin to weep or cry. While we during lockdown could maintain the online setting regarding session times, fees, and holidays etc. the room was not there. Like a depression can lead us to deeper areas in ourselves, the lack of physical presence can in a deep analysis cause the setting to weep. This may eventually lead to a better understanding of the role of the setting in analysis and to take this understanding back into face-to-face analysis in our "own consulting rooms, where the setting may previously have been mute and insufficiently considered" (ibid., p. 807).

Conclusion

The pandemic forced me to revise my initial, too one-sided optimism regarding online analysis. I had to admit that despite its many advantages too much online work and no physical contact with my patients made me slightly depressed. The unstable connections, the looser boundaries, the occasional delayed sound, and frozen pictures etc. have in itself been exhausting and no doubt part of the reason. But besides this there was a feeling of sadness and loss where the formulation 'the sessions began to weep' made sense.

I am now back to the 'old normal,' albeit not entirely. A few of my patients and a number of my supervisees are still entirely online; most of my patients and some supervisees are back face to face, but there is a group of patients who are much more flexible than before regarding whether they, depending on their other schedule, ask to see me online or face to face. And for me this feels natural which it would probably not have done before the pandemic.

References

Lemma, Alessandra (2017). *The Digital Age on the Couch*. London: Routledge.

Mathew, Marilyn A.F. (2021). Together – apart: in touch in a time of separation. *Journal of Analytical Psychology* 66 (3): 463–483.

Merchant, John (2016). The use of Skype in analysis and training: A research and literature review. *Journal of Analytical Psychology* 61 (3): 309–328.

Merchant, John (2021). Working online due to the COVID-19 pandemic: A research and literature review. *Journal of Analytical Psychology* 66 (3): 484–505.

Wiener, Jan (2012). Reflections on the role of the analytic setting in the light of COVID-19. *Journal of Analytical Psychology* 66 (4): 793–812.

Chapter 2

Are You There? *Dis-connection* Entering the Analytical Space

Olivia del Castillo

In her work, Olivia del Castillo delves into her experience on the changes in the analytical framework up to the lockdown due to the global pandemic. Ethical doubts arose in the face of continuous alterations due to the imperatives of life under those circumstances. People have continuously transferred in other homes, equipped with more and more advanced facilities offered by technology. According to her the risk is that the analytical experience adapted to technological resources may remain superficial. On the contrary, this situation presents a deep emotion that cannot be ignored: the mourning for what has been lost. Not ignoring the mourning for the lost can change the nature of what is found anew. The inspiring mythical image of Dionysus – the God who does not want to be ignored – offers to her as a suggestive image, leading to the emotion that creates the difference between a superficial approach and a deeper experience of transformative change, about what we are living through and is about to come.

> *This is the dramatic immediacy …is in which the Dionysiac spirit and its tremendous excitement make themselves known. No suffering, no ardent desire of the human soul speaks forth from out of this excitement, but the universal truth of Dionysus, the primal phenomenon of duality, the incarnate presence of that which is remote, the shattering encounter with the irrevocable, the fraternal confluence of life and death.*
> (Walter Otto, *Dionysus: Myth and Cult*)

Years ago, when patients moved from the city they lived in and I had my practice, we prepared for our farewell by considering contacting another analyst at the location they have moved. The interruption of their analysis forced us to face separation and mourning. I would say that something happened through this experience, which affected both of us. We were facing an end, an announced death that led to a new stage of life and a transformation in both analyst and analysand. Through the mourning assumed by the end of the analysis, we internalised what each one of us represented inside the other, and left space for another analyst to dialogue with the patient's psyche. This would lead to a new development in their process.

DOI: 10.4324/9781003266402-11

Years later, things began to change. Some patients had to move temporarily because of their job, but they did not stay in another place permanently either. Thus, it did not make sense to look for another analyst to follow their process. The fact that they had to move and cross geographical boundaries so often, challenged the limits of the analytical framework. It was like a hurricane that threatened the possibility of an ongoing process of the analysis, which meant a threat of dis-connection: no farewell, no mourning to open the door to a new beginning. Therefore, we began to consider staying connected and organising the sessions remotely, by telephone or internet. With scepticism, ethical doubts, and many efforts, we tried to build a "stable framework." Nevertheless, this framework seemed to be continuously in danger to be diluted by the hurricane. It was a matter of arranging appointments between disparate time slots, finding intimate places, respecting the ritual of the sessions, and dealing with the devices that became part of the framework.

I remember the case of a patient,[1] who was a classical ballet dancer and travelled with the ballet company in Eastern Europe. She stayed in hotels, where the internet connection was very insecure. Thus, the feeling of "connecting and disconnecting" entered the scene. We strived to stay connected, accepted difficulties, and appreciated the advantage of not interrupting the analytical process. The devices – computers, iPads, and smartphones – became very important to us. Once, we had a session in which the patient was located at a hotel reception in Serbia. There some guests were talking loudly and singing. I could barely hear her, but I felt her. I asked myself: what are we doing? We had many difficulties: time and space were losing their containing essence, and technology was becoming sharply and noticeably embedded in our analytical relationship.

Considering how the therapy with this patient progressed, I deduced years later that this dismembering madness made sense. She was there, and I was there too, virtually. Probably, this saved her from deep depression. Everything was dark inside and outside, but we were still holding our sessions, undisturbed despite the difficulties.

At that moment, I wondered if the transferential relationship that she established with me, and I established with her was also virtual once we met in person. In any case, the possibility of creating a sense of "being there," seemed to have an effect, even though the encounter was virtual.

Preserving the work that connected for fifty minutes – the time of the session – kept the *flame of the candle* burning within the analytical relationship, recalling the metaphor of Gaston de Bachelard (Bachelard, 1988)

The situation we lived during the lockdown began a long time ago with the hurricane that moves women and men defying time, space, the presence of the body, and the experience of death: the death of one possibility of life so that another can be born authentically, which is something hard to conceive without living "the shattering encounter with the irrevocable" (Otto, 1965, p. 351) and the sacrifice of omnipotence.

We are standing in front of the unknown. I wonder what the recognition of the hurricane with the shape a threatening virus, which locks us down, brings us: a new opportunity to share and give birth again to us in order to save Dionysus? Or a mutation of humans into hybrid beings, fascinated by the ease that technology offers us?

Dis-connection

We are virtual to a certain extent. We were virtual even before the technological era. Everything that seems to be and is not has always existed. It acts both when we are sharing space in person and when we meet through the screen. However, technology has made what is virtual gigantic. Now technology nourishes the virtual with an accumulated body absence. The virtual becomes a giant that can suffocate emotion, "the dramatic immediacy" of Walter Otto's speech (Otto, 1965, p. 351).

The Internet rescues us from the face-to-face disconnection of nowadays' hurricane. However, perhaps the disconnection that really entered analysis is the disconnection from the experience of the body, from death and transformative mourning, which results in a mutation that increasingly brings closer to the artificial intelligence. The phantasy is that at some point, this intelligence, the artificial one, will replace the therapist. It remains to be seen whether the therapist will become a robot or whether the robot will be embedded, implanted in the therapist. Let's see it. Let's keep us open to the unknown. Let's keep us open to welcome what is yet to come. Let's make room for the *image* to expand our imagination, to be able to develop our own ethics that governs our lives while we navigate the situation.

I am afraid of getting caught in an everyday mechanism in which the care of my consultancy (the space, the arrangement of the elements in it, the lack of devices) may be reduced to "having a good computer." I fear that traveling by train to attend my practice in Madrid every week will no longer make sense. This journey is a kind of ritual of connection between two worlds, Barcelona and Madrid, which means a lot to me. I fear that the time will come when I will no longer see the need "to be there" in person. As long as my body holds out, I do not intend to give up the weekly ritual, just in case I mutate into a highly hybrid being that loses eros and desire towards my work as an analyst.

What we Experienced during Lockdown

As soon as we recognised what the hurricane of the virus was manifesting, we put our work in a safe place during the quarantine and found shelter in a frame that we could feel as "the cave". Some of my analysands had a liberating experience. They were able to return to a state which made them free from being exposed to the world: the pressure of face-to-face interactions, the sometimes-needed distance from the analyst. In these cases, the experience allowed to go deeper into their need to distance themselves from others. "The cave" made them feel contained and able to talk about it. Certainly, this made them improve. One of my patients took advantage of the lockdown to disconnect herself from the analysis – her place in the space we shared was left empty. I am safeguarding it until a farewell takes place. I predict that the farewell will take place inside me after a while, but it will be necessary to happen. In the meantime, our WhatsApp chat still exists: another virtuality that keeps the connection-disconnection in the air.

Most of the analysands accepted and were grateful that we found a way to continue the analysis, including the experience of restlessness of the moment. It was a rich experience. Not denying that we were in a tunnel that would lead to something unknown. This brought something new to the process and opened many viewpoints. Being there, living the dis-connection imposed by the lockdown and pandemic, robbing the lacking-bodily-presence hybrid nature of our encounters: without smell, without touch, only virtual through the activation of audio-visual mirror neurons (Merchant, 2016, p. 315). At least this allowed us to connect with the new and the unknown.

Mourning has been the common thread of this stage. It was not only the death of the many people who died alone – buried without even a ritual. It was also what was dying within us due to the pandemic's imposition. This experience and emotion prevented us from being annihilated by the imperative of the Internet, which fascinates us for the advantages it offers, both virtual and mechanical, and therefore archaic and distant from the experience of movement and the journey from one place to another. In my opinion, if we lose sight of this, we will lose the opportunity to discover what this moment brings to us and to accept what we would never have accepted. Therein lies the drama to which we must surrender ourselves.

As soon as possible, I started travelling with a safe-conduct from Barcelona to Madrid – back and forth – on Thursdays and Fridays every week. The wagons were almost empty, the stations deserted. There were only a few of us who moved from one city to another. The police asked us for our identity cards and the certificates justifying our journey.

Once in Madrid, I saw some patients, who agreed to attend the session in person, with open window, masks, and keeping extreme distance. I remembered the experience I once had with a Lacanian psychoanalyst when I was very young. She told me to sit down at the other end of the room. I was not too fond of that excessive distance. Now, I have seen that in this extreme distance, many living elements can be activated.

Even though I travelled from one city to another, I continued to do online sessions. We decided in each case how we would do the session, respecting each one's sensibility and the action of the Titan of the pandemic which is still there. We recognised the Titan, but we also recognised what we are capable of to do while facing him. Going back and forth by myself on the train, I wondered if, in this way, I have kept in mind the physical presence of the analytic relationship with the analysands. Something was pulling me intuitively, and I let me to be guided.

Gradually, we are now returning to meet most of the patients in person. Perhaps after the next holiday break, we will already have crossed a certain threshold in order to enter into another time and breathable atmosphere. It seems clear that we will always use the online resource when the tension arises between the possibility of coming to the consulting room and staying at home, in "the cave," to do the session from there. I imagine this will be a new intense experience of continuous ethical decisions, that will not spare us the emotion of what is imposed on us in each coming moment of *tremendous excitement* (Otto, 1965, p. 351). How will affect this the process of each of my analysands? How will it affect me? Something is already affecting me. Something reaches me: the value of walking on the street and moving, and the desire to assimilate and imagine the possibilities that are to come. I want to be aware of time passing by. Confinement has made me stop and observe to see what is there without further pretension. Now I feel like adjusting what is there, measuring it to adjust it. As León Febres-Cordero (2020, p. 25) points out:

> This is not a question of optimism versus pessimism. It is a question of seeing what is there, to measure it, adjusting it… measuring and adjusting it to present living, so as to include in that living the shreds of the body remaining to us. Because this is all about saving the body, and moderating the destruction inflicted by the Titans – those violent collective forces unleashed…. Our remedy will be to give birth to ourselves. This is about saving Dionysus.

Note

1 I explain the following episode with the patient's permission.

References

Bachelard, G. (1988). *The Flame of a Candle*. Dallas: Dallas Institute Publications.
Febres-Cordero, L. (2020). *Histeria Colectiva Universal. Sobre la Naturaleza Virtual*. Madrid: Fundación CITAP.
Merchant, J. (2016). The use of Skype in analysis and training: A research and literature review. *Journal of Analytical Psychology* 61 (3): 309–328.
Otto, W. F. (1965). *Dionysus: Myth and Cult*. Bloomington and London: Indiana University Press.

Chapter 3

One *Other* Contagion in the Time of Coronavirus

Dan Cross

During the coronavirus pandemic, one notices a trend in which science is increasingly doubted or rejected in casual, off-handed ways. This brief study looks at one quotation as representative of this trend, and offers a psychological interpretation of the attitude of mind that it reflects. The quotation is "I was thinking that I should get vaccinated, but I'm not going to, because they [the vaccines] haven't been tested. This is just a big experiment on people. I'm not sure the virus is even real anyways. You know, science doesn't really know much." Internal contradictions between the explicit and implicit aspects of the quotation are discussed phrase by phrase, culminating in an overall interpretation that sheds light on an attitude of mind and its functioning and real related meanings.

In this brief study, I'd like to explore a phenomenon that has become more pronounced and frequent during the coronavirus epidemic. In the consulting room, on the news, and in conversations on the street, one notices an increasing trend in which once-unquestioned assumptions of the scientific worldview are doubted or rejected in casual, off-handed ways. Consider the following example, from a university-educated, government worker in his 50s, who told me in passing,

> I was thinking that I should get vaccinated, but I'm not going to, because they [the vaccines] haven't been tested. This is just a big experiment on people. I'm not sure the virus is even real anyways. You know, science doesn't really know much.

This sort of comment, while not mainstream, is far from unusual. And unlike serious, reflective criticisms of science, such as may be found in the work of some critical culture theorists, this "attitude of mind" (Jung 1926, para. 629) comes across as ungrounded, even conspiratorial. How can we understand such a statement? Should we approach the statement as rooted in the individual who made it? Or, should we rather look at the way of thinking that just happens to have found expression in this particular person? After all, as Jung observed, "we are so in the habit of identifying ourselves with the thoughts that come to us that we invariably assume we have made them" (Jung 1928, para.

DOI: 10.4324/9781003266402-12

323). The implication here is that, in fact, we often do not create our own thoughts. So, where else could they come from? Jung clarifies that "an attitude or frame of mind ... more often owes its peculiarity to mental contagion, i.e., to example and the influence of environment" (Jung 1926, para. 630). Indeed, we find clues in this direction when we ask people, like the government worker that I have quoted, what they mean by what they say. How have they come to such conclusions? What are their reasons? What is their evidence? Typically, responses to such questions are clouded, full of contradictions, and reveal the reality that the people expressing such an attitude of mind have only a limited understanding of what they are saying. To be sure, the actual words are voiced by the person, but the background or style of thinking comes from outside the person, from "the crowd" (Jung 1925, para. 255).

So, we find ourselves in an interesting situation: faced with the reality that *the way of thinking* – rather than the individual – is where the action is. Therefore, in the following pages, I will delve into the quotation I have provided, as a typical example of this attitude of mind, and attempt to interpret it psychologically. It will serve as our specimen for study, so to speak. We will try to make sense of its inner contradictions, and reveal its true meaning, that is, what is *really* expressing itself in this attitude of mind.

As a method, we will look at the interplay among (a) the explicit, or *what* is being said in a more or less literal way; (b) the implicit, or *how* the ideas are put together; and (c) the contradictions we find between these explicit and implicit aspects. The explicit aspect of the quotation is conscious to the speaker. If we repeated the words aloud to the speaker, he would recognize the words, and consider them his own. This is true because they overlap with the "subjective attitude" of the speaker (Jung 1948, para. 388), even as they reflect an unconscious, collective pattern of thinking, below the surface. On the other hand, the implicit is mostly, and sometimes entirely, unconscious to the speaker. Like the meaning of a dream, it only becomes clear with psychological attention and reflection. It is, in fact, already there in the quotation, but only implicitly so, looming almost invisibly between and around the words themselves. It would probably surprise its speaker to hear our reflections on this aspect of the quotation. It would seem foreign to the speaker, and in a very real way it is, since it corresponds not to his subjective attitude but to "public opinion, to the time-spirit, or the original, not yet human, anthropoid disposition which we also call the *unconscious*" (Jung 1948, para. 388).

Now, let us dive into the quotation, taking it phrase by phrase. At the end of the discussion, I will attempt to draw some conclusions, but for now let's stay close to "the text." For the reader's ease, here is the quotation again:

> I was thinking that I should get vaccinated, but I'm not going to, because they [the vaccines] haven't been tested. This is just a big experiment on people. I'm not sure the virus is even real anyways. You know, science doesn't really know much.

The first phrase of the first sentence displays reflection ("I was thinking that ...") and an imperative ("I should get vaccinated"). The real, concrete option of getting vaccinated is on the table, or at least it recently was. In the explicit words, things are pretty straightforward so far. And the same is true for the meaning implicit in how the ideas are put together. Moreover, there are no contradictions between the explicit and the implicit, and so not much catches our attention just yet. With the second phrase ("... but I'm not going to get vaccinated"), things become more interesting psychologically. What is happening here? Explicitly, it seems like a concrete choice has been made to not get vaccinated, but implicitly we sense something else going on. After all, a real choice regarding vaccination would involve a consideration of the options, weighing out their respective merits, and so on. This doesn't happen, and so we have to think about what the mentioned "choice" really amounts to. What is going on implicitly? Looking more closely, we see that the choice about vaccination has been replaced by a choice *to not make such a choice* in the first place. In other words, this attitude of mind does not *really* make a choice about getting vaccinated or not, but rather it sidesteps the process of thinking through the options. Explicitly, as we will see, the attitude appears to go on referencing vaccination, but implicitly it has switched its agenda to not-thinking and not-choosing. Next, with the final phrase of the first sentence ("because they [the vaccines] haven't been tested"), a record of poor diligence is assigned to a bad actor, that is, whoever failed to do the testing. Responsibility for real choice, already shirked off by this attitude, is now displaced altogether and becomes the (ir)responsibility of some imagined other.

Before looking at the quotation's first sentence as a whole, we need to briefly touch on the psychological meaning of vaccination. What does it symbolize? On a literal, practical level, vaccination is an act that penetrates the body, and injects a substance (i.e., the vaccine) in order to bolster one's ability to fight off a virus coming from without. The vaccine familiarizes, and thereby better prepares, one's immune system to deal with something that it may have to face in the future. Symbolically, therefore, vaccination is the act of consciously allowing oneself to be altered beneath the threshold of consciousness, and especially in regards to dealing with an *expected* threat, by becoming more familiar with that threat. It symbolizes the act of consciously allowing one's thinking to be reached and altered at a deeper, unconscious (i.e., implicit) level.

Now, bringing together the entire first sentence of our quotation, along with the symbolic meaning of vaccination, we can psychologically interpret the first sentence as follows: The attitude of mind expressed in our quotation does not want to be penetrated by, nor made familiar with, a threat that it itself (at least implicitly) perceives: the threat of having to seriously think through a difficult decision. It does not want to risk an alteration to itself, which would call for a reckoning of the dissociation between its explicit and implicit meanings, and would return the responsibility for a real choice on vaccinations to the attitude itself. Instead, it establishes, through the expression of a denying choice ("I'm not going to ..."), a self-inoculation against having to consider such a choice at all. It turns away from thinking things through.

The next sentence of our quotation reads, "This is just a big experiment on people." The neurotic[1] contradiction between explicit and implicit meaning continues, causing us to sense something uncanny or strange. A conspiracy is vaguely invoked, further shifting responsibility to an imagined other, a "they" without anything substantial to fill out the reference. No efforts are made to describe who "they" are, and instead an appeal to emotions (*e.g.*, suspicion and outrage) is made. Here we catch the psychically contagious aspect of this attitude of mind reaching out its tendrils. After all, nothing is so contagious as emotions cut free from logic and reflective thinking (Jung 1949, para. 701).

To grasp the full meaning of this sentence, we also need to consider the symbolic meaning of experimentation. Literally and practically, experimentation is the application of a structured, impersonal intervention designed to ascertain the factual answer to some question. Its goal is to bring something – perhaps suspected (i.e., hypothesized), but not yet known – to light. An experiment is meant to reveal the actual facts, or a truth of sorts. Symbolically, therefore, experimentation evokes notions of truth, dealing with concrete reality, and dispelling mistaken assumptions and illusions.

Bringing these insights together, we can interpret the second sentence of our quotation as follows: This attitude of mind is dodging responsibility for discovering the truth about itself and the situation it faces, instead making an emotional appeal to see some vague other as the problem. It effectively says, "*They* are trying to find something out, but not *me*. I'm just caught up in this situation, that, by the way, seems a bit fiendish."

The next sentence reads, "I'm not sure the virus is even real anyways." Explicitly, this sentence is rather straightforward. It simply states the opinion that the virus may not be real. The implicit meaning, however, is what accounts for the forgivable reaction some may have upon hearing such thoughts: scratching their heads in confused consternation. After all, the reality of the virus is surely not a matter of opinion, but of established facts, based on widely verifiable evidence, and unequivocally accepted by relevant authorities, such as virologists and epidemiologists, from around the world. So, what is going on here on the implicit level? An important clue is the fact that the virus is first explicitly mentioned only now, *after* the attitude of mind has neurotically dissociated its own explicit and implicit meaning. The previous sentences set the stage for mentioning the virus directly – they *inoculated* the attitude of mind against taking responsibility for its own grounded thinking, choice, and consideration of the truth. Thinking about vaccination and the virus symbolically, we can now interpret this sentence of the quotation as follows: This attitude of mind, already (implicitly) having some sense of the challenge it faces (i.e., to responsibly think through a choice, considering the actual facts), metaphorically *vaccinates* itself against "the virus" of this challenge. The implicit agenda and duplicity of this attitude of mind becomes clearer:

it avoids thinking and the truth, and in this very move reveals that it (implicitly and neurotically) "knows" what it is doing. Its own inner contradictions reveal an unconscious *"mise en scène"* (Jung 1912, para. 364; Giegerich 2013, p. 28). And, like someone angrily shouting, "I'm not angry!" the ironic self-contradiction belies an implicit recognition of the truth, as well as a refusal to accept it.

The last sentence in our quotation reads, "You know, science doesn't really know much." On the explicit level, "you know" are just filler words, similar to "um" or "well." But, implicitly, they address an audience and therefore insinuate some agreement between the attitude of mind and whomever may hear it. We again catch the attitude attempting to psychically "infect" anyone listening, trying to find new minds in which to perpetuate itself. And then, "... science doesn't really know much." Science, already prefigured by the idea of experimentation, now comes into the foreground. On the explicit level, the mysterious "they" that was alluded to before is now revealed to be the discipline of science, in personified form. Science is the bad actor. Meanwhile, on the implicit level, the responsibility for thinking, choice and consideration of the facts, is given its final displacement away from the attitude of mind. Therefore, we can interpret this sentence as follows: the attitude of mind lays responsibility *for its own shortcomings* at the feet of science. And with that, we have looked at each phrase of our quotation in turn.

Now, what can we say about the quotation as a whole? Bringing together our insights regarding each phrase, we can interpret the entire quotation as follows: this attitude of mind sees the challenge of thinking through a practical decision on vaccination as a threat. Rather than making a considered choice on the topic, it neurotically dissociates itself, and then appeals to suspicious emotionality as a way to spread itself among unsuspecting members of the collective. At the same time, the attitude "vaccinates" itself against the "virus" of considering the actual facts and truth about itself and its choice, and places the blame for its own shortcomings on science. What does this reveal to us about the trend mentioned at the outset of this paper? It seems to represent an unconscious and contagious trend in which the difficult task of thinking is avoided, responsibility is displaced, and some other is blamed. It's important to see that the issue here is not *really* about vaccination, but rather about seriously facing the burden of thinking through just one of the realities in this difficult time.

Note

1 The contradiction is neurotic because it involves a dissociation (Giegerich 2013, p. 212). The attitude of mind is divided within itself (between explicit and implicit meaning), this inner-contradiction undermines any potential to deal with the real, practical issue with which it started out (i.e., actually *choosing* whether or not to get vaccinated).

References

Giegerich, W. (2013). *Neurosis: The Logic of a Metaphysical Illness*. London and New York: Routledge.

Jung, C. G. (1912). The theory of psychoanalysis, in H. Read, M. Fordham and G. Adler (eds) *Collected Works of C. G. Jung*, vol. 4. Princeton, NJ: Princeton University Press. (Hereafter CW).

Jung, C. G. (1925). The significance of the unconscious in individual education, in *CW*, vol. 17.

Jung, C. G. (1926). Spirit and life, in *CW*, vol. 8.

Jung, C. G. (1928). The relations between the ego and the unconscious, in *CW*, vol. 7.

Jung, C. G. (1948). The phenomenology of the spirit in fairytales, in *CW*, vol. 9/1.

Jung, C. G. (1949). The significance of the father in the destiny of the individual, in *CW*, vol. 4.

Chapter 4

Covid-19

Impressions, Sidelights, and Thoughts from the Psychotherapeutic Practice

Renate Daniel

During the first lockdown in March 2020, many patients canceled their appointments in face of fear for infection. The office became more empty. Some patients, however, did not want to interrupt their treatment under any circumstances, for instance because the psychotherapy session was the only way to escape domestic conflict or domestic violence, at least for a short time. Others, however, experienced their therapeutic process as very important and fruitful, and were unwilling to give it up.

But with the pandemic, psychotherapeutic work changed in terms of the external framework as well as the content issues.

Already the welcoming, common in the western world, had to be done in a different way. What has become almost a matter of course for us after 1 1/2 years of the pandemic, namely not shaking hands, was an irritating experience in March 2020. An age-old ritual was suddenly unwanted. Some patients were happy about this, because they no longer had to be ashamed of their sweaty hand, which showed how stressed they were. Others, on the contrary, missed this gesture or continued to involuntarily stretch out their hand for the greeting for a long time. We then reminded each other to avoid doing so for mutual protection. The disinfection of, say, door handles or chair arms was also a new behavior to be practiced, drawing attention to the invisible threat at the beginning or end of the session. With these precautionary measures, one suspected the virus very concretely in the room, which is why it was unavoidable to also deal with it in terms of content. Which person could infect me? Does a patient or therapist constitute a danger? Which object is contaminated with viruses? Who or what should I stay away from? And is it therefore better to avoid a physical meeting altogether and see each other digitally instead?

Such questions and the careful behavior derived from them happened and still happen with the intention of keeping the risk of infection as low as possible. But a minimal risk remains; despite all our efforts to be cautious, we cannot completely control the risk of infection. With this remaining risk, fear of infecting another person emerged in some patients. Many felt a responsibility to protect others from this disease. In concrete terms, this meant: Can I

DOI: 10.4324/9781003266402-13

visit my grandmother even though I cannot be 100 percent sure that I will not infect her? Can I continue to attend school or university even though my father is a high-risk patient and an infection would be very dangerous for him? These questions were accompanied by fear and guilt, which were new in this form. Before the pandemic, when we met people with influenza – an infection that is also not entirely harmless and that kills a great many people every year – we usually kept a certain physical distance, but hardly ever consciously thought about whether we could infect someone. We didn't feel guilty if, as virus carriers, we had infected other people. That has changed since the pandemic. This was very stressful for some people because they could never forgive themselves if they infected a beloved person. Because of this concern, many have minimized physical contact to what is absolutely necessary, switching to video calls, privately and in therapy.

With video sessions in psychotherapy, the head became the center of attention, because only the head was visible, no longer the whole person. This fits symbolically with the age of neuroscience with its fascination and focus on the brain. In the video sessions, smell, major parts of gestures, the physical presence and atmosphere in the room were missing. Even the voice is altered. It is hard to describe and capture what a joint presence in a room does or triggers, but that it does something to us, that is for sure. But in the virtual world, not only were familiar things lost, but new experiences were gained. Thus, for the first time, one was given a glimpse into the homes of patients, for the first time one could or had to intrude into their privacy, as long as the patient did not choose an artificial screen background. The psychotherapeutic vessel was no longer a room chosen and provided by the therapist, in which one would sit together. Now the therapeutic space was separated into two locations. In the virtual session, one was physically distanced, but somehow also closer than before due to the insight into private rooms, and this involuntarily triggered fantasies. Especially since the patients themselves now had to choose their room for the therapeutic session – more or less consciously or because of the spatial possibilities. Some sat in the kitchen, others in the bedroom, on their bed, sometimes the pet was present, or a person could be seen walking by in the background. These very concrete phenomena have also a symbolic meaning, they are a challenge for the therapeutic process because, among other things, it is a question of whether this should be addressed and in what way. Among other things, there was the question of whether the patient could sufficiently protect the therapeutic conversation or the therapeutic process and himself or herself under the given domestic circumstances. Interestingly, some patients experienced the physical separation as an opportunity to talk about shameful or other stressful topics for the first time. They experienced themselves as more courageous, more free. So there are many facets of the two-place situation. One of them is that in a video session neither therapist nor patient had to wear a mask and thus each other's emotions remained visible. In contrast, in the face-to-face encounter, mask-wearing was required for many months. The face and its facial expressions were no longer perceptible, and patients who had to wear a mask in the initial contact I later did not recognize at all without a mask; it took some time until I could become familiar with their face. The patients had a similar experience. Unconsciously, we had images about the respective concealed face and had to correct them when we saw it for the first time in its entirety.

In psychotherapy, it also became clear that in the first months of the pandemic, the soul was almost a non-issue in public discourse – attention and worldview were materialistic. Fear of physical infection and physical death took center stage. There was hardly any discussion in the media about the importance of the psyche in terms of the infectious disease in the sense of psychosomatic interrelationships. However, panic as well as months of stress or severe worries have an impact on the human immune system and the predisposition to infection. This was shown, among other things, in a study in which 420 healthy women and men aged 18–54 were infected with cold viruses. The more stressed the subjects were at the beginning of the study and the less socially integrated they were, the higher the probability of catching a cold and the more pronounced were the clinical and immunological signs of a cold. Only one month of prolonged, stressful conditions doubled the likelihood of contracting the illness (Schubert 2015, p. 75). Based on these and other findings of psychoneuroimmunology – a research on the interaction between the immune system and the psyche – physician and psychotherapist Christian Schubert is convinced that increasing chronic stress, economic crises and global panic reactions in Western industrialized nations are partly responsible for the pandemic spread of infectious diseases.

Fear of a potentially fatal viral disease, as well as watching the horrific images of ventilated Covid-19 patients, weakens our immune system and has been shown to increase vulnerability to viral infection. In concrete terms, this means that it is not only the quantity of viruses to which we are exposed that determines our likelihood of falling ill and the severity of the course of the disease, but our mental state, including the quality of our relationships. This could explain why so many nurses, geriatric caregivers, physicians, and others working in so-called system-relevant professions have fallen ill with Covid-19. They were exposed to enormous physical stress (long working hours, protective clothing, etc.) and mental stress (anxiety, feeling overwhelmed, having to witness how terrible the disease is, etc.). However, trusting relationships, the feeling of being protected and the associated reduction of stress are important in the healing process of physical illnesses. Von Franz (1997, p. 25) reports that when a surgeon in the 1960s began to have a conversation with his patients the night before each surgery, the mortality rate of his operations dropped significantly. A recent scientific study was able to show the immunological phenomena of this phenomenon: the saliva samples of patients and therapists after a therapeutic session usually had less stress hormones and more immune activating substances (Schubert & Amberger 2019, p. 217).

These few examples show that we have a broad and well-founded knowledge regarding psychosomatics, but in view of the real danger of death caused by the pandemic, much has been forgotten or suppressed.

Even the World Health Organization (WHO) has now recognized that we have paid too little attention to fundamental mental needs, even if they have a significant impact on physical health. In March 2021, it sounded the alarm about the danger of restrictive pandemic rules for newborns and premature babies. Indeed, it has been proven for at least 30 years that premature or underweight newborns who are allowed to snuggle and cuddle on their mother's or father's bare chest for several hours a day reduce their risk of death by about 40 percent. The loving skin contact is extremely important emotionally and physically. Physical health is not possible without the soul and emotional safety.

Now, however, this meaningful behavior has been banned in the delivery departments of many countries during the pandemic – for reasons of infection control. However, according to the WHO, the risk of death for these newborns due to the ban on cuddling is at least 65 times higher than the risk of getting a deadly corona infection through contact.[1] Not only newborns, but also children, adolescents and young adults have been "forgotten" to some extent in the pandemic. For example, when they were expected to learn virtually, without considering that learning happens in relationships, in exchange, in dialogue and with each other. Children are not just hard disks that can be fed with data. Children, adolescents and young adults have made many sacrifices during the pandemic, often willingly, to protect their parents and grandparents. After a year and a half of the pandemic, their suffering becomes visible: many struggle with depressive symptoms, hopelessness and suicidal phantasies. The physical distance required by the pandemic not only eliminated the ritual of shaking hands in the Western world, other rituals were also banned or placed under very restrictive conditions: Baptismal celebrations, wedding parties, birthday parties, saying goodbye to a dying person in the hospital, or funerals. All this became quite different, and quite suddenly. Now, philosopher Martin Hartmann assumes that we all – without even pondering about it – trust in the permanence of this world and simply assume that tomorrow everything will not be different from today (2020, p. 48). The lockdown showed that this is not the case. This has disturbed many people and caused considerable mental suffering. For example, a 20-year-old patient wept bitterly because he was not allowed to attend the funeral of his beloved grandfather. He doubted the correctness of this restriction. He saw no sense in it. An 85-year-old patient who lived alone felt the same way. She was not willing to sacrifice everything to minimize the risk of infection. She did not want to put her physical health first over her quality of life. Despite the ban of contact, she had invited her three closest friends because they felt a deep need to celebrate her birthday and thus life together, especially in these difficult times. They deliberately took this risk because they did not know if they would still be alive a year later. Each could die before the next birthday, and not just from Covid-19 but from any illness. To them, the focus of the public debate on Covid-19 patients seemed inappropriate. Incidentally, the four women were denounced by a neighbor and punished with a high financial fine. The denunciation shook the four friends more than the fine.

The threat of death has aroused in many people the need for orientation and understanding: people want to know where the virus comes from, who or what is responsible for the pandemic. A look at the medieval plague epidemics makes it clear that there have always been collectively accepted hypotheses about the causes of disease. At that time, people blamed God, were convinced that God punished sinful people. God had the power to make people suffer terribly. Few people in the Western world would accept such an explanation today. It is no longer a collectively accepted idea since the Age of Enlightenment. Now, science is primarily responsible for explaining the world. According to this, the pandemic is first of all a natural phenomenon, triggered by a transmission of pathogen germs from the animal kingdom to humans. This description does not satisfy everyone. Why? It is hard for some to bear that a pandemic, like other diseases, can just happen, that it is simply part of nature. For many, this is not enough; they have a psychological need for a narrative that makes sense, a narrative in which there are reasons, responsible parties, and guilty parties. Whereas in the medieval religious worldview such power was assumed to reside only with God, in the current secular worldview it has recently become imaginable that individual people like Bill Gates have the power to steer the destiny of the world. What used to be in God's hands is now at the disposal of people. This is indeed the case in some areas of life; mythologically speaking, promethic theft is not a one-time act, but an ongoing process. Mankind is stealing more and more from the gods, gaining more and more opportunities to intervene in natural processes.

Among other things, the pandemic makes visible a crisis of trust and a spiritual crisis: Some people can no longer trust scientists or experts – even if the facts are correct. Perhaps this is also because the experts, as specialists, no longer take into account the reality of life of the average person. However, it has been proven that the willingness to trust is based less on data and facts than on moods and atmosphere – thus on emotions and emotional needs. And if people no longer feel that they are being taken seriously and valued, it is difficult for them to trust the theory of an expert.

World explanations provide orientation, support and security, and that is very precious. World explanations stabilize our mental balance, they are indispensable, no one can live without a world explanation. And if an expert cannot convince us, we involuntarily and usually unconsciously look for other theories that seem plausible to us. Then we experience ourselves sustained. For philosopher Markus Gabriel, the scientific worldview is one religion among others. In his opinion, the concept of religion has become too close to the concept of superstition (2015, p. 158). These provocative theses allow to stay in dialogue with followers of so-called conspiracy theories, instead of rejecting them in a generalized way. On the one hand, because no world view or world explanation is only rational, but is based on mostly unconscious and unquestioned basic assumptions, on the other hand, because the need for stability connects us across all different world explanations. And if we look into history, we still do not know which worldview comes closest to reality. We do not know exactly why we favor a particular world view; it is not chosen by the ego, but by the unconscious. Of course, it is not a matter of accepting conspiracy fantasies, but of being able to take up and question fears lying behind them, in order to enable a critical and constructive dialogue also in the psychotherapeutic practice. At best, this can help to maintain the relationship of trust between patient and therapist.

Note

1 www.geo.de/wissen/gesundheit/weniger-kuscheln-wegen-corona–who-sieht-fruehchen-in-gefahr–30436012.html

References

Gabriel, M. (2015). *Why the World Does Not Exist*. Polity Press.

Hartmann, M. (2020). *Vertrauen. Die Unsichtbare Macht*. Frankfurt: S. Fischer,

Schubert, C. (Ed.) (2015). *Psychoneuroimmunologie und Psychotherapie*, 2nd edn. Stuttgart: Schattauer.

Schubert, C., & Amberger, M. (2019). *Was Uns Krank Macht, Was Uns Heilt. Aufbruch in Eine Neue Medizin. Das Zusammenspiel von Körper, Geist und Seele Besser Verstehen*, 6th edn. Munderfing: Fischer & Gann.

Von Franz, M. (1997). *Archetypal Patterns in Fairy Tales Studies in Jungian Psychology by Jungian Analysts*. Inner City Books.

Chapter 5

Poetry as a Personalized Lockdown Therapy

Roula-Maria Dib

This chapter explores the soothing effects and boundary-breaking role of poetry during the recent times of global crisis. Since the beginning of the pandemic, more and more poets from around the world have been sharing their work, experiences, and ideas with each other on creative online platforms. By interviewing several well-established poets who have had their poems featured in and read during virtual poetry events of the literary and arts journal Indelible, this work will look at the therapeutic side of poetry, which arose during the unfolding of a literary community. It was a healing ritual for many; this chapter seeks to highlight this aspect, shedding light on some of the poets and on their poetry, which helped themselves and others to cope with the pandemic. The results of the interviews came to show how writing poetry became a healing practice, one that offers an outlet for thoughts and feelings to be explored, as well as expressed.

While I am in no position to prescribe poetry as a therapy, I can confidently say that I have been witness to its soothing effects and boundary-breaking during this unprecedented global crisis of the Covid-19 pandemic. People need distractions, hope, diversions, reflection, contemplation, positivity, and most of all, they need to articulate and share the expressions of the fear, confusion, hope, and effort they are going through. As founding editor of literary and arts journal *Indelible*, I have observed the unique therapeutic power of poetry. I discovered that although I thought I had known about poetry's healing effects, I actually hadn't – until I was able to directly experience the unfolding of a community whose members were able to support each other through the beauty of embodying thoughts and feelings into words. Before Covid-19, when *Indelible* was in its first year, there were no virtual events that helped bring contributors together. Then, a few months into a pandemic-stricken world, came the idea of getting to know the faces and voices behind the words and images featured in the journal. And that was only the beginning of *Indelible Evenings*, an online series of poetry events in which poets from around the world get to share their craft and ideas with other like-minded people. And yes, for the lack of a more accurate term, I

DOI: 10.4324/9781003266402-14

would say it was "therapeutic" for many; after the first virtual event in June 2020, I started receiving emails from many people who attended and/or contributed to the session, asking me to fix regular poetry meetups. And so it happened; one year after the launch of *Indelible Evenings*, I decided to interview some of the contributing poets and ask them about how poetry has helped them cope with the pandemic.

Apparently, the exponential increase in the number of poetry submissions showed that people seemed to be writing more poetry. Through some *Indelible* interviews, I learned that writing poetry became a therapeutic practice for many of the poets; it became a routine that offers an outlet for thoughts and feelings to be explored, as well as expressed. For many, such as the poet Ralph Earle, poetry as a practice has helped in understanding the new feelings brought on by the pandemic: "The act of writing poetry helps me make sense of my experience as a human being, more so during times of stress, and especially during the pandemic." Sharing poetry with others, however, whether through publication or via live Zoom readings, offers the opportunity to connect, and the chance for comfort and reassurance at a time when everyone became incredibly isolated almost overnight. According to poet Debra Kaufman,

> First the shock of it, and then recognizing that this was an unprecedented phenomena, I decided to be more intentionally present.... Reading and writing poetry connected me to something larger than me, and reminded me of the beauty of the souls of others.
>
> (Dib et al., 2021)

While the outer world is something people needed to shut themselves away from because of its danger and inaccessibility, poets tend to further connect with their inner worlds during lockdown. Poet Yahia Lababidi shared his experience by saying "yes, reading and writing poetry is typically how I self-medicate – reducing anxiety, spreading me – and this has been doubly important during dread of pandemic which has felt like a period of enforced mass meditation and intangible *momento mori* …," which resonates with Susan Rowland's notion that "Covid is a kind of alchemy, a transformation of the collective in us in a dark nigredo state where we are forced to get to the prima materia, the core of our existence, the essence of ourselves" (Carpani, 2020). This "enforced mass meditation" or the enforcement of getting "into the prima materia" is actually the poetry during a time of creative darkness – a *katabasis*, or descent into the underworld, after which creativity and transformation take place. Some poets, like Florence Nash, worked through creative chaos and tried to pin it down by writing more structured forms of poetry: "this year has prompted a number of pandemic-related poems (which all seem to arrive in sonnet form – maybe indicative of a need for structure in a disordered world?)" (Dib et al., 2021). Out of chaos emerges beauty, as well as structure, and to return to Susan Rowland's comment that covid is an alchemy, we find that resonating in many poets who were able to materialize their psychic images through the language of poetry, creating both beauty and healing. Christine Murray, poet and editor of *Poethead*, acknowledges this:

> While we need history books, we also need human witness and art during times of turbulence and global cataclysm. Poetry teaches us that the human voice in all of its vulnerability and in the face of trauma can and will create beauty.
>
> (Dib et al., 2021)

Furthermore, poet Bernard Pearson states that the pandemic had a fruitful impact on his writing: "the disquiet in the world has been the backdrop to creativity" (Dib et al., 2021). And "social" virtual poetry events have given people the chance to connect with the inner worlds of each other through sharing articulations of the same experience. This delivers a soothing self-therapy, an escape during a claustrophobic time of lockdown, when it feels like the walls of the world are closing in. Pearson further relates to this by adding:

> I felt a genuine connection across culture, life experience, and creative ability. I have never felt anything quite like it before, despite these occasions being virtual, they had a profound effect on me in a way that other 'in the flesh' networking however enjoyable had not. My horizons had been widened and my understanding of what writing really is about expanded.
>
> (Dib et al., 2021)

Moreover, the willingness of the wider poetry community to meet and share the reality of our unreal experiences together in an online open mic event solidifies the notion that people needed poetry as much as they needed to be joined together by poetic experience. To speak about the global anxiety through the connective language of symbols and metaphors also confirms that – at least according to what the poets believe – poetry itself has a therapeutic effect, and meeting together on the poetry plane in real time, from different time zones, represents the shared global experience that we were in; we all wanted to express ideas we wished we could speak about in regular language. Hence the emergence of *Indelible Evenings*, an almost-weekly digital series of poetry readings, conversations with guest poets, and discussions of creative writings. And people always showed up – they were there for the poetry and the energy it released and invoked in them. Poet/artist/depth psychologist Carole Mora claims:

> The surreal challenges of the recent year or so have thankfully been tempered by opportunities to also listen to readings of poetry by others, bringing a refreshing sense of reorientation, tethering, and needed connection to sensibilities and qualities of being that really matter. These

gatherings have provided an additional sense of mooring during these stormy, pandemic times.

(Dib et al., 2021)

These newly emerging feelings toward an unprecedented uncertainty needed to be articulated and understood through a medium that does it justice; consequently, "Inchoate feelings, that are cognitively unspecified, require metaphors" (Modell, 1997). With so much reflective time spent alone or in isolation in a seemingly silent world, the language of poetry (and thus, heightened use of metaphors) has helped many people to connect with the world in trying to understand it. According to literary scholar and poet Susan Porterfield:

> In a time of covid and social distancing, when so much has not happened or has stopped happening, for me, writing poetry, which is itself an isolating, lonely activity, has strangely connected me more to the closed-down world. 'It survives,' and by doing so, helps me (us, the world?) to survive. It truly is 'a mouth,' a way to interact in a still, more muted world.

(Dib et al., 2021)

But it was not only about expressions made in solitude – it was about overcoming loneliness by sharing these expressions and experiences of solitude together. There was a need not only for metaphors, but for sharing this metaphoric process of *translating experience* with others, for making this connection in "socially" sharing these experiences on the affective and imaginal levels. People needed reassurance that they were not alone in this frightening new situation. They needed to share ideas, images, and metaphors, which is really an exchanging of lenses that are actually looking at one and the same problem. This type of "breaking bread" by sharing a global ordeal through poetry has a profoundly comforting effect, breaking the boundaries of distance through creative connectivity. Poet Carly Brown reflects on this notion:

> Poetry and specifically poetry events definitely have helped me cope with the pandemic. At several events, such as *Indelible* readings, I've seen fellow poets share their work, or even just their thoughts and musings, on the pandemic itself. Hearing this has on many occasions reminded me that I'm not alone in what I'm feeling: confused, uncertain, lonely etc. It's really contributed to my sense of connectivity with other writers and other people generally, and that is a great help at a time of isolation.

(Dib et al., 2021)

Similarly, editor of *The Ekphrastic Review*, poet/artist Lorette C. Luzajic comments:

The pandemic was unique as an emergency because it was truly universal, and that truth contributed to my thoughts and my writing. Being able to connect with others through poetry readings or similar Zoom events has been a really important way to bond with other writers and to grow as a writer in a frightening circumstance.

(Dib et al., 2021)

And of course, it was not only the poets themselves who attended these events – so many people sought poetry for solace, whether they practice writing it professionally or not; for it is not a requirement to be a poet or to cognitively comprehend the literal meanings of poems (if there is such a thing) in order to enjoy its comforting effects. Many listeners, poets or not, take solace from the lyricality of verses, regardless of their literal meanings. Through such events, poetry has proven itself to be an embodied experience, requiring the human voice, eyes, and outpour of emotion – it is meant to be felt, not understood, by the listeners.

It is worth remembering that *The Red Book*, which Jung wrote during his period of personal crisis between 1913–1915, can be viewed as an inspiring paradigm displaying the healing metaphorical processes of the psyche. Comparably, poets nowadays are utilizing the imaginal domain to articulate and cope with an unprecedented experience. This deepened exploration of the inner world during times of global crisis renders the poet more expressive and comprehensive of the collective unconscious, since poets

> voice rather more clearly and resoundingly what all know [...] The mass does not understand it although unconsciously living what it expresses; not because the poet proclaims it, but because its life issues from the collective unconscious into which he has peered.

(Jung 2009, p. 191)

Images emanate from the unconscious and, through active imagination, materialize into the figurative language of poetry. And metaphors are the translation, articulation, and transformation of emotions and archetypal content into the domain of language. This centrality of metaphor is also asserted by Jung:

> An archetypal content expresses itself in metaphors as such a content should speak of the sun and identify it with the lion, the king, the hoard of gold guarded by the dragon or the power that makes for the life and health of man; it is neither the one thing nor the other, but the unknown third thing that finds more or less adequate expression in all of these similes. Even the best attempts at explanation are only more or less successful translation in the other metaphorical language.

(Jung 2014a, I, par. 267)

In his *Red Book*, Jung paradoxically aligns reason with what he calls "unreason": "We recognized that the world comprises reason and unreason; and we also understood that our way needs not only reason but also unreason" (Jung 2009, p. 404). Jung zeroes in on *a-rationality,* or "the greater part of the world [that] eludes our understanding ... part of the incomprehensible, however, is only presently incomprehensible and might already concur with reason tomorrow" (Jung 2009, p. 404). In a time when reason and confirmed truths are still in a trial phase behind the obscurity of uncertainty and fear, the unreason of poetry may yield a few answers. The active imagination involved in the conversations poets may have with themselves (or with the world around them) offers this therapeutic effect – perhaps in the same way that the *Red Book* had helped Jung cope with his crisis by resorting to the imaginal. I was particularly struck by the reflection of poet Steve Pottinger, who, without using the term "active imagination," expresses just that in his description of the role poetry had played for him during the pandemic:

> Primarily, I'd say poetry helped me in that it allowed me to articulate my response to what was happening, and – as always – what I wrote often came as a surprise, an expression of a truth or an attitude that I'd not have been able to come to in everyday conversation. This was, and still remains, invaluable. I think poetry does that a lot. It's one of the things I love about it – it's like a conversation with myself in which I'm always learning.
>
> (Dib et al., 2021)

It is a time of transformation, to be broadcasted to the world through poetry, which in itself is a transforming act. However, the way poetry is being handled and shared nowadays has also undergone a major change, especially with the arrival of virtual poetry get-togethers, which I believe are here to stay. This is because the need for poetry, the need for answers, and the need to reach out to one another have all made us perceive technology through a new light. As Susan Rowland had stated: "people are starting to individuate their technology ... our relationship to it is being forced to change (so we can be with each other)" (Carpani, 2020). And this of course rings truth under the umbrella of poetry and the pandemic, resonating with poet Hedy Habra's reflection:

> It has been extremely rewarding to make new friends and get to know a diversity of voices through these virtual gatherings that offered a network of support and solidarity. I think that the poetry we created during the pandemic enabled us to transcend the quotidian by living in alternate worlds and redefine ourselves. It is as though poetry allowed us to see ourselves reflected in these collected, disparate fragments as one would in an ever-expanding stained glass, creating a harmonious whole, encompassing time and space.
>
> (Dib et al., 2021)

It is indeed a transcendence beyond the ordinary and quotidian; a transformation and redefinition of ourselves through sharing our own inner worlds with the inner worlds of others (made possible through technology). It is what Rowland may see as a "re-membering of Dionysus" through the collection of "disparate fragments" that Habra mentions, in order to create a new, harmonious whole. It is alchemy.

References

Carpani, S. (2020) Covid-19 and the suspension of certainties: Susan Rowland in conversation with Stefano Carpani. Online at: www.youtube.com/watch?v=7U89L_4aqUs (accessed 30 May 2021).

Dib, R. (2021) Poetry as food for the soul (various *Indelible* poets). *Indelible*. Online at: https://indeliblelit.com/2021/06/13/poetry-as-food-for-the-soul-various-indelible-poets/ (accessed 27 June 2021).

Jung, C. G. (2014a) *The Psychology of the Child Archetype*, ed. and trans. by Gerhard Adler and R.F.C. Hull. Princeton: Princeton University Press.

Jung, C. G. (2014b) The problem of types in poetry, in *The Collected Works of C.G. Jung*, vol. 6: *Psychological Types*, ed. and trans. by Gerhard Adler and R.F.C. Hull. Princeton: Princeton University Press.

Jung, C. G. (2009) *The Red Book: Liber Novus*, ed. by Sonu Shamdasani, 1st edn. London: Norton and Company.

Modell, A. (1997) The synergy of memory, affects, and metaphor. *The Journal of Analytical Psychology* 42: 105–117.

Chapter 6

Presence and Absence of the Body in Psychotherapy During Lockdown

Paolo Ferliga

This contribution focuses on the changes implied in distance therapy in relation to the role of the body which very important in what he calls the co-transference, the relationship between therapist and patient. During lockdown the encounter between patient and psychotherapist is no longer a meeting of two psyches/ bodies, but a meeting between two images, two partial, superficial representations of the body: the representations of the faces of the two protagonists, therapist and patient, on a monitor. From the very first moment the contact between the two bodies, in the author's habits mediated by a handshake, is dissolved, cutting away an important implicit aspect of the meeting for communication. In the same way, for a therapist the possibility of seeing a patient as a whole, observing his body movements and perceiving his smell, is lost. After describing the problems generated by this deprivation of sensory features of the encounter, the author shows the role that mindfulness and active imagination can play in fostering communication and exchange in the analytic couple.

The full lockdown imposed by Covid-19 in Italy for a period of more than two months, from 9 March to 18 May 2020, and the following months characterized by partial and differentiated restrictions in different regions of the country have radically changed our way of doing therapy.

From meeting in person – mine usually initiated by a handshake – we have moved on to the virtual meeting that begins with a click.

Everything changes from the outset.

Before and after the lockdown, on the other hand, the meetings with the patient took place at my practice, which is a few kilometers from my home. The sound of the bell announces the patient's arrival. I get up from the armchair and welcome them at the door, shaking their hand. This physical contact gives me important information from the very first meeting. The temperature of the hand, the intensity, duration and depth of the grip, say something about the patient and symbolically represent the first moment of the relationship that at this level we could define as *co-transference*, according to the terminology introduced by the Jungian analyst Kay Bradway (1991). During the course of the therapy it is then possible to notice that the way in

DOI: 10.4324/9781003266402-15

which the two hands meet and clasp, changes. If things go well, the squeeze tends to become longer and more intense: you feel that the communication has deepened. Even the expression of the face and the emotional quality of the gaze, captured from the first meeting on the threshold, change over time. Sometimes the facial features relax and, instead of a questioning look, a smile appears. If you pay attention to your body countertransference, you also feel a continuity between the facial features and the handshake.

The first meeting then continues in my room, where the patient sits opposite me. There the words take on a fundamental role for the meanings they convey, but also the tone of the voice and the posture of the body say something. Once seated, I can observe the position of the body and see if the patients let themself go on the chair or maintain a contracted position. At the end of our session I accompany the patient to the door and, in the corridor, I see them walking in front of me and I can observe the rhythm of their step. When I then go back to my room, something of them remains, their smell or perfume they had put on.

From the very beginning, therefore, the encounter between therapist and patient is mediated by the body and sensory perceptions. Attention to perceptions is important to grasp aspects of the transference relationship that anticipate words and sometimes they reveal what words don't say. As Merleau Ponty writes in *Phenomenology of perception*, we cannot in fact ignore the body in order to "understand" others and the world outside us: "Our own body is in the world as the heart is in the organism: it keeps the visible spectacle constantly alive, it breathes life into it and sustains it inwardly and with it forms a system" (1958, p. 235).

It is what Edmund Husserl calls, in his phenomenological research, the living body (*Leib*) understood as the perceptive organ of the subject who makes the experiences (1913).

During lockdown, but then also afterwards, to comply with the safety restrictions imposed by the pandemic, the first contact, mediated by the hands, disappeared as well as the possibility of observing the body in its entirety and perceiving its smell. Instead of the warm sound of the bell, the meeting begins with the more mechanical Skype or WhatsApp tone, and there is no physical contact between the analyst and the patient.

The encounter is no longer between two psychic-bodies, but between two images, two partial, superficial representations of the body: the representations on the monitor of the faces of the two protagonists, therapist and patient.

In fact, we usually only see the patient's face and shoulders when meeting via the Internet. We cannot thus observe the body in its entirety. We miss the movements of the hands, the way they sit, the position of the legs, the signs of the body that we usually notice in face-to-face sessions. I remember a young man who, for about a month, sat on the edge of an armchair, never relaxing and maintained a strained posture with his head sunk into his shoulders and tilted forward. He seemed to defend himself from the relationship with me and this was also clear from the few words he uttered during the session. At the beginning of the second month I was able to observe that his posture in the chair was changing little by little and that he was assuming an increasingly comfortable position. In parallel, the flow of words also became more fluid. In this case it seemed to me that his position changed not only in relation to my words, but also in relation to the position I assumed in the chair, which was decidedly more relaxed than his.

In remote sessions, on the other hand, the "living body" disappears, replaced by a partial image on a monitor. During the lockdown period, therefore, in search of contact with the patient, my attention was focused on the features of the face, on the patient's gaze and on the tone of their voice. In the absence of touch and smell, only sight and hearing come into play. The absence of the body therefore invites me to a new exercise. In addition to how words resonate in me, I try to "feel" what relationship there is between the patient's words, their image and the tone of their voice. It is an exercise that forces me to refine my attention, to focus on the patient's face and voice. In fact, the voice also plays an important role. Unfortunately, sometimes the sound is modified by the *medium*, by the personal computer, but if you have known the patient for a long time, it is not difficult to hear the different tones that their words take on, depending on their emotional state. The image of the face and the voice thus take on greater importance than they had in face-to-face sessions. In my personal experience I have noticed that this greater ability of attention has remained active in me even when we returned to face-to-face sessions.

Regarding the importance of the voice, I remember that in the past, on some occasions when a patient had moved away for work, I had continued the therapy by telephone. There was still no Internet and video calls were not possible. In those cases, only the voice kept us in touch and the attention turned to its tone, the speed with which the words were pronounced, the duration of the pauses, the alternation of sound and silence. For me, who use the face-to-face setting, that situation led me to imagine sessions with the couch, where the gazes of therapist and patient usually do not meet. Using the phone, I felt the lack of that encounter mediated by the gaze, but I must admit that the intensity of the emotional exchange did not diminish.

Then, when the patient returned to our city, we could meet again in person and the body contact reappeared with all its richness, but also with its ambivalence. Comparing face-to-face sessions and telephone sessions I had the impression of grasping some important differences, which can never be considered one-fits-all, but are always linked to the individual case, to the type of transference relationship with the patient. On the phone, for example, a greater distance is established between the two subjects of the therapy. This distance can favor the work of *reverie* and the use of *active imagination*. The imagination seems freer and the recounting of dreams, even perturbing ones, is less difficult for the patient. In the absence of the body, however, interpersonal communication risks losing the relationship with the experience of the limit, of which the body is the bearer, which is indispensable for the definition of the identity of the subject. Interpersonal communication can then move onto a level of idealization and projection, which makes an authentic understanding of the transference dynamics more difficult. The encounter in presence, on the other hand, if it sometimes makes the game of imaginative fantasy more difficult, allows a livelier contact, thanks to the presence of the body, with the Shadow. As we have already said, precisely sensory perceptions provide the coordinates in which words can take on a more authentic meaning. Only once Jung speaks of the body as a Shadow of the Ego,

> The body is a most doubtful friend because it produces things we do not like; there are too many things about the body, which cannot be mentioned. The body is very often the personification of this shadow of the ego. Sometimes it forms the skeleton in the cupboard, and everybody naturally wants to get rid of such a thing.
>
> (Jung 1976, 18, par. 40)

After my therapeutic experience during the lockdown, I think this is an intuition to be valued.

But let's go back to the virtual meeting that is established at a distance thanks to Internet technologies. In truth, the encounter is not between two images, that of the other that each of the two sees on their respective screens, but between four images. In fact, not only does the image of the other appear on the screen, but also one's own image on a smaller scale. This presence, the image of my face next to that of the patient, disturbed me for a certain period. I noticed that my gaze sometimes left the patient's face to turn to mine, perhaps prompted by an unconscious narcissistic movement.

I remember once that because of a particular screen quality, my nose appeared red, although it really wasn't so. I was in the same situation as the protagonist of Pirandello's novel, *Uno, nessuno, centomila*, when he is caught by his wife looking at his nose in the mirror. When she points out that it is leaning to the right, he feels anger and irritation at the discovery of a physical defect, and for a while he can think of nothing else. In that situation I began to think that the patient might believe that I had been drinking and to fear that I was drunk. It took me a few minutes to abandon the idea that had formed in my mind, starting from the image sent back to me from the screen. On other occasions I have observed that my hair was dishevelled or that the collar of my shirt was out of place. I would have liked to eliminate that image which, as a double of my ego, replaced my body and disturbed me, distracting me from the relationship with the other. I then discovered that in group meetings it is indeed possible to hide one's image and I tried to do it. In seeing my image disappear, however, I felt a slight sense of anguish, as if that image were the last potential contact with my body. I couldn't resist for long and put it back on the monitor. It seemed to me that in this situation the images take on an autonomous life that our ego struggles to govern.

I also wondered how much the patient can be disturbed by the appearance of the image of their double on the screen. Sometimes I seemed to catch moments of distraction in them too, signalled by a look that moves to the side or by some gestures: straightening their back, fixing their blouse, arranging their hair.

My impression is therefore that the duplication of the image favors the emergence of some narcissistic traits, both in the therapist and in the patient, because it places both of them in a situation similar to when we look at ourselves in a mirror.

In fact, the characteristics of my image that appear on the monitor are the same as those I capture when I look at myself in the mirror. If I move my left hand, for example, on the monitor I see moving what appears to me as the right hand. This situation reminds me of Jacques Lacan's famous definition of the "mirror stage," according to which the child recognizes the image in the mirror as their own at the age of six months. This is a particular situation, functional to the identification of the ego, before their relationship with the other. On the other hand, when we look in the mirror as adults we could say that the mirror urges us to turn our attention to ourselves, in a sort of enjoyment similar to that experienced as children.... If you are enchanted by the mirror, however, you risk remaining prisoner of a narcissistic dimension which distracts the ego from the relationship with the other. It seems to me that in the case of remote communication, this process is favored precisely by the absence of the body which always remains off the screen. The comparison between the images takes place in a sort of "non-place," as Marc Augé would say, devoid of identity and relationship, a virtual space, forbidden to the body.

Faced with the annoying presence of my image on the screen and observing some of my patients' behavior, I wondered how I could put the body back into the equation, even in the situation of remote therapy.

I learnt to listen to my body and feel what it was communicating in countertransference during my years of training with Martin Kalff, whose method is outlined in the book *Old and New Horizons of Sandplay Therapy: Mindfulness and Neural Integration* (Routledge 2021). The practice of mindfulness learnt from him has been of great help. During remote therapy, I found that if I brought my attention to bodily perceptions through breathing, the disturbing power of my double image on the monitor diminished, and I could better concentrate while listening to the patient.

I therefore also suggested to patients, in some cases, to start the session with a few minutes of meditation, closing their eyes and bringing their attention to the body through the breath. I have been able to observe that when the patient manifests fatigue and difficulty in attention, a few minutes of mindfulness under the guidance of the therapist can help them.

I also lived this experience in some supervision groups on dreams and active imagination, which I lead with some Italian colleagues. Our meetings usually take place at the end of a working day, in the evening after dinner. We all feel tired and sometimes find it hard to keep our attention alive. Moreover, in front of the monitor fatigue and sleep increase. In these cases I have found that a moment of mindfulness, at the beginning of the meeting, helps to leave the worries of the day behind, helps to relax and allows you to enter into a more attentive and open relationship with the other members of the group and with the images that are presented in the meeting.

To conclude my critical observations on distance therapy, focused on the problems generated by the absence of the body in the relationship, I would like to point out two positive elements. First of all, thanks to the Internet, I was able to continue to see and support patients who would have been severely damaged by a sudden interruption of the therapy. As for the method of analytic psychotherapy, precisely the absence of the body has taught me to recognize its value even more, and to pay more attention to the symbolic value that sensory perceptions assume in the transference relationship between therapist and patient.

We have gone through a difficult period, which does not appear fully concluded yet, but, in this period, we must admit that also due to the Internet we have been able to exploit the potential of images coming from the unconscious; we have also learnt to distinguish between *virtual images*, those coming from the monitor, and *real images*, those of our dreams and imagination, which nourish our soul.

References

Bradway, K. (1991). Transference and countertransference in Sandplay Therapy. *Journal for Sandplay Therapy* 1 (1): 25–43.

Husserl, E. (1952 [1913]). *Ideen zu einer reinen Phänomenologie und phänomenologischen Philosophie Zweites Buch: Phänomenologische Untersuchungen zur Konstitution*. The Hague: Martinus Nijhoff.

Jung, C. G. (1976 [1935]). The Tavistock Lectures. On the theory and practice of analytical psychology, in *Collected Works*, vol. 20. New York: Princeton University Press.

Merleau-Ponty, M. (2005 [1945]). *Phenomenologie of Perception*, translated by Colin Smith. London and New York: Routledge.

Chapter 7

What Does the Virus Do to the Analytic Container?

Thoughts on the Frame in Times of Pandemic

Daniela Eulert-Fuchs

Taking the unexpected and sudden termination of an analysis by a patient as a starting point, the author asks what impact the pandemic had on the analytic space and, in particular, on patients with early relational trauma.

The author speculates that the re-inscription of early experiences the therapy aims for not only happens at a verbal level, but also implicitly at a non-verbal level. Her hypothesis is that the formation of new relational representations demands, at certain – vulnerable – points in analysis, sensory perception and presence. She suspects telecommunication does not allow for this in the same way as traditional in presence setting. She also questions whether the analyst's analytic ability may have been reduced due to her unconscious fear of the virus and reflects on the possible impact of this factor on the analytic process.

She questions herself on the theme of the analytic space and feels that, in particular in times of the pandemic, it is important to create a symbolic "vas" that can stand fear and destruction, creating the container that helps to allow the rhythm and the melody of a therapy to develop, that is unique and characteristic of each analytic pair.

For one and a half years now, we have collectively experienced a time of serious threat with unclear outcomes.

Also, as a society, we are at risk of regressing to earlier mechanisms of coping, and of creating myths in order to banish our fears. But any crisis also creates potentials. After all, analytical psychology and psychoanalysis have always moved with the context of their time. And we may surely assume that they will not remain the same when this pandemic finally comes to an end.

One key fact in this is the switch to digital media. Up until recently the subject of controversial discussions (cf. Braun, 2013; Roesler, 2017; Lemma & Caparrotta, 2014; Russel, G. I., 2015; Ehrlich, 2019), they were widely used due to Covid.

Many of our colleagues have had positive experiences with "tele-analysis" (Roesler, 2017), and in some cases, the medium led to an intensification of the process (cf. Sedlacek, 2021, p. 435; Merchant, 2016, p. 321–322; Roesler, 2017, p. 373).

DOI: 10.4324/9781003266402-16

I myself was already used to using video calls as well as the telephone.

Like others (cf. Merchant, 2016, p. 321–322; Zalusky, 1998), I had learned that we can use counter-transference on the virtual level, and that transference can be interpreted, which allows us to continue the analytical process in a satisfactory manner.

Now I would like to reflect upon a female patient for whom this transition to telecommunication did not work out so seamlessly. I experienced a termination that caused me much concern. Therefore, this is a painful reflection, an attempt to consider many open questions and my own personal dismay, hoping to understand more and in more depth.

I would like to take you on this inner journey, and maybe, in the end, we will be able to justify Jung who said that we can only learn from failures (Jung, 1929/1966, p. 64, §73).

What Changed with Covid?

One obvious change concerns the frame: due to legal provisions, we had to switch to digital media in our analytical practice at short notice several times.

Normally, we act on the assumption that the frame means a certain safety for the analytical pair, that it structures and safeguards our work (cf. Will, 2017).

"One must observe the proper rites," the fox says to the little prince (Saint-Exupéry, 2010/1946, p. 59).

Safety and stability are as important for the analytical process as is the ability to endure not-knowing, the negative capability (cf. Bion, 1970/2004).

Structure is important on the intra-psychic level, for one's relation to the unconscious, as well as interpersonally, for the development of the analytic relation.

So the fox says to the little prince: "If, for example, you come at four o'clock in the afternoon, then at three o'clock I shall begin to be happy." (Saint-Exupéry, 2010/1946, p. 59).

Only by experiencing dependability we can trustingly enter into the venture of needing others and allowing them to become significant for us.

With Vio, my young analysand, I had already travelled a long – and sometimes challenging – path along this route.

Vio had been referred to me as a young girl in a serious, life-threatening crisis. In this contribution, I cannot go into the details of Vio's traumatic past. They are irrelevant for my meditations anyway.

Vio caused me concern and much thought.

But soon after we had begun our work, she stopped self-harming, or taking risks with drug abuse and many other things, and went back to school.

I asked myself why Vio lost her symptoms so soon but remained unable to think about them for a long time.

We had worked for five years with great regularity twice weekly sitting down.

The initial speechlessness only changed slowly.

But in the meantime, Vio was able to allow painful memories to reach her consciousness and to think about them with me.

The telephone had tided us over the first lockdown; after that, we worked wearing masks with the windows open. Then came the second lockdown, and after the Christmas break there was only a curt cancellation, and after this, nothing.

What had happened?

Up until this moment, the analysis had taken an unremarkable and regular course. The analytic relation and frame seemed stable.

But they did not hold.

How is this to be understood?

It is to be expected that changes in the frame can be endured less the more intense the necessity to resort to the physical presence of the other for one's own regulation. This is all the more true the lower the ability to take the other inside or represent them.

Vio was able to emotionally invest in the analyst, she needed her and benefited from the analytic space.

But how much was rooted in her?

We surmise that the analytic relation, too, slowly leads to changes in the relational representation.

Marianne Leuzinger-Bohleber links this process to neuro-biological insights: She writes that neuronal strands stemming from the trauma will not be deleted in the context of therapy, but that alternative new paths can be established, with both initially existing side by side. New formations have to be inscribed in many repetitions, and only when these are more or less stable, both will be connected with each other (cf. Leuzinger-Bohleber, 2014, p. 945).

Early representations form in continued interaction with the primary objects. These are mainly mirroring processes which are well researched today (cf. Fonagy et al., 2004). They serve to develop an inner image of oneself and others, to anticipate the future, to tolerate reasonable absence, and to regulate affects.

Saint-Exupéry describes this process in a both vivid and poetic way: the fox says that the golden colour of the wheat fields will remind it of the golden hair of the little prince, even though wheat is of no use to it (Saint-Exupéry, 2010/1946, p. 58).

Here, the wheat fields not only stand for the interiorization of sensory experience, the inner image/ the representation of the little prince's hair, but also for the memory rooted in emotion, and therefore for feelings that can also be thought (Damasio, 2013, p. 121ff.).

But Vio's early life was severely unsettled.

She had not experienced an environment in which she could learn to interiorize experiences and use them as inner objects (Winnicott, 1971, p. 101ff.) It rather seemed as though she had to grapple with an inner emptiness that was the result of an unbridgeable absence and abandonment and the rejection of intrusive violence.

As traumata cut off parts of the emotional and symbolic development (cf. Kalsched, 1996, 2013, 2015), feelings and words are lacking, experience is dissociated.

Vio had been busy getting herself to safety and fending off the trauma; her psyche was unable to picture and represent the other, she needed to ward off the pain and the emptiness, and often also to numb it.

But Vio had made progress.

After the summer recess in 2019, she was first able to talk about the fact that she had missed analysis and the analyst. Until then, she was unable to discuss separations and painful feelings of abandonment.

Vio also said that she had remembered the sessions in the holidays, and that some things had helped her cope with difficult situations.

What does this mean?

Was Vio beginning to open herself to the possibility, and the risk, of the analytic relation?

Had the analytic work begun to leave traces in her?

The fox tells the little prince that the wheat fields would continue to remind it of the prince when they would no longer be together.

From this, we understand that the fox now carries the little prince inside itself, that he is rooted, or represented, in its interior. Now the fox can think of the little prince when seeing the wheat fields. It can miss him and remember beautiful moments, shared experiences and feelings.

The representation is thus also the basis for being able to say goodbye, for not denying a farewell, but mourning it and continuing to carry the other in one's interior and thus remaining connected to them.

We know that with Vio, this development – which had only just started – was preceded by a long process.

The analyst was needed in a concrete manner – as a present, regulating object and as a figure of transference that accepts and processes the transference. In this way, she allows the analysand to modify or form representations. Assumably this does not only happen verbally, but, as in early development, through implicitly and nonverbally interiorized experience.

This physical-sensory experience, or the "symbolisation primaire" (cf. Roussillon, 1999) needs the experience of being together in one place.

Ogden describes how the holding function of the setting worked for a female patient with massive, diffuse anxiety: regulating the room temperature created a shared sensory surface – "as if I had physically touched her and held her together" – and caused her to calm herself (Ogden, 1989, p. 34).

My hypothesis is that unconscious pre-verbal processes of harmonization are harder to communicate in the digital format.

The pre-symbolic-sensory dimension does not exist in the same form in virtual contact, as Ogden's example shows. But in my opinion, it is precisely what plays a significant role in the formation of representations.

Another, added handicap were the sudden and unforeseeable changes in the frame.

José Bleger (1967) describes the frame as the constantly operating background against which the analytic process unfolds. As long as the frame is stable, it remains unnoticed. If for whatever reason it is disrupted, Bleger says, it turns from a mere background into a figure, i.e. a process. Bleger writes that very early parts of the personality are deposited in the frame, remaining in it silently until there is a disruption. These parts of early relation experience survive, similar to Bion's psychotic part of the personality, in the form of an agglutinated nucleus. Bleger calls the fear linked to this a "fear of confusion."

I am asking myself how Vio experienced the abrupt change to the telephone in a time of such great inner change and exterior insecurity.

I think that Vio was in a vulnerable phase.

The change happened when the shock of early traumatic experience revived and, at the same time, the defence (against dependence and relation) was weaker. Winnicott calls this a phase of a high degree of dependence (Winnicott, 1965, p. 141), which is decisive for analysis.

Vio would have needed stability at this time, also regarding the space.

She had dared a tentative opening, but what she had hoped to gain, namely trust and safety, eluded her ... the changes in the frame and the loss of stability caused her to become distressed and therefore she "held off" and was thus in danger of falling back into chaos and former coping strategies.

I suspect the essential thing is the timing:

Not the mental structure per se is decisive in whether the process is successful, but at what time of the therapeutic process we had to transition to tele-presence.

But how does this have to do with Covid?

One important characteristic of the frame is that it delimits the reality outside of it from the one inside (cf. Milner, 1952). Parsons (2007, p. 1442) compares this with a theatre or a playground. Beyond the threshold, we find ourselves with different principles and expectations. In the analytic space, too, reality is suspended, thinking is free and at the same time sheltered, which allows access to deep unconscious levels.

But in the pandemic, the treatment room, too, becomes a space of potential danger. The threshold is unable to banish the virus. Both analysand and analyst are equally vulnerable. Did this affect the inner setting? The space in the analyst's psyche that should enable her to examine everything that is happening for its unconscious meaning, and to maintain an analytic attitude under any circumstance (cf. Parsons, 2007, p. 1445)? Was the inner frame of the analyst (cf. Parsons, 2007) affected by the "real threat"?

Already in 1915, Freud wrote surprisingly ageless words in his *Thoughts for the Times on War and Death*: "We showed an unmistakable tendency to put death to one side, to eliminate it from life." On the effect on life this attitude to death has, he says: "Life is impoverished, it loses in interest, where the highest stake in the game of living, life itself, may not be risked" (Freud, 1915, p. 290).

Could it be that a part of the analyst was – as Freud put it – "dead to life" in the analytical sense, i. e. to her feelings of counter-transference, fantasies and anxieties because she had shut out death? Had the fear remained so unconscious that the handling of the setting was submitted to the existing rules without examining them for their unconscious meaning? And even more – was the possibility to be unconsciously available constrained?

In particular when transference proceeds silently and negative feelings are not (yet) uttered, it is likely one needs particular concentration to "awaken" them in the therapeutic space: on the one hand the ability to sense unconscious negative feelings of transference, and to address them, but on the other hand also the stability and readiness to engage with these archaic affects in order to hold aggression and destructivity and work with them.

This needs psychic space.

All "thinking" on earlier experience happens with a mental apparatus that the infant did not have at its disposal.

An approximation of pre-linguistic-unconscious suffering is like enduring in the dark. Seeking out the traces demands dedication to the early pain, to impotence and hopelessness.

I am asking myself if the readiness of the analyst to open herself to these feelings and to bring them to her mind in body and soul was compromised by fear and insecurity.

But what does this do to (negative) transference?

It seems likely that Vio was unable to become conscious of her affects – in particular anger and shame – and to bring them into the conversation.

A vulnerable analyst cannot be burdened.

I remember many mother-child-pairs I have seen and accompanied. How good it felt when a mother was able to hold her baby with her gaze, her voice, her touch ... how it settled down. I also remember how babies reacted to this contact being interrupted: first by attempting to regain the mother, then with the attempt to regulate themselves and – when it collapsed – with despair and finally resignation.

Vio's form of resignation probably was her disappearance.

Two days ago:

I move to a different platform changing trains. As chance has it, I am on the way to Vio's hometown. My telephone rings, a flat, diffident voice at the other end.

"Excuse me. I wanted to make it by myself, but I need help, may I come again?"

I am in a hurry, but I stop in my tracks.

I know the voice. It is Vio's ...

Vio, who I had thought of so much in the past months.

Is there a connection?

I don't know, and it may remain unnamed and inexplicable.

But as "something that actually happened" (Hogenson, 2009, p. 184) it strengthens the hope that the inner work of the analyst, her reflections, are not in vain.

For Vio's withdrawal could also be perceived in a teleological-final way:

When Vio "slammed" the door shut, she "woke up" her analyst. She made her think, and revived her analytic function and the reverie. Has Vio reconquered this space in the analyst through her absence and thus expressed her primary, archetypal hope (Eulert-Fuchs, 2020) to be finally understood after all?

Maybe this text was also my attempt to maintain a connection to my analysand. Maybe it is not only the unconscious (cf. Jung, 1948, § 754), but also the unconscious communication and the scale of the analytic field that cannot be measured in meters (cf. Cwik, 2021).

This manner of understanding points towards an emergent, final dimension of the analytic process, a dimension that helps us – in spite of all our shortcomings – to find meaning.

In particular in times of the pandemic I feel it is important to create a symbolic "vas" that can stand fear and destruction. Not by sealing them off, but by attempting to reflect upon them. Our Jungian examination and theory formation is one way to deal with and contribute to this. I am asking myself whether the reflection of the analyst, her attempt at understanding and at maintaining contact to her inner world, creates the container that helps to allow the rhythm and the melody to develop that is unique and characteristic of each analytic pair. This trust would allow for a flexibility that could stand disruptions of the frame and simultaneously would allow to work on them. In this way, the analytic space can remain the instance that provides safety that – even in times of great threat – offers comfort and shelter.

References

Bleger, J. (1967). Psycho-analysis of the psycho-analytic frame. *International Journal of Psychoanalysis* 48: 511–519.

Bleger, J. (2013 [1967]). *Symbiosis and Ambiguity: A Psychoanalytic Study.* London: Routledge.

Bion, W. (1970/2004). *Attention and Interpretation.* Oxford: Rowman & Littlefield.

Bovensiepen, G. (2019). *Die Komplextheorie. Ihre Weiterentwicklungen und Anwendungen in der Psychotherapie.* Stuttgart: Kohlhammer.

Braun, C. (2013). Ist da jemand? Beziehungserfahrung, Individuation und Cyberspace. *Analytische Psychologie* 173 (3): 304–320.

Cwik, A. J. (2021). The technologically-mediated self: Reflections on the container and field of telecommunications. *Journal of Analytical Psychology* 66 (3): 411–428.

Damasio, A. (2013). *Selbst ist der Mensch. Körper, Geist und die Entstehung menschlichen Bewusstseins.* New York: Pantheon Books.

Ehrlich, L.T. (2019). Teleanalysis: Slippery slope or rich opportunity? *Journal of the American Psychoanalytic Association* 67: 249–279.

Eulert-Fuchs, D. E. (2020). The other between fear and desire. *Journal of Analytical Psychology* 65 (1): 153–170.

Fonagy, P., Gergely, G., Jurist, E. L., and Target, M. (2004). *Affect Regulation, Mentalization and the Development of the Self.* London: Karnac.

Freud, S. (1915). Thoughts for the Times on War and Death, in *The Standard Edition of the Complete Psychological Works of Sigmund Freud,* vol. XIV (1914–1916): *On the History of the Psycho-Analytic Movement, Papers on Metapsychology and Other Works*, pp. 273–300.

Hogenson, G. B. (2009). Synchronicity and moments of meeting. *Journal of Analytical Psychology* 54: 183–197.

Jung, C. G. (1929/1966). The Aims of Psychotherapy, in *Collected Works*, vol. 16, 2nd edition. Princeton: Princeton University Press, pp. 61–83.

Kalsched, D. (1996). *The Inner World of Trauma. Archetypal Defenses of the Personal Spirit*. Hove: Routledge.

Kalsched, D. (2013). *Trauma and the Soul. A Psycho-Spiritual Approach to Human Development and its Interruption*. Hove: Routledge.

Kalsched, D. (2015). Revisioning Fordham's 'Defences of the self' in light of modern relational theory and contemporary neuroscience. *Journal of Analytical Psychology* 60 (4): 477–496.

Lemma, A. and Caparrotta, L. (eds) (2014). *Psychoanalysis in the Technoculture Era*. London: Routledge.

Leuzinger-Bohleber, M. (2014). Den Körper in der Seele entdecken Embodiment und die Annäherung an das Nicht-Repräsentierte. *Psyche – Zeitschrift für Psychoanalyse* 68: 922–950.

Merchant, J. (2016). The use of Skype in analysis and training: A research and literature review. *Journal of Analytical Psychology* 61 (3): 309–328.

Milner, M. (1952). Aspects of symbolism in comprehension of the not-self. *Int. J. Psychoanal.* 33: 181–194.

Parsons, M. (2007). Raiding the inarticulate: The internal analytic setting and listening beyond countertransference. *International Journal of Psychoanalysis* 88:1441–1456.

Ogden, T. (1989/2006). *The Primitive Edge of Experience*. Northvale, NJ and London: Jason Aronson.

Roesler, C. (2017) Tele-analysis: the use of media technology in psychotherapy and its impact on the therapeutic relationship. *Journal of Analytical Psychology* 62 (3): 372–394.

Roussillon, R. (1999), *Agonie, Clivage et Symbolisation*. Paris: PUF.

Russel, G. I. (2015). *Screen Relations: The Limits of Computer-Mediated Psychoanalysis and Psychotherapy*. London: Karnac Books.

Saint-Exupéry, A. (2010/1946). *The Little Prince*. BN Publishing.

Sedlacek, S. (2021). Herausforderung Fernanalyse (Klinische Werkstatt). *Psyche – Zeitschrift für Psychoanalyse* 75, 434–444.

Will, H. (2017). Wie der rahmen den analytischen prozess organisiert und schützt, in Unruh, B., Moeslein-Teising, I., and Waltz-Pawlita, S. (eds), *Grenzen*. Gießen: Psychosozial-Verlag, 101–116.

Winnicott, D. (1965). *The Maturational Processes and the Facilitating Environment: Studies in the Theory of Emotional Development*. London: The Hogarth Press.

Winnicott, D. (1971). *Playing and Reality*. London: Tavistock Publications.

Zalusky, S. (1998). Telephone analysis: Out of sight, but not out of mind. *Journal of the American Psychoanalytic Association* 46: 1221–1242.

Chapter 8

Lockdown Therapy
What the Virus Gives and Takes Away

Roberto Grande

The author emphasizes how psychotherapeutic work at the time of total lock-down brings about enormous changes for both therapist and patient. Covid-19 pandemic magnifies existential anxieties, related to the impossibility of planning one's life and controlling the unpredictability of existence. The setting of analysis and psychotherapy change radically for adults, children, individuals and groups. The online work, and the compulsory wearing of a mask, highlight the sensory limitation and therefore the value of it in the therapeutic relationship. Grande believes that, in order to get out of the pandemic and the climate risk, it is necessary to reflect on the irrational collective components that prevent more advanced forms of psychic and social functioning. The author concludes stating that, paradoxically, the pandemic, by highlighting isolation and sensory deprivation, can push us towards a new sense of community, a cooperative mind and towards a more effective fight for survival.

Working Online

September 2021, I'm writing. I remember well how I entered the pandemic: exiting the Italian NHS in December 2019, greeting my colleagues, unaware of future events.

I would have dealt with professional life differently from then (after all, for years I had been dividing myself between public and private clinical work, teaching activities, writing) but I did not imagine how much it would be.

Since February 2020, the epidemic has forced me to take long months of physical social isolation,[1] but not emotional or spiritual. At that time, Stefano Carpani's idea was born, together with other dear Jungian friends, of free psychological support for health personnel, who had been overwhelmed by the situation.

I felt lost and guilty for having left my travel friends in the public service, in the pandemic ... I had a really good timing! I knew it was synchronicity, and that fate was telling me something. A Yiddish saying goes: "If you want to make God laugh, tell him about your plans."

After all, my business has continued unabated since then. Even before Covid, working online was part of my daily professional activity. For

DOI: 10.4324/9781003266402-17

example, I was already doing clinical supervision online for colleagues who live far from me. But the supervision activity has a different value and specificity from the analytical work: the supervisee's story refers to others, the analyzed person says it in the first person. It is as if for me online supervision could, in some way, do more without physical presence than psychotherapy work does.

My online work with patients has increased, but it has not become mandatory for me. When the Covid vaccines were not yet available, according to the Italian Board of Physicians, people could have medical examinations in case of urgency only.

A young woman I have been following for years, refused to do online sessions, not having privacy at home (she lives with very intrusive mother and sister). She was very sorry. Only after the administration of the vaccine (June 2021) did she come back, proving that the relationship remained strong.

Another woman, in the impossibility of privacy, chose to do sessions online, from the car: luckily for her it was summer, and she had a quiet place to concentrate.

Fabrizio, an engineer who fights panic attacks, told me of the suffering, of the loneliness felt, since he lives alone.

My schizoid or socially impaired patients, in general have been happy to be allowed to stay indoors.

A form of psychotherapy, group psychotherapy, has (to date) been almost canceled by Covid, because it is impossible to carry out online without losing much of its effectiveness.

Therapists who, like me, have learned analytic psychodrama (I did a personal analysis and a didactic analysis of Jungian psychodrama), know what a precious resource is the physical presence in the role play, as a substantial part of the transference and of the countertransference in group sessions (Yablonsky 1976, pp. 118, 126). During group meetings (for example in the staging of a dream, an episode of life), the participants immerse themselves in the role play, in the role that the protagonist-subject of the event has given them. They do it first of all emotionally and physically, unconsciously. They don't think; they subsequently reflect, at the end of the game, on the sensations and thoughts, thus clarifying, guided by the conducting analyst, the projections and meanings.

These components are also of great importance in individual sessions. In online work, the patient and analyst lack physical perceptions, body language, a useful psychological work tool; the gestures are reduced, focused on the face, on the voice; you are at the mercy of technology, of pixels; disturbs us and hinders the latency of the audio and / or video signal, which makes communication more difficult.

Working online, what do I lose from eyes, from an emotional mydriasis, or from the wrinkling of a forehead …? Of shaking hands on the armrest, of nervously moving a crossed leg …?

Although the online signal is on high definition, it will never be as sensitive as a glance caught in the other glance, like the refinement of a sudden intuition that comes from a gesture, from an expression.

In Presence, Masked

In face-to-face activities, the use of a mask has become mandatory. I do not know the face of some patients, because they arrived after February 2020; of others, of their faces, I have a distant memory. People "in presence-masked therapy" are forced to be far away, also because the face is fragmented. We know how important the mother's face is in the mother-child relationship (Stern, 1985, p. 92).

A patient, after many sessions, talking about how she feels about me, her good relationship with me and the need to cope with life, confessed to me with gratitude: "Doc, so yes your eyes laugh, and your gaze comforts me."

Another patient, who had gone to the dentist, was told, after a demanding implant operation: "For a month only use your teeth to laugh."

What about the complex of having an ugly mouth, the symbolism of the seduction of the lips? If you put on dark glasses to hide your gaze and an emotion that passes into your eyes, what happens with the mask, what passes and what does not pass anymore?

Certainly, at least, hopefully the virus will not pass.

The annoyance of having an itchy nose risks distracting, losing the thread. One should count how many times one touches or adjusts the mask, even in moments of counter-transference (when I don't understand, when I'm bored, when I get irritated, when I get aroused).

Sensory Deprivation

First the digital universe, then the pandemic, deprived us of many sensory stimuli. The online sessions and the face-to-face sessions with the mask each remove something from the pre-pandemic analytic relationship. The first takes away the body and the physicality of the relationship; the second the completeness and recognition of the face, and facial expressions.

Perhaps the external setting of Jungian analysis was most affected by the pandemic? In sessions of classic psychoanalysis, analyst and patient (lying on the couch), do not look at each other.

The pandemic asks us to turn our attention to the importance of the sensory matrix. What would have changed Jung, of his *Psychological Types*, in particular of the Extraverted Sensation Type, in the light of the epidemic? (Jung, 1971, par. 604–609, 792)

Today's children, who don't see their peers' faces in school, lose sensory skills. As a result, they will have different emotions, different relationships and different brains from pre-digital and pre-Covid children.

A child is on the beach, playing with the sand. The sea is in front of him. He digs a hole, carries water in a bucket, puts some shells around the edge. He adds sticks and algae, as if it were the palisade of a protected fortification. A stick does not want to stay up, the child tries to coordinate his fingers, he manages to plant it, then he looks satisfied at his work.

At the same moment another child, in his apartment in the condominium overlooking the same sea, moans in amusement in front of his portable console. On the screen, tanks go up and down a hill. The fingers frantically press the keys, skillfully switch from one to the other. Tanks explode in front of his eyes, chasing movements faster than ever.

Both children play, both have fun. Both, through play (the most serious thing they know and can do) build their brains. But different areas are activated in their brains, as they perform different activities. Looking at a screen, pressing the buttons of a joypad or playing in the sand are different activities building different brains. And this also applies to the difference between sitting in the presence of someone (even with a mask) or online.

> The media change our brain irrespective of content, and he [McLuhan] famously said: 'the medium is the message' ... Erica Michael and Marcel Just of Carnegie Mellon University did a brain scan study.... They showed that different brain areas are involved in hearing speech and reading it, and different comprehension centers in hearing words and reading them ... each medium creates a different sensory and semantic experience.
>
> (Doidge, 2007, p. 308)

According to Pattis (2011, p. 23), "The vegetative nervous system is the first to react to this. Children who loose their stutters or their nervous tics, or ask for the toilet after just half a session of working intensely in the sand are very simple examples."

Imposed Setting, Rule within Rule. The Phantom of Freedom

The pre and post Covid settings are abysmally different.

We are undergoing a dramatic sensory deprivation and consequently a huge distortion of the setting occurs: the analyst's room, with its colors, smells, intense or soft light, its rituals, is far away. The journey to the practice, the departure from the session is distorted: online, you can prepare yourself halfway, from the torso up; from the waist down, it is informal; from the waist up the mask, the *Persona:* "The term derives from the Latin word for the mask worn by actors in classical times. Hence, persona refers to the mask or face a person puts on to confront the world." (Samuels, Shorter and Plaut, 1986, p. 107). It is like television busting. We have the session without the half which, not only symbolically, is more instinctual.

I have an ancient memory. I had to phone my analyst, Giancarlo Durelli, esteemed Jungian analyst and psychodramatist in Turin, who: "with Santuzza Papa had founded the Rebis, Jungian study center for analytical psychodrama" (Romano, 2017, p. 260), because I wanted to propose working together with him by forming a psychodrama group with children. I was so excited and focused that, despite being at home, I got all dressed up.

I thought that one important occasion deserved an important dress. I brought into the psychodrama group that episode, which I felt was a liturgy. It was my search for the sacred, the initiatory, the religious ritual.[2]

What does it mean to stand in front of a screen and talk in your underwear? Why in an online seminar, among many, do people appear listening to the speaker while eating chicken? Isn't this perhaps a sign that the relationship is lax, distant, less involving? Physics teaches us that electrical dispersion rise if there's an imperfect isolation. If freedom turns in dispersion, its creative essence is lost.

When the sensory stimuli increase, the difficulty of their processing sends into a tailspin attention and procedural memory.[3] Following a lesson on the video, having many other stimuli around, facilitates dispersion. As it happens in ADHD,[4] the person is too sensitive to extraneous stimuli (DSM-V, 2013, pp. 59, 61).

An analyst or trainer, who is faced during online work with people who eat and do gymnastics, must raise the question of the meaning of freedom and relationship.

What makes a person freer, who calls by flushing the toilet freer?

Collective Phobic and Persecutory Thinking

If psychoanalysis was born as a tool to fight against the individual's lack of freedom, not as an instrument of power, I confess that I am uncomfortable when patients (many) spend entire sessions talking about the vaccine and the Green Pass.

No-vaxes take it out on those who manipulate us, the others insult the conspiracy theorists.

Couples fall apart because one is pro-vax and the other against. Social relations are ideologized. In place of the struggle against a common enemy, division emerges. Symbol means put together (greek *sunballo*); on the contrary, devil means to divide (greek *diaballo*).

Covid has triggered an unconscious and irrational collective reaction that pertains to the laws of the collective psyche. The suggestion, not recognized, feeds reactions of panic terror.

For example, I find very stupid to rely on the irrationality of countless booster doses, and not to extend vaccinations to poor countries, Asia and Africa, still without vaccines (September 2021). From there the variants will also arrive in civilized countries.[5] Humanity behaves like that child who, playing hide and seek, covers his eyes convinced that others will not see her/him.

According to Jung: "Thousands of miles lay between me and Europe, mother of all demons" (Jung 1989, p. 264).

It is as if a huge previously hidden collective emotion had come to the surface, stimulated by the viral epidemic. Was there no terror before? Was it born from the virus? No, it was triggered by the virus. It was just hidden in the folds of our oldest collective brain, mimetic as the virus itself does, in order to survive.

The coronavirus carries deeply ancestral symbolism, to be the cause of the psychic contagion we have witnessed.

A girl I helped at the age of 14, due to relationship difficulties, returned in October 2020, at the age of 18, suffering from a first psychotic episode; she had a persecutory delusion of contamination from Covid. We went on until July 2021 with antipsychotics and weekly sessions, luckily avoiding hospitalization.

We should begin to deal with people's mental health, before it crumbles in such situations. Perhaps, never as now, we should consider not only individual psychodiagnostics categories but collective too, imposed by collective *noxae* (such as the coronavirus), involving social psychic reactions; this would help people, the polis and the collapsing economy.

Western collective thought, under a thin veil of scientific rationalism, is following the coordinates (more phobic than rational) of the all-out defense, to protect itself from an elusive enemy, depending on the circumstances identified with black, yellow, the virus, the fool, the pagan … the different and the stranger, in short. Always lurking to avoid dealing with the alien that dwells in us; the one who can save us if we do not make it dangerous by ignoring it; what Jung called Shadow.

Thus, for decades, we have been induced to disinfect the thoughts of our children to remove aliens from the family circle and to defend ourselves from the virus of other people's ideas.

Yet, in the literary and historical context, the term *contamination* is widely used, and it has a clear positive value. For example, we say "contamination of ideas, of cultures." I call it an attitude of openness and fight against prejudice; it is the ability of contact with insecurity and the precariousness of existence. These are the psychic antibiotics that would help us not to get sick with depression and a thousand physical symptoms.

Instead, we have developed a psycho-antibiotic resistance to altruism; we are immune to the beneficial action of the other and we do not tolerate uncertainties.

Many phobic are fine, these days, because they have learned to understand that their fears are irrational and exaggerated; they accept them and work on their interiority.

Therefore, they laugh at those who are seized by Covid-panic.

I conclude this reflection by saying that I bear the anti-Covid rules (mask and distancing) as a new religion; I am bored by the liturgy of the disinfection of handles, armchairs between a patient and another, which I practice as an *entre-neuse* after every intercourse with clients. I look at the Coronavirus as I look at a part of me that I did not know and that I have recently discovered: with distrust, with wonder, trying to understand what it can do *for me*, possibly not *to me*.

Basically, I try to remain myself and use the best possible working method.

If "The medium is the message" (McLuhan, 1964, p. 19) and if "Every psychotherapist not only has his own method – he himself is that method" (Jung, 1970, par. 198) then no medium and no method (online, face to face, behind the bed) is *a priori* the best or the worst.

The virus has given us more limits and made us more aware of what we already had, and what we have lost.

Once again, in Thebes, the epidemic sent by the Gods can be a punishment for humanity but also a signal of possible awareness and improvement.

Notes

1 The lockdown to which I refer was the first 'total lockdown' in Italy: from 9 March 2020 to 4 May 2020.
2 Religion comes from *re-ligere*, gathering of formulas and rituals.
3 Procedural memory is a type of long-term memory involving how to perform different actions (riding a bike, tying your shoes).
4 ADHD, Attention Deficit Hyperactivity Disorder.
5 I'm curious what the situation will be like in 2022 when this book will be published.

References

Doidge, N. (2007). *The Brain That Changes Itself: Stories of Personal Triumph from the Frontiers of Brain Science.* Penguin Books Limited, Group USA.

American Psychiatric Association, DSM-5 Task Force (2013). Diagnostic and Statistical Manual of Mental Disorders (DSM 5). American Psychiatric Publishing Inc.

Jung, C. G. (1970). *The Practice of Psychotherapy in Collected Works*, vol. 16, Bollingen Series XX. Princeton, NJ: Princeton University Press.

Jung, C. G. (1971). *Psychological Types in Collected Works*, vol. 6, Bollingen Series XX. Princeton, NJ: Princeton University Press.

Jung, C. G. (1989) *Memories, Dreams, Reflections.* New York: Vintage Books.

McLuhan, M. (1964). *Understanding Media: The Extensions of Man*, critical edition. Corte Madera, CA: Ginkgo Press.

Pattis, E. (2011). *Sandplay Therapy in Vulnerable Communities: A Jungian Approach.* Routledge.

Samuels, A., Shorter, B., and Plaut, F. (1986). *A Critical Dictionary of Jungian Analysis.* Routledge.

Romano, A. (2017). *L'inconscio a Torino.* Nino Aragno Editore.

Stern, D. (1985). *The Interpersonal World Of The Infant – A View From Psychoanalysis and Developmental Psychology.* London: Karnac

Yablonsky, L. (1976). *Psychodrama. Resolving Emotional Problems through Role-Playing.* New York: Basic Books.

Chapter 9

How Are You?

The Mystery of Communication between Alone-nesses[1]

Emilija Kiehl

The coronavirus pandemic forced psychotherapists to swiftly move their practice online. We had to find ways of working without the very particular role that our consulting rooms play in this kind of work. The psychosomatic aspects of the interactive field, of the transference and countertransference, cannot be "transported" from a shared physical space into cyberspace. A form of Keats' negative capability is needed to work under unconscious pressure to compensate for what is missing and forge a new, unknown ingredient. "How are you?" clients ask me sometimes, and this is no longer just a question for analytic interpretation but a confirmation of our shared reality. In this new reality, new themes are entering the analytic space. This chapter explores the emergence of these themes in the altered internal and external environments that our patients and we now occupy. The author asks crucial questions that call our attention with the utmost urgency. An increasing number of people, mostly young, are questioning the moral integrity of the "might is right" attitude, whether socially, economically, politically, or towards animals and nature.

> *"Yes, it is the in-between world, the pathless, the manifold, and dazzling. I forgot that I had reached a new world, which had been alien to me previously. I see neither way nor bridge"*
>
> (Jung, The *Black Books*)

On his travels through the turbulent, often perilous realms of his unconscious, Jung encountered figures and places co-existing on different levels of his inner landscape. He recorded these experiences in *The Black Books*, later adding the powerfully vivid images, which then became his *Liber Novus* or the *Red Book*.

In the above citation, Jung arrives at the ontological "place" where the soul dwells – a place beyond the reach of his brilliant scientific mind. Jung's model of the psyche emerged from these travels and took shape through the interplay between his consciousness and the unconscious, where the spirit of the depth and the spirit of the time mingle, and the human mind can get a glimpse into the vicissitudes of the immensely rich life of the psyche.

DOI: 10.4324/9781003266402-18

As psychotherapists, we strive to provide/be the bridge Jung struggles to see in the above passage, by accompanying our clients on the travels that Jung accomplished on his own and came back to tell us of his findings.

The shape and size of our consulting room with all its objects, lights, colours, smells, positions of chairs and the couch (if the couch is used), fabrics, textures, views from our windows, together create a vessel we occupy together with our clients. Within this vessel, another one is weaved, out of our body-to-body communications, bodily postures, the pheromones, our voices, words and glances we exchange. In the safety of this multileveled container, the interactive field between client and therapist can be planted with seeds for change. Our consulting room has an irreplaceable function in this process.

And then, the coronavirus forced us to swiftly move our practice online and find ways of working without this function. A shift in boundaries. I kept my schedule intact so that, although we no longer occupied the same space, my clients and I continued to occupy the same time. This calendar continuity and the fifty minutes of the analytic hour, in what Bergson (1886) calls the objective or "clock time," was now a container for the living inner continuity in the experienced time or the Duration, where change happens. Duration is for Bergson qualitative rather than quantitative and can be measured only when symbolically represented in space. In this "organic whole," past, present and anticipation of future coexist, and here we can grasp our clients' inner world through intuition. With a mixture of awkwardness and relief, my clients and I were able to recognise this "place" online and find each other anew.

My computer screen gave the same view of my consulting room to those who already knew it and those I met only online had a visual idea of what it would be like if we were in the room together. However, the psychosomatic aspects of the interactive field, of the transference and countertransference, cannot be "transported" from a shared physical space into cyberspace. A form of Keats' negative capability is needed to work under unconscious pressure (the "Zoom fatigue"), to compensate for what is missing and produce some new, unknown ingredient. "How are you?" clients ask me sometimes, and this is no longer just a question for analytic interpretation. It now feels like a confirmation of our shared reality.

George, (not his real name) found that, although it felt different, online work did not diminish the quality of the connection we had established working person-to-person. Furthermore, this was not an entirely new experience for us as we had already worked online when George was away on business. So, we continued, comfortable enough in the uncertainty about when we would be back in my consulting room. However, as months went by, George began to notice that he was missing something: his journeys to and from my consulting room, the thoughts and feelings arousing before and after each session, the physical movement in and out of the potentially transformative space of the analytic hour. They were lost in the quick sequence of tasks around connecting and disconnecting online.

The "clock time" and the duration can be out of sync.

A native man Jung met on his travels through Africa was offered a lift in a car. Half an hour later, the man asked if the car could stop. He stepped out and stretched himself on the ground. "Did the car drive make him sick?" someone asked. "No," the man replied, he felt fine but just had to wait for his soul to catch up. It had remained behind because the drive was too fast for it (Jung 1961, quoted in Sabini 2002).

A client I have worked with entirely online described a long- term inner struggle with a terrifying, often mocking "attacker." We connected quite quickly and safely enough for the client to notice and let me know when I appeared as the "attacker." At one such moment, having made an important disclosure, the client revealed feeling fear and regret in expectation of my judgement (attack). Would this have been less terrifying if we were together in the room? I asked.

"Quite the opposite!" the client replied. "If we were in the same room, I wouldn't have had the energy to say any of this – I would be trying to break through a barrier just to connect with you. This 'space' feels safe, I feel your presence, and I can think and breathe freely."

The immensely informing density and richness of the body-to-body communications in a shared physical space can be overwhelming. Online therapy can then provide a safe space of a different kind. The facilitating aspects of the online interactive field are yet to be explored and understood by both therapists and clients.

A client I had worked with for many years on the manifold impact of severe relational trauma often travelled for work, "taking me with him" in his laptop. During the lockdown, we continued to tread carefully through the calamitous, at times terrifying, and utterly lonely inner terrain that had become his dwellings. Online, he was always on time, which was a struggle when we worked in person. Our connection acquired a new depth and closeness, accelerating our work towards the crossing between what Melanie Klein terms the paranoid-schizoid and the depressive positions. I wondered if the virtual container had the capacity to sustain this turning point and carry the work to the "other side." As it happens, it did not. My client returned to the previous developmental position and I am left with a feeling that, in this case, the absence of a whole array of invaluable body-based pointers for navigating the process of this profound psychological change made the crucial crossing impossible. At least for now.

These brief sketches outline some of my experiences so far. The full effect of the changes that our patients and we are having to adjust to are yet to emerge. Together, we are the pioneers in the ongoing development of this work. A new approach to the mystery of communication between alone-nesses, a new paradigm for the way we think and work, may be in the making.

In the presence of death, we all live in a city without walls.[2]

Looking at each other on computer screens, confined at home, our patients and we were faced starkly with our common vulnerability towards something outside the safe analytic space. We were together and alone in the world which seemed to have come to a standstill. The governments of the wealthiest and most powerful countries, leaders of the "free and developed world," were shown to be incompetent, unreliable, often corrupt. Who can we trust to sort this out? The reality, integrity and the cost of our apparent progress came into focus and began to be questioned in analysis. Jung warned us about times like this when he wrote:

"But our progressiveness, though it may result in a great many delightful wish-fulfilments, piles up an equally gigantic Promethean debt which has to be paid off from time to time in the form of hideous catastrophes" (Jung, 1959/2002, par. 276).

The pandemic has cast a shadow of death across the globe, at the same time revealing many socio-economic and political ills that had for centuries been plaguing the world we have created for ourselves and have forced on our fellow creatures on the planet. Senselessly exploiting human, animal and other natural resources in our, seemingly unstoppable march toward ever-lasting "growth and prosperity" (for some), we have forgotten about responsibility and our own vulnerability towards the nature we have, in phantasy conquered. Despite the warning signs that had been around for a long time, we were surprised when circumstances beyond our control forced us to stop what we were doing and, startled by the fear of death and "the end of the world as we know it," shut ourselves in our homes (those of us who have homes, that is) and work out how to hold on to bits of what was hitherto considered our "normal" lives. Many aspects of the shadow of the "normality" we want to return to were exposed: what is "normal" about it and for whom? Back in 1941, Jung saw that:

the breathless haste, superficiality, and nervous exhaustion with all the concomitant symptoms – craving stimulation, impatience, irritability, vacillation etc. [...] may lead to all sorts of other things but never to any increased culture of the mind and heart.

(Jung 1941, par. 1343).

The current gradual opening of the lockdown comes with ethical questions about our future. Where do we go from here? Is there such a thing as a collective rite of passage and, if so, what does it involve, individually and collectively?

In an interview for IAAP, Heyong Shen tells us that the Chinese character for "crisis" also means "opportunity" (Shen 2020).

Murray Stein sees thus this momentous time for humanity:

The image that comes to my mind is an *Umbra Mundi*, a world shadow hovering over us and infecting our psychic lives. I see this shadow spreading over the globe like a solar eclipse. The alchemical term for it is *nigredo*. The sun is covered by the shadow of death. It is the familiar stage that signifies the beginning of significant transformation. We are being asked to walk through the valley of the shadow of death. It is biblical. The question is: will we be able to use this experience for individuation? Or will it just pass like a bad dream of the night that when we awake, we are happy to be free from?

(Stein 2020)

The ever-widening socioeconomic divide championed and enforced worldwide by the conservative and neoliberal governments alike can no longer be ignored. Anticipating globalisation and the unstoppable rise in socioeconomic inequality, comments were made in the 70s that one day the gap between the rich and the poor may become so vast that we will no longer recognise each other as the same species and will begin to eat each other. The currently rising awareness of the dark side of the "success" of globalisation came mainly through the much-maligned social media, forcing the establishment media to begin to report on what they would typically ignore, blackout or ridicule. The unbridgeable chasm between those who can and those who cannot work from home; the basic living conditions, let alone the working conditions of millions of people in the United Kingdom, found their way into the mainstream media. It transpired that over 3.8 million children in the UK live below the poverty line and would go hungry without free school meals during the lockdown. The blatant exploitation of the underpaid health workers, who were in the middle of the deadly pandemic offered a pay rise of 1%, while the military received 4%, brought into the public domain broader questions of values in the world ruled by market forces. The ethics of the "real world" that we believe we (and our clients) should comply with, entered the public discourse and discussions about creating a more humane society are no longer confined to those on "the radical left" or dismissed as "dreaming of Utopia."

And the discourse doesn't stop there. An increasing number of people, mostly young, are questioning the moral integrity of the "might is right" attitude, whether socially, economically, politically, or towards animals and nature. Does human evolution require that we depart from this attitude of dissociated exploitation and disregard for the suffering we cause? Is it possible for us to approach the difference in socioeconomic class, gender, race, and species beyond the usual categorisation into superiority and inferiority?

The possibility that the coronavirus came from the Chinese "wet markets" revealed the horrific conditions animals are kept in before they are slaughtered in front of the customers who want their meat "still warm." Another cultural practice in China then came into focus: "Yu Lin dog meat festival" where dogs are dragged through the streets and tortured to death in front of cheering spectators who believe that dogs' body parts taste better if they are terrified before they die. In response to these revelations, other cultural practices and methods of killing animals, such as kosher and halal, were also scrutinised, followed by questioning the "advanced" money and time-saving industrial animal killing techniques in the "developed" countries. The increasingly vocal movements for ecological awareness and humanity for animals challenge the ethics of raising animals in order to kill them for the pleasure of eating their body parts and wearing their skins on our backs and feet. The growing scientific evidence that we do not need to eat animals to be healthy and that animals value their lives and feel the pain and fear of death just as humans do challenges the justifications for killing them. Furthermore, the undeniable impact of industrial animal agriculture on climate change has led to the demand for video cameras in slaughterhouses so that the public can make informed rather than dissociated dietary, fashion, and ecology-aware choices. As expected, the mighty animal slaughter industry is doing all it can to prevent this conscious choice, and the disturbing images of animals' suffering and deaths are censored in the corporate media.

The speed of our material progress has blinded us to the unsustainable impact of our ego-led actions, with our consciousness (and conscience) lagging behind, like the soul of Jung's acquaintance in Africa mentioned earlier.

Jung had anticipated the challenges we face when he wrote:

We are very far from having finished completely with the Middle Ages, classical antiquity, and primitivity, as our modern psyches pretend. Nevertheless, we have plunged down a cataract of progress which sweeps us on into the future with even wilder violence the farther it takes us from our roots... [This] has given rise to the "discontents" of civilization and to such a flurry and haste that we live more in the future and its chimerical promise of golden age than in the present, with which our whole evolutionary background has not yet caught up.

(Jung 1963, p. 263).

Similarly, in his book *Carl Jung, Darwin of the Mind,* Thomas T. Lawson writes:

Like a child, we seem, collectively, both wilful and oblivious to the consequences of our acts. We have, in modern times demonstrated a capacity to affect our life-supporting planet that has radically outstripped our understanding of how either to control the effects of what we do or to regulate our actions so as to be able to limit or avoid those effects.

(Lawson 2008).

My clients are becoming increasingly interested in social and environmental issues, and some are planning to or already are becoming actively involved. Our work now includes concerns for our collective future on the planet. Much of the "normal" we want to return to has brought about the crisis we now face. As professionals and citizens, we have a responsibility to allow the vital questions about the ethics of the way we live into psychoanalytic work and explore with our clients the links between the personal and the collective evolution of the psyche in the world we create and the environment we dominate. Jung had already addressed this complex task when he wrote:

"'But why on earth,' you may ask, 'should be necessary for man to achieve, by hook or by crook, a higher level of consciousness?' This is truly a crucial question, and I do not find the answer easy. Instead of a real answer, I can only make a confession of faith: I believe that, after thousands and millions of years, someone had to realize that this wonderful world of mountains and oceans, suns and moons, galaxies and nebulae, plants and animals, *exists.*" (Jung, 1959/2002, par. 177).

Notes

1 Abraham Maslow quoted in Rosemary Gordon (1993).
2 Epicurus, Letters. Quoted in De Masi (2004).

References

Bergson, H. (1886) *Time and Free Will*. Kindle edition

De Masi, F. (2004) *Making Death Thinkable*. London: Free Association Books.

Gordon, R. (1993) *Bridges: Metaphor for Psychic Processes*. London: Karnac Books.

Jung, C. G. (2020 [1913–1932]). *The Black Books*. WW Norton & Company.

Jung, C. G. (1941/1953/1991). The Symbolic Life: Miscellaneous Writings. In *CW*, 181–20. Routledge & Keagan Paul.

Jung, C. G. (1963) *Memories, Dreams, Reflections*. Fontana Press (HarperCollins).

Jung, C. G. (1959/2002). 'The Psychology of the Child Archetype'. In The Archetypes and the Collective Unconscious, *CW*, 9i. London: Routledge.

Lawson, T. (2008) *Carl Jung, Darwin of the Mind*. London: Carnac Books.

Sabini, M. (2002) *C.G. Jung on Nature, Technology & Modern Life*. Berkeley, CA: North Atlantic Books.

Shen, H. (2020). Interview of Heong Chen (China), by E. Kiehl. Iaap.org.

Stein, M. (2020). A world shadow: COVID-19, interview by R. Henderson, online at: https://chironpublications.com/a-world-shadow-covid-19/

Chapter 10

Psyche and the Speed of Life
Jungian Reflections on the Pandemic

Milena Sotirova-Kohli

This chapter presents some reflections on the impact of the Covid-19 crises on the life style of people and values in the Western society. Life slows down, the world freezes, news of death, suffering, insecurity, helplessness, confusion come on all channels, through all media. Life shifts at home and in the vast space of the internet. What has the unconscious to say to what is going on in the world? Jung believed that psyche is a self-regulating system. Under all circumstances the human psyche strives at achieving inner balance, and dreams are the natural reaction of a self-regulating psychic system. Considering the results of small-scale exploratory research on dreams conducted by the author and Arthur Funkhouser after the onset of the pandemic, Kohli argues that the pandemic and the measures introduced to stop the spreading of the virus lead to a slowing down of life and provide the possibility of a return to oneself. In this sense, and in resonance with the ideas of the German sociologist Hartmut Rosa, she sees in the current situation both a danger and a chance for Western society, and describes her discovery of the possibilities and difficulties of online therapy sharing her clinical experience.

I would like to dedicate my reflections to all those who suffered loss, who selflessly helped others, and to the memory of all those who departed this life during the pandemic without having a chance for goodbyes.

December 2019

The news circulates of a new virus that kills people in Wuhan, China. I am shocked, but it all seems to be far away. My schedule is so full, I have the feeling life turns around checking off appointments.

January 2020

The virus is already in Europe. Would it come closer to Bern? My agenda is still so full, I know I must change something.

February 2020

The first cases of the new virus are detected in Tessin, Switzerland. Can that be? My agenda is still full.

March 2020

DOI: 10.4324/9781003266402-19

The world shuts down. For the first time since the second world war the federal government in Switzerland takes over and orders a nationwide lockdown. Is this all real? Ah, the agenda, it does not matter.... Appointments are cancelled one after the other. Am I sorry about this?

Life slows down. The world freezes, news of death, suffering, insecurity, helplessness, confusion come on all channels, through all media. Life shifts at home and in the vast space of the internet.

How does the psyche react I ask myself as a Jungian analyst; what has the unconscious to say to what is going on in the world?

***

Jung believed that psyche is a self-regulating system. Under all circumstances the human psyche strives at achieving inner balance. And "dreams are the natural reaction of the self-regulating psychic system" (CW 18, p. 110, par. 248) according to Jung. For Jung dreams

> arise spontaneously without our assistance and are representatives of a psychic activity withdrawn from our arbitrary will. Therefore, the dream is a highly objective natural product of the psyche from which we might expect hints about certain basic trends in the psychic process.
>
> (CW 7, para 210, p. 131)

Furthermore, dreams "add to the conscious psychological situation of the moment all those aspects which are essential for a totally different point of view.... In dreams occur all those aspects which during the day were insufficiently appreciated or totally ignored." (CW 8, p. 345, par. 469).

I decided that if I want to know how the psyche reacts to the current circumstances, I should study the dreams people are having. Dreams would best demonstrate how the unconscious reacts to the stresses of these times.

Together with my colleague, the Jungian analyst Arthur Funkhouser, I decided to conduct an exploratory research under the form of an online anonymous survey asking people about their experience with dreams and dreaming during the pandemic. The survey was administered in German and English online via survey-monkey. It consisted of ten questions. Demographic data as to the age and the gender of the participants was collected. We assessed for change of socioeconomic status since the beginning of the pandemic, whether oneself or significant others had been infected or died due to Covid-19, and the attitude of the respondents toward dreams and dreaming. We inquired whether participants in the study observed any changes in their experience of dreams after the onset of the pandemic and whether there were dreams that left a strong impression on them since the onset of the pandemic. If so, what were the dreams about and how did the participants feel in the dreams. The survey did not look explicitly for dreams with images related to the pandemic. We were interested in those dreams that were evaluated by the participants as significant to them in this time. We believed that these dreams would demonstrate best the compensatory reaction of the unconscious in the current situation. The results were modest and somewhat interesting.

There were 40 participants in the English survey and 27 in the German one. We need to point out that this was not a representative sample of the general population. Most of the respondents in both groups were people with an interest in dreams which existed before the pandemic (90% in the English group, 86% in the German group). People in both samples were predominantly in the 18 to 64 years of age age-group and were not greatly affected by the pandemic with regard to their health or their socio-economic status. Most of the respondents have noticed no change in their dream life (58.62% in the German sample and 57.50% in the English sample). Just 27.5% in the English sample and 38% in the German sample reported having had more vivid dreams since the pandemic (which is contrary to the current wide-spread belief that in the pandemic people have more vivid dreams). Of the respondents in the German group, 65.52 % reported having had no impressive dream since the pandemic began while, however, 65% of the English respondents reported having had a dream that made a big impression on them since the pandemic began. The majority of those reporting having had a dream that left strong impression on them since the pandemic reported experiencing a change in their life since the dream occurred. In the English sample 32.6% of the people reported having negative emotions in their dreams that they qualified as important to them, 28.26% experienced positive emotions in their dreams that left big impression on them, 28.26% did not answer the question. In the German sample 55.5% did not write any answer to the question regarding dream importance, 25.92% experienced negative emotions in their dreams that left strong impressions on them and 11% deemed the emotions from the dreams that left big impressions on them to be positive.

The first publication of dream research on dreams in the times of the pandemic was in June 2020. Deirdre Barrett, a Harvard dream researcher, published her work on pandemic dreams. Barrett's research is widely quoted in the media. According to the researcher, dreams after the onset of the pandemic were more vivid than before, there were specific recurrent themes in dreams and people tended to remember more dreams (Barrett, 2020). This research was followed by a series of studies from different countries, most of which confirmed these findings. Most studies found a predominance of negative affect in people's dreams during the pandemic.

The results of the survey Arthur Funkhouser and I conducted did not confirm the finding that people have more vivid dreams after the onset of the pandemic. In a sample of people predominantly interested in dreams from before the onset of the pandemic and people who were not affected strongly by the pandemic, the majority of the participants observed no change in their dream lives and experiences of dreams during the pandemic. How shall we understand this fact? Is it that after the onset of the pandemic the quality of dream life changed, or can one explain these findings differently? Did the dreams of those affected closely by the pandemic and the measures to stop the spreading of the virus become more vivid? Or was it that the pandemic led to slowing life down and people had more time to observe their dreams? Those who were interested in dreams from before the pandemic report obviously no change in their dream-lives. Can it be that by virtue of having space to pay more attention to one's dreams there is a sense of dreaming that is more vivid? I remember a member of a dream group I lead who during our first meeting reported she was taking part just out of curiosity and that she actually never dreamt. At the next session the same participant came all excited and told the group how. since she was in the dream group, she now had the most remarkable and vivid dreams.

The impact of the lockdowns is supposedly also the reason for the observed increase of dream recall reported by people in the times of the pandemic (Barrett, 2020).

Furthermore, the English-speaking respondents reported more significant dreams in the time of the pandemic than the German speaking respondents. Can it be that the country of residence and respectively the intensity of the pandemic crises have led to stronger unconscious reaction to the situation expressed in the form of significant dreams?

Our survey was very small scale, unfortunately too small scale to be able to make any statistically significant conclusions. But the data we collected raised some questions for me.

Overall, it made me ask myself if the pandemic and the resulting lock-downs led to a return of people to themselves.

Obviously, people react in a different way to the pandemic depending on the country they live and the degree to which it was affected by the pandemic, but also depending on who they are and what their values in life are or were at the onset of the pandemic, as well as how their life was affected by the pandemic and the measures introduced to stop the spread of the virus.

However, it is undeniable, that the worldwide lockdown slowed down life and thereby put the brakes on to its ever-growing speed. For a moment, we just were, and the world was not predictable and secure anymore. We were forced to stop taking the order of things we were used to as the Order of things. We were forced to search for stable ground outside the appointments in the agenda or the meetings and achievements at work.

The German sociologist, Hartmut Rosa, proposed that modernity has been marked by an ever-growing acceleration of life resulting from the develop-ment of technology and being associated with the fact that, even though people live busy lives, many experience a sense of frustration with life (Rosa, 2013). According to Rosa the very intensity of our lives and our schedules leads to this feeling of frustration. In the ever-increasing speed of life and the ever-growing possibilities we live with create the impression that we are never up to date, we constantly have to catch up with more recent developments.

The constant flood of experience leaves no time to assimilate these, hence we are left feeling empty even though we seem to have busy lives. In a certain sense this intensity of life estranges us from ourselves. Is this feeling familiar to you? And at the same time, mindfulness is full in trend.

In this hectic of life, as Prof. Rosa pointed out in an interview with the German newspaper *Der Tagesspiegel* in March 2020, Covid-19 works as a radical decelerator. The lock down functioned as a break and reminded people of the unpredictability of life. Prof. Rosa saw two possible outcomes of the current situation – continuing to do what we have always done in trying to control the situation, or to start listening to ourselves and the world, and thus enter again into resonance with the world and ourselves. Thus, according to him, the current crisis holds not only danger but also a chance for us.

Being restricted to the own apartment or house transferred much of life online. This is another controversial topic. In much of the literature the virtual world is associated with dissociating from the here and now of daily reality and is often treated as having negative impact on people when over-used (ex. Toronto, 2009, Schimmenti & Caretti, 2017, Korte, 2020). The message of much of the literature on this topic seems to be: Do not spend too much time in the virtual world; it is not good for you. Most scholars bring rather negative messages about the consequences of over-indulging there. However, it seems to me it is far more important to understand what makes virtual reality so appealing. In a life of ever-growing speed and ever-growing demands, in which one is never up to date due to the very principles of organization of modern societal life (Rosa, 2013), virtual reality seems to be an escape and retreat, a compensation in Jungian words. One would think we just need to slow life down and people can return to themselves in the here and now of their bodily existence. However, the lock down proved it to be different, demonstrating at the same time the multifaceted compensatory possibilities of the virtual world.

As Hartmut Rosa pointed out in his interview in the time of the lock down it was acceleration itself that was shifted to the virtual world. Most of our appointments, meetings, conferences, discussions shifted online. Even therapy for the most part shifted to the online modus.

Had someone asked me two years ago to conduct online therapy, I would have declined. My conviction was that it was not possible to have the intimacy necessary online for a good therapeutic relationship and effective therapy. Interestingly enough, research demonstrated the opposite was true. The working alliance in an online therapy is not only not worse but can be even better than in in-person therapy (Cook & Doyle, 2002) and a meta-analysis of studies on the effectiveness of online therapy demonstrated no difference in effectiveness between face-to-face therapy and online therapy (Barak et. al, 2008).

In March 2020, the authorities of the Kanton of Bern cancelled all in-person therapy sessions for group therapies in the cantonal Psychological Services. There were many adolescents in the group for adolescent girls that I lead there. Before the lockdown most of them felt isolated and appreciated the exchanges with peers in the secure frame of the group therapy. Losing this support in times that were anyway challenging seemed to be associated with a high risk of worsening of their mental states. I was faced with the challenge of finding a way to support them. So, I very quickly decided to conduct the group online. We met every week online for one hour at the times when the group would have taken place physically. And I learned from session to session. With time, a form for the group sessions evolved which provided a framework for the participants and rules for the setting from which each girl logged in. We learned together, we cooperated, the girls, me and the psychology students that helped with conducting the group. And I had the impression that for the girls being able to support us with the technical difficulties in the beginning of the online phase was important and strengthened their sense of self-worth. The reactions that the girls had to the news that we would conduct the group online differed, from joy and excitement that something was going on in a time in which they felt isolated to fear of online sessions.

One of the participants who was registered to be in the group declined participating. She felt insecure taking part in an online form of therapy. With others I could observe marked changes over the course of online sessions. A girl with selective mutism started to take part in the discussions. At first, she spoke very quietly, then more often and louder. Later she gave the feedback that she felt more secure since she could log in for the sessions from her room in the family flat. Overall, in the online sessions, the girls showed the tendency to be open much more quickly in the discussions and to share more personal information than in the in-person sessions. This was not just my observation; it was also the feedback that the girls gave me after the online phase of the therapy was over.

This effect was observed and described by the American psychologist Suler in 2004. Suler described it as a disinhibition effect demonstrated by people taking different forms of online treatment. The physical absence of the therapist in the immediate physical environment and the fact that the therapy takes place in a familiar and secure environment of the client obviously lead to the fact that people tended to share thoughts and experiences which otherwise were not so readily shared. This effect is related also to a form of intimacy specific for online therapy which Weinberg (2019; 2020) calls e-intimacy. Weinberg describes e-intimacy as all that people can share with one another when they do not have a body (2020). In my experience e-intimacy in therapy has the potential to bring about depth and is related to openness on both sides.

The experience of clients of teletherapy was in my experience influenced greatly by the technical means they had at their disposal for the sessions. Participants who logged in with their smart phones for the online group therapy reported being less able to follow the session and enjoy the process. The speed of the internet connection and the ability to retreat in a quiet place during the sessions also impacted their online session experiences.

Some patients when switching to online sessions reported being happy to be able to see the face of the therapist since we did not need to wear masks.

It was interesting to observe the transition from online back into the in-person setting. A patient with whom I had online therapy sessions over a longer period of time reported, after we returned back to the in-person sessions, finding that she needed to readjust to the new setting. She felt it was easier to open up and speak about herself when online but she found that the reassuring messages from her therapist when shared in an in-person setting had larger impact on her.

In all the above cases of online therapy I knew the patients personally. I discovered that this has a big impact on the online therapy process as well. Bringing with me the physical impressions of the patient facilitated my understanding their situation and what the patient was sharing with me. Later, I made the experience of working online with patients from different countries that I did not personally know. Having never met the patient in person affected my ability to appropriately adjudge the patient and his/her situation. Seeing the gait of the patient or the way the patient dresses and looks already provides a big deal of information about the state of mind of the patient which was missing when meeting the patients exclusively online. For example, in the case of a patient from a distant country with whom I worked for a while online, it took four or five sessions until I understood the degree of her obesity, a fact I would have in in-person therapy sessions realized right away.

Undoubtedly, the online mode of working did reduce the speed of life. A fact that not only I enjoyed. In a group supervision session members of the group shared reluctantly that they enjoyed the lockdown, secretly they were hoping for further such times of low speed of life.

So, how do we come out of the times of the pandemic? Which way from the two possible options that Prof. Rosa spoke about are we about to take – do we speed up and make up for the lost time, again accelerate and alienate us from ourselves and the world, or do we continue to listen ever deeper to ourselves and the world?

***

June 2021

We have new variations of the coronavirus. The topic of the Covid-19 is part of daily life, so much so that wearing a mask is now routine. My agenda is full. The appointments are one after the other.

July 2021

It is summer. I can hear the cow bells from the nearby field. Children in the neighbor's garden are playing in the swimming pool. France introduces stricter measures trying again to stop the spreading of the Covid-19 virus. And the agenda …

I would like to thank Arthur Funkhouser for editing my English.

References

Barak, A., Hen, L., Boniel-Nissim, M., & Shapira, N. (2008). A comprehensive review and a meta-analysis of the effectiveness of internet-based psychotherapeutic interventions. *Journal of Technology in Human Services*, 26 (2-4): 109–160.

Barrett, D. (2020). *Pandemic Dreams*. Oneiroi Press.

Cook, J. E., & Doyle, C. (2002). Working alliance in online therapy as compared to face-to-face therapy: Preliminary results. *Cyberpsychology and Behavior*, 5 (2): 95–105.

Jung, C. G. *Collected Works*. Princeton University Press.

Korte, M. (2020). The Impact of the Digital Revolution on Human Brain and Behavior: Where do we stand? *Dialogues in Clinical Neuroscience*, 22 (2): 101–111.

Rosa, H. (2013). *Alienation and Acceleration. Towards a Critical Theory of Late-Modern Temporality*. Suhrkamp Verlag.

Rosa, H. (2020). Das Virus ist der radikalste Entschleuniger unserer Zeit. *Der Tagesspiegel*.

Schimmenti, A., & Caretti, V. (2017). Video-Terminal Dissociative Trance: Toward a psychodynamic understanding of problematic internet use. *Clinical Neuropsychiatry*, 14 (1): 64–72.

Suler, J. (2004). The online disinhibition effect. *Cyberpsychology and Behaviour*, 7 (3): 321–326.

Toronto, E. (2009). Time out of mind: Dissociation in the virtual world. *Psychoanalytic Psychology*, 26 (2): 117–133.

Weineberg, H. (2020). *Online Group Psychotherapy Course*. Zur Institute, USA.

Weinberg, H., & Rolnick, A. (ed.) (2019). *Theory and Practice of Online Therapy: Internet Delivered Interventions for Individuals, Groups, Families and Organizations*. New York, Routledge.

Chapter 11

To Touch and To Be Touched

On affection, infection and contagion. An analysis of the analytic ethic reimagined through coronavirus

Tiffany Houck-Loomis

The convergence of the global pandemic caused by the novel Coronavirus, the raise of hate crimes across the globe and the exposure of structural racism and white supremacy inherent in every aspect of daily life in America, call for a radical reconceptualization of the ethical responsibility of the analyst in and out of her office. The author proposes that one ethical response to our changing world is in a new formulation of the old analytic dictum, "The patient cannot go where the analyst has not gone." Rather, she recognizes a dual asymmetry in the analytic relationship where the patient, affected by the events in the world, takes the analyst where the analyst unknowingly needs to go but has not yet been able to go, pressed further into the unknown as analyst and patient experience the events of the outer life contiguously, side by side. By interweaving the collective reality of the outer world with clinical vignettes, I offer an analytic ethical response to the trauma through which we are all living.

The work of analysis turns on the heels of affection. Allowing oneself to be affected by the other in front of us, the other within us, and the dance between the two in the context of global events that affect us both, is what allows for transformation within our work. Transformation within the analysand and analyst alike. What does it mean to be affected by the world, by the other in front of us and within us? What does it feel like to affect the other? And what of infection? What does it mean to be infected by the catastrophes of the world, Real and imagined? And to be infected by or with the other in front of us, the other within us, the novel other invading our planet and everyone who comes into our consulting rooms simultaneously but not in the same way as we had once believed?

The gods of the old world, the patriarchy, and the principles upon which they structured society and the ruling principles of progress, capitalism, and individualism, are dissolving before our eyes. Simultaneously, the rush in the collective to carry on "as normal," turning a blind eye to the global and irrevocable consequences we are suffering, accentuates dysregulation, fragmentation, and simply feeling, "not well." "What am I doing wrong?" is the pervasive question amongst the majority of my patients nearing the end of

DOI: 10.4324/9781003266402-20

this current pandemic. Though the context out of which this question arises varies greatly from patient to patient, Hillman (1982) describes this as the realistic effects of the external world somatized within each individual patient.

How has this global moment affected the analytic endeavor? The convergence of the global pandemic caused by the novel coronavirus and the raise of hate crimes across the globe over the past year and a half, have exposed the inherent structural racism and white supremacy in every aspect of daily life in America. To me, this global moment, and the way it has affected the city in which I live, and the lives of the patients I work with in a predominately lower income neighborhood, call for a radical reconceptualization of the ethical responsibility of the analyst in and out of her office. I propose that one ethical response to our changing world is in a new formulation of the old analytic dictum, "The patient cannot go where the analyst has not gone." I propose, rather, a dual asymmetry in the analytic relationship where the patient, affected by the events in the world, takes the analyst where the analyst unknowingly needs to go but has not yet been able to go. Pressed further into the unknown as analyst and patient experience the events of the outer life contiguously, side by side.

For many years at the beginning of my training and throughout my first analysis, I held onto a conviction that real change may not in fact be possible. That the most we could hope for, that I could hope for, is for better alignment or adaptation to the inner and outer life. The work was to make conscious one's personal unconscious repressed material and to begin the lively process of deeply relating to contents of what Jung terms the collective psyche, aspects of Self that have not yet come into being. I know there is a Jungian perspective that holds that we are not working with individuals but rather, with objective psyche, and therefore the question of change is already the wrong question. However, once I began to see a full practice of individuals over the course of several years and then began a new analysis, myself, I was again haunted by the question of change. I began to feel that change was in fact possible even if I struggled to articulate how and if this desire to articulate how is, in and of itself, a betrayal of the analytic process.

I theorize that change is indeed possible and its possibility, the mutative agent, lies within the space between the intrapsychic processes of the analysand and analyst and the shared interpersonal relationship where consciousness about one's intrapsychic process becomes possible. The two, imaged initially in Jung's Personality #1, the interpersonal or the personality in the world in relation to others and to ideas, and Personality #2, the intrapsychic or the life of the inner world of the individual, inevitably influence one another, and are often substituted or one used as a displacement for the other, sometimes causing erasure, until a space is created between the two, through consciousness for both to exist in dialogue and in relation (Jung, 1989, pp. 87–88; Saban, 2019, pp. 5–30).

I understand the challenge in trying to hold this space between the interpersonal and the intrapsychic lives in one's relationship to hope. The space between the intrapsychic process of the patient and the intrapsychic process of the analyst collapses when the interpersonal experience in the transference gets identified with the projections or rigidified around an attachment to a particular outcome based on the analyst's hope. I have named this dynamic, or attachment to a particular outcome, as the seduction of hope. And I believe it is this seduction that may influence the analyst away from believing in and working toward the possibility of change.

If we did not have hope in our work, I am not sure we could sit with our analysands day in and day out. Especially during as dire a time as was during the height of the pandemic. And yet, hope can itself become a kind of stalemate to the work if held to as an ideal. If the satisfaction of hope is attached to a particular representation, without acknowledgment of the unknown, without acknowledgement of the mystery of becoming, it can lead to a stillbirth in the analysis. The hope many people put in the vaccine effort proved to be a similar such example. The hope that the world would open, and everything would go "back to normal," is what kept many people, those who were responsible for reporting information around the pandemic, from confronting the catastrophe that the global pandemic unveiled and kept pointing toward with one cultural example after another. The catastrophe that we, in America, have been functioning over for four centuries. With the push of the vaccine effort, America has become even more deeply divided and suspicious of one another and of those responsible for making decisions around daily life.

People seek treatment in the hope of healing, of feeling better, in an effort to change. Similarly, the analyst is often drawn into this vocation for these same reasons, to offer help, hope and healing. However, this eagerness, perhaps even desperation in the face of the other who sits in front of us, can pull the analyst out of her analytic stance. We can get seduced into a desire to help or to heal, a desire to help alleviate suffering. We can get seduced at the interpersonal level, seeking a representation of the satisfaction of our desire or an attachment to a particular outcome, foreclosing another kind of knowing that emerges through suffering. This desire, I suggest, might be a displacement of the analyst's own desire to feel, if not useful, at the very least relevant to the process of healing in the patient. This desire may also be born out of the real difficulty that comes with sitting in the unknown space, sitting with the mystery that is herself, sitting with her own infiniteness that threatens to swallow whole and ultimately betrays the radical otherness of the other in front of her and subverts the passion both necessary and spontaneously initiated from within the analyst toward the mystery of the subjectivity sitting before her.

I proffer, building on my previous work, illuminating the work of *yonic knowing* in contrast to *phallic understanding* as the source of another kind of knowing that has been pathologized, marginalized and called borderline, is a womb knowing predicated on not knowing or knowing from another source that is namely from the body and from the wordless, nameless place, the unknown space of becoming (Houck-Loomis, 2021). Yonic or womb knowing also holds a space for potential without possessing it or claiming the capacity (or right) to know (Chetrit-Vatine, 2004, p. 843). What Chetrit-Vatine (2004, p. 845) names as, "a space for her in me: a matricial space." Matrice meaning womb. What I have called the capacity for a womb of one's own (Houck-Loomis, 2021).

It is in this space the passion of the analyst seduces the patient deeper into his/her/their own process of becoming, into a relationship with the Self, the transcendent other that is both personal and beyond the personal. It is simultaneously this same space that the analyst, if open to her ever unfolding and becoming, is affected by the patient and taken down deeper into her own process allowing for mutual penetration, and individual becoming. As Luce Irigaray (2019, p. 11) says,

> To assume our particularity, we create a void which does not correspond to a lack but to that which allows us to shape a place of our own thanks to which we can open up to the other without relinquishing ourselves. It needs such a void to take place in us, and between us, in order that we should permit the other to appear as other and our presence to one another…. Desire reopens the place which was allocated to us by the world into which we came.

The capacity to literally and concretely bear life within me has informed my own clinical work and my own thinking about change in this specific way. When another life is being incubated within, a life that has both happened upon me and simultaneously been chosen by me, it evokes a host of associations, fantasies, and emotions. In analysis we can think of this as the initial call or email from 'out of the blue' and the acceptance of the new patient, agreeing to take her on and in. Who is this other life growing within me? What is my relationship to it? What will become of it in me and of me in it? What will become of us? Or not? Gestating another life brings with it a profound and enduring hope, a passion informed by desire, and an ethical responsibility to this other in me.

My ethical responsibility to the other, as I understand it, is to gestate hope for the potential within, without possessing an attachment to a particular fantasy about its becoming. Another way of saying this is that my ethical responsibility is to be expectant of the other's becoming without claiming knowledge of her, without "knowing her." It is a hope without an object, it is a void that is not lack but is potential. It is close to what Chetrit-Vatine (2004, p. 843) articulates using Levinas's (1998a, p. 156) idea of the caress. "The caress is not there to compensate or repair. It allows pain to free itself by itself. It allows the opening of a window. It points toward the existence of a future, a future that is forgotten in the moment of pain." As Levinas (1998b, p. 82) says, "The caress is awaiting that pure future with no content." As soon as I have a fantasy about what the other inside of me is going to be or become, I risk robbing it of its very own becoming. This is the betrayal of being known.

Having, myself, carried four pregnancies – two healthy children to term, one who came prematurely and did not survive and one who implanted in the tube and thus miscarried early on, and of these four only one was actually intended, sought and tried for – I know of the experience of gestating a potential, even an unexpected potential, of incubating the hope for this potential always with the knowledge that this potential may abort or terminate prematurely, or experience a still birth.

Incubating hope, in love, for the potential without robbing it of its own mystery and subjectivity, without betraying its capacity to know, be known, and not be known, in my view, is the work of the third, the space between the intrapsychic and the interpersonal, the space where the mystery lives and thrives in its own way and on its own time. This space, enabled by the interpersonal relationship between analyst and analysand, when held and not collapsed, allows for the analyst other to be affected within, in her own intrapsychic process by the intrapsychic process of the patient. The life that is within me, that I have made space for, is both of me and completely alien to me and what it will become, *if it will become*, is a mystery unto the both of us, a mystery that illuminates my own mystery of becoming. Fundamental in this experience is the capacity to equally hold onto life and death at the same time.

Perhaps there is no other moment than now to write about such things. At the time I am writing this, it has been one and half years since a foreign virus invaded our planet. An unknown content that has threatened life as we have thus known it, upending fantasies of invincibility and invulnerability amongst white people in the west, rattling our perceived organization around and by rationality. To hold both the symbolic and the literal, the intrapsychic phenomenon and the literal and concrete interpersonal phenomenon without collapsing the space in between without merging one with the other, I believe, enables the capacity to mourn and suffer the terror the most recent pandemic has elicited. *The capacity to hold life and death together, enables an incubation of hope without collapsing into an attachment for a particular outcome.*

It is the paradox that is illuminated each morning after my ashtanga practice as I chant, "May all beings be free from suffering, May all beings be free of disease, may all beings know happiness," while consciously holding in mind and heart the reality that at the height of the pandemic in NYC death tolls soared above 800 a day and also holding in mind another fact that became more apparent and highlighted throughout our shutdown, that is, the atrocious rate at which Black bodies are the subject of police brutality. It is paradoxically holding the knowledge that our world was being ravaged by this virus, vast amounts of people were and are suffering from this disease and the economic consequences of this disease, and the racial inequality that this disease has brutally illuminated. My chanting that all beings be free from suffering does not preclude suffering, but rather it holds the paradox that allows for the third space wherein meaning is made, healing may be found in the active work of mourning, and a way forward coagulated. A space for the other has been made in me but the way that this other will affect me and be affected by me is not yet known. Its future is yet untold.

While the literal and psychic reality of contagion is real, and the stamina and aggressiveness of this particular virus is unmatched in comparison within our recent recorded history, this reality is met with significantly substantial fantasies of invincibility or immunity on the one hand and paralyzing fear met with complete isolation and quarantine on the other. Intra-psychically we may individually encounter the foreign element of the unconscious, that which penetrates us, silently, unexpectedly, and throws our entire life's course off its previously perceived trajectory, in a similar way. This is what Jung (2009, p. 264) refers to as our incapacity, the unknown element that invades us and demands our attention willingly or not. One tries her best to ward off such unwelcomed encounters by making plans for a future, plans that align with her conscious intentions, Personality #1. Unknown to her are her own depths, or Personality #2, that beckon her attention.

As Jung (1960, par. 130) says about the unconscious, "it is not this thing or that, it is the Unknown as it immediately affects us." When the alien element, that which is unknown and threatens death, literal perhaps, but symbolically a death to her former way of life, her previous world order is thrust into oblivion. What to make of one's previous intentions when life has been completely upended? How to hold the opposites now – life and death – together. How to hold this paradoxical space for the intrapsychic phenomenon of the moment while also attending to the real interpersonal, concrete reality that we are now seeing all of our patients virtually, that our patients are suffering physically as well as emotionally, financially, and psychically. How to hold this paradox when particular vulnerable communities are now even more vulnerable due to the literal threat of a literal virus ravaging communities who do not have access to the kind of quarantine space needed for safety not to mention adequate health care, testing or adequate food supply? How to hold hope for a healing from the suffering while acknowledging the devastation and inevitability of the suffering?

Interpersonally, what does this moment allow for us to see, how does it allow us to know differently? Considering the concrete reality of the external suffering, how do we, in the privacy of our own homes, allow ourselves to be affected by the intrapsychic reality of the patient through the screen without an attachment to the outcome of his/her/their treatment? I end this article with a series of questions rather than answers. For me, Jungian analyst, teaching faculty, writer, and single mother of two children at vastly different developmental stages during this pandemic, what became forever altered during this time, is the fantasy of analytic anonymity. The dual asymmetry, allowing myself to be taken where I had not known to go before, becoming both infected and affected simultaneously by the patient in front of me and by the events that occurred all around us over the past 18+ months, has opened new pathways of sitting with the other within me and the other in front of me paradoxically holding and letting go of hope for what may come.

References

Chetrit-Vatine, V. (2004). Primal seduction, matricial space and asymmetry in the psychoanalytic encounter. *International Journal of Psychoanalysis,* 85: 841–856.

Hillman, J. (1982). Anima Mundi: The return of the soul to the world, in *The Thought of the Heart, and, The Soul of the World*. Ashland, Ohio: Spring Publications.

Houck-Loomis, T. (2021). A womb of one's own: Trauma, the transcendent, and the transference in the borderline phenomenon. *Journal for Studies in Gender and Sexuality* 22 (1): 16–27.

Irigaray, L. (2019). *Sharing the Fire*. Cham, Switzerland: Palgrave Macmillan.

Jung, C. G. (1960). The structure and dynamics of the psyche. In H. Read, M. Fordham, G. Adler, and W. McGuire (eds), *The Collected Works of G. G. Jung* (Vol. 8).

Jung, C. G. (1989). *Memories, Dreams, Reflections*. New York, NY: Vintage Books.

Jung, C. G. (2009). *The Red Book*. New York: W. W. Norton & Company.

Levinas, E. (1998a [1948]). *From Existence to Existing*. Paris: Librairie Philosophique.

Levinas, E. (1998b [1947]). *Time and the Other*. Paris: PUF.

Saban, M. (2019). *'Two Souls Alas': Jung's Two Personalities and the Making of Analytical Psychology*. Asheville, NC: Chiron Publications.

Chapter 12

Jungian Analysts' Experiences of Working Online

John Merchant

Involvement in the IAAP's formulation of its 2020 questionnaire to members concerning the Covid-19 pandemic gave Merchant the opportunity to canvas the experiences of colleagues from around the world about working online. This chapter overviews their very personal responses which have been grouped thematically following a qualitative analysis. One common issue was the understandable adjustment to working online, especially if not an analyst's personal preference. Other experiences included a noticeable exhaustion factor with online work, particular ways of using the screen, the need for patients to find a confidential space for online sessions, adjustments to patients' personal preferences and how to respond to new referrals online. Overall, the analysts found that online work does not have to preclude a genuine analytic process (including transference and countertransference) and that often the "online disinhibition effect" actually enabled troublesome emotional material to be disclosed more easily online. It is encouraging that these personal experiences all align with previous research findings. Most importantly, the online experiences of colleagues indicate that a good enough analytic process can unfold so long as practitioners are aware of the media peculiarities involved and the adjustments these require.

As part of the IAAP's formulation of its 2020 questionnaire to members about the Covid-19 pandemic, I received input from 24 colleagues worldwide about their personal experiences. Following a qualitative analysis of this very engaging material, I grouped their answers thematically. One common issue was the (understandable) adjustment to working online. As USA1 said, "I have found it to be an adaptability curve," and adjustments included "patients seeing their analysts on the screen in a different environment" alongside "what happens to silence?" (Aust6); "being alone in the room with yourself" (Aust11); "the absence of body" and "[patients] showing me their rooms, homes and animals and that is interesting in its effect on them and on me!" (Aust5); plus "a different distance between myself and the patient" (Aust10). Hence Italy1 said,

> At the beginning of the lockdown, I needed to stop a short while, to understand what was happening in the world all around, to remain in the

DOI: 10.4324/9781003266402-21

silence of my home, to think and to find a way to go on with my practice. I needed time to think about how to arrange a new setting

adding later that "Skype analysis is a quite different kind of analysis, for me." And USA1 added,

At first, I couldn't 'feel' my patients emotionally. The main reasons, then, were the lack of actual eye contact and secondly the inability to see their whole bodies in motion. I realized how much I use my observations of and their somatic experience (in real time) as part of analytic communication. Then, I learned to slow way down and better pair my intuitive function more closely with my visual acuity. That made things flow infinitely better as I could see the more nuanced aspects of our interactions. That is to say, I began to 'feel and read' my patients, myself and our interactions – what a relief for both of us. By now, it's pretty seamless and rich.

The online process is undoubtedly "changing the way we conceive of analytic work," as Aust12 put it, but critically Aust6 highlighted it "does work" despite being "a very different experience."

The Screen

A further issue commented upon was seeing oneself on the screen. As Aust1 said,

A question I think worth exploring is the difference between platforms where the two participants are visible on the screen – that is there are two images – one of oneself, one of the other, on the screen simultaneously. I think this does a brain scramble, we are not used to processing relational connection this way [that is] looking at yourself and looking at the other – a sort of techno splitting.

As a practical response, Aust1 has been using the Coviu platform which is encrypted to protect privacy and has a "waiting room" with the option to turn off one's own image.

Further to, Italy1 said,

[Skype analyses] require a bigger effort in order to keep under control the various 'disturbing factors' that interfere with my listening, with my attention to what the patient brings. For example, looking at my image, inevitably catch[es] my attention and it happen[s] that I could think 'Oh, Gosh, what bad hair I have today!'

Aust2 went further, saying they "only do tele-analysis because the screen is not just off-putting, but is experienced as 'aggressively intrusive' [Ladson

Hinton's 2020 phrase]." They were uncomfortable closing their eyes while sitting in front of a close screen for it interfered with their reverie.

Similarly, NZ3 said, "I find it challenging and a little disconcerting to have such close proximity to the on-screen other as the usual physical distance in the consulting room is much greater than that of face-to-face online." And Aust12 said "I can concentrate better when using the phone" because the phone does not have "technical glitches such as bad reception, pixilation, people looking in the wrong direction" or the disjunctive angles of the client's screen. In a similar way Aust5 found, "reverie and silence can be marred by – 'are they still there?'; 'have we been cut off?'" In terms of the "glitches," Aust8 emphasised the need for "a few back-up plans."

Related to the "brain scramble" Aust1 mentioned, USA2 only works by phone,

> [I] find that Zoom is simply too confusing – the images are not quite 'right.' The data my brain is collecting – body language, tone of voice, etc. is untrustworthy. It has the illusion of eye contact, but of course, it is not actual eye contact. It is a video watching a video. This situation makes me feel more and more dissociated. All of this is fine, if exhausting, for a meeting … but I am not offering video analysis to my analysands because I would have to continually adjust and remind myself that the visual information is off and then my focus would be in the wrong place. Or, worse, I would be reacting to a false image and then I would be off in the analysis itself…. Perhaps this is because I am a visual person, perhaps it is that I depend to a large extent on the actual feelings in the transference field in the room. Whatever the personal situation, I am only working by phone. That is also not ideal of course, but it is much easier for me to concentrate and there is an intimacy that several of my analysands have spoken about that is useful.

These comments highlight that the screen can have a sense of "illusion" to it and that one's own image can be distracting. Participants' adjustments become required, either by opting for tele-analysis or activating alternate platforms like Coviu where screen images can be monitored.

Exhaustion

It is noticeable that USA2 (above) used of the word "exhausting" in relation to Zoom, an experience not that uncommon, for Aust6 also said "it's exhausting" and Aust5 said, "working online is demanding in all sorts of ways. At the end of the day I am done in." Furthermore, NZ2 said, "I find that using the phone or other online mediums is more demanding on my energies and discernment; and more difficult to foster and respond to silence than in an embodied encounter."

It would appear, however, that the demand on energy is not limited to screen work, for USA2 also said,

While working on the phone, I find it harder to remember the sessions and I have to take extensive notes, unlike in-person. I am sure this has to do with the total experience of in-person work being simply more memorable, as all the senses are activated and the interpersonal field phenomena in the transference is so alive.

So online fatigue is likely to be another issue about which analysts need to be aware, and therefore to include appropriate arrangements in their schedules.

Personal Attributes/Preferences

Another issue USA2 highlighted (above) is the place of the personal attributes of the analyst (as in "I am a visual person"). On this theme, Aust3 who had been doing tele-analysis for decades said,

> I am aided in working by phone by being a trained musician with a very responsive ear, so the duration and intensity of an intake of breath conveys something to me just as does a pause mark on a music score.... I sometimes work for short periods with my eyes shut because the voice, breath and possible silences tell me far more than the body arrangement or movement.

Furthermore, Italy1 said, "Skype analysis can – likely – be useful, efficient, but often, for me, it involves a lack of information and requires, at the same time, a greater effort to control factors of disturbance, [it] clearly depends on Psychological Types!" And also "I suffered listening to many of my colleagues who had been able to do a sudden switch from the traditional setting to Skype," again indicating the place of personal preferences.

The personal preference of patients in terms of the screen (or not) was also noted by a number of analysts. Such preferences need to be explored to determine the best modality for them. Patient preferences could possibly be due to the "respective character of each therapeutic alliance" (Aust3) but also to the nature of previous in-person sessions (as in use of the couch or chair) for noticeably, Italy2 said their patients "preferred to use the telephone instead of Skype, perhaps because most of them were used to the couch, so we didn't look in each other eyes." In fact, two of their patients said they preferred the telephone "because they felt freer without my gaze on them."

Despite personal preferences, individual adjustments can be made as Italy1 said,

> I know, by doing some Skype analysis, that I can also work switching on other modalities: this requires a different perspective from me, a different way of listening – in these cases, working on images is, absolutely, the main instrument I have.

Patients can also adjust as Italy2 added, "soon ninety per cent of patients were enthusiastic about remotely working" and one of their patients, "At the end of lockdown, proudly smiling said [they] had improved [their] relationship with the telephone" which had previously been negative. For many patients, adapting to online work has probably occurred because lockdowns have required it in their own occupations. As Aust4 succinctly stated, "Many [patients] have also shifted to working online themselves so it has been useful that this transition has been so prevalent, the shift has been normalised" adding that "most people are surprised how well the process goes."

The Positives

The above comments highlight that online analysis can be productive, which aligns with previous research (Merchant, 2016; 2021). Indeed, NZ1 said their online work with an overseas patient was "profound and effective," mentioning the patient's "readiness" and the "chemistry (transference/counter-transference)" between them which

> resulted in a series of dreams, and intra/inter- psychic shifts that have significantly transformed [the patient's] life. Words fail to convey the magnitude of what has unfolded. I do believe psyche itself, lives through us. It is not confined by the limitations of the temporal world, including distance. This is truly Jung!

Similarly, USA2 (above) said "there is an intimacy [in tele-analysis] that several of my analysands have spoken about that is useful." And previous research has shown that such intimacy can foment disclosure, what Suler (2004) calls the "online disinhibition effect." As an example, Italy1 said,

> unexpectedly, during a Skype session, a patient talked, for the FIRST TIME, of a very important part of [their] childhood, never mentioned before. From that moment, a new path opened for us.... I guess that Skype, by keeping us in distance, could reassure that patient about the managing of the affects connected to [their] telling the story.

Italy3 found something similar in that "the modality of the therapy (phone vs presence) had a huge impact on the analytic material – over the phone, [the patient] expressed bursts of rage towards [their] family members," which had never occurred in-person. In a related way, NZ2 said of one patient "Over the last three sessions by phone this person has broken through a significant trauma which was constellated by the phone experience." Significantly, one of Aust12's patients said with tele-analysis they felt as though "'I was really inside [their] head' which gave [them] a strong sense of being received and attended to and this enhanced the relationship." Furthermore, Aust5 said "I actually prefer the intimacy of the phone and find my countertransference much more available there."

These comments align with research findings, for online analysis can facilitate positive outcomes through communication of primitive affects and it does not preclude transference/countertransference. Noticeably, Ann Casement (2021, p. 148) confirms this in her new book *Jung: An Introduction*,

> From my long experience over many years of using Skype, Zoom, and/or the telephone for sessions … there has been no difficulty whatsoever in experiencing alchemical transformation by these methods. In other words, alchemy and tele-analysis are completely compatible as technology is no hindrance to the production of *regression, incestuous longings* and *transference-countertransference*.

Indeed, online "alchemical transformation" was also experienced by Aust9,

> I am finding the symbolism of alchemic process to be helpful in amplifying the predicaments of isolation, confinement and pressured constriction, as well as the heating up of psychic life. Alchemy's analogies with 'movements of the soul' are useful. The continuities of analysis, and its sealed vessel (even via Zoom), have become more explicitly containing.

Importantly, there has been a suggestion from colleagues that the pandemic could have aided analytic work, even if done online. As Italy1 said,

> I have seen that the dreams my patients brought in analysis, during this period are definitely deeper, richer in significant and more powerful images. I wonder if the threat and the danger for life that daily was/is around us could help patients to be more open to their unconscious world.

Similarly, Aust9 found that "an *intensifying* of the work has been one notable effect of the switch to phone/online sessions for more than half the people I see…. Dream life has revved up. People are more amenable to/keen on active imagination." And NZ2 said, "the current restrictions provided an acceleration of their process" whilst Italy2 noted that "the lockdown was for me and my patients a great opportunity to experience ourselves in extreme situations and to use our creativeness."

Confidentiality

Confidentiality was a further issue colleagues raised. Aust7 said, the "most significant issue for me (and clients) is the security of whatever platform one uses." However, more colleagues commented on patients having to organise their own private/confidential space, as Aust4 said,

Most clients are unconcerned about confidentiality of the platform – they are more concerned about confidentiality in their own homes and lots of people are sitting in their cars talking to me.

Italy1 said during their lockdown "Most of my patients had difficulties to find a private space at home, or they felt not at ease with Skype." Similarly Aust5 said that organising a "private space in the house is sometimes difficult" and Aust8 has "one or two patients who find it hard to find a private place at home." As such, Aust10 has noticed patients' "inability to feel completely private."

These comments highlight the need to work with our patients, not only in finding a confidential space from which to make online contact but whether it would be preferable to use a platform like Coviu which encrypts and protects confidentiality.

New Patients

Regarding new patients, Aust4 said "newest clients are the most difficult to work with remotely. The embodied holding is more fragile." However, USA2 who is only doing tele-analysis said, "I even began a new treatment by phone – rather amazing!" and this seemed to be working. It would appear this issue could be patient specific.

Conclusions

We are currently in challenging times. The Covid-19 pandemic has been ongoing since early 2020 and Estes and Thompson (2020) maintain we could be in "a collective continuous traumatic stressor" (p. S31). Significant adjustments have thereby been required of analysts both in their personal lives and in their capacity to work online. Working online is not just a flow-on issue due to enhanced technology for in the pandemic it has become a necessity, even for those analysts who do not prefer it. Noticeably from the themes summarised above, many analysts have not only had a similarity of personal experience but these themes do align with findings from previous research. Most importantly, the online experiences of our colleagues indicate that a good enough analytic process can unfold so long as practitioners are aware of the media peculiarities involved and the adjustments these require.

Acknowledgements

I am extremely grateful to my Jungian analyst colleagues who so willingly shared their experiences that underpinned this chapter. They are Dr Sue Austin; Annie Boland MD; Dr Stefano Benegiamo; Patrick Burnett; Dr Glenda Cloughley; Amanda Dowd; Rachael Feather; Jacinta Frawley; Dr Sheena Gallocher; Dr Chiara Giubellini; Andrew Gresham; Dr Sally Kester;

Margaret Klenck MDiv; Anna Mangion; Julia Meyerowitz-Katz; Joy Norton; Dr Judith Pickering; Dr Susan Pollard; Lorraine Richards; Joy Ryan-Bloore; Adj. Prof Les Stein; Andre Zanardo and Luisa Zoppi.

References

Casement, A. (2021). *Jung: An Introduction*. Bicester, UK: Phoenix Publishing House.
Estes, K. & Thompson, R. (2020). Preparing for the aftermath of Covid-19: Shifting risk and downstream health consequences. *Psychological Trauma: Theory, Research, Practice, and Policy* 12: S1,S31–S32.
Hinton, L. (2020). Personal communication.
Merchant, J. (2021). Working online due to the Covid-19 pandemic: A research and literature review. *Journal of Analytical Psychology* 66 (3): 484–505.
Merchant, J. (2016). The use of Skype in analysis and training: A research and literature review. *Journal of Analytical Psychology* 61 (3): 309–328.
Suler, J. (2004). The online disinhibition effect. *Cyberpsychology & Behavior* 7 (3): 321–326.

Chapter 13

Saying "Goodbye" over Zoom
On Termination During Covid

Jon Mills

In a most personalized narrative, Jon Mills reflects on his career as a psychologist and psychoanalyst in his final days of terminating with his long-term analytic patients after he decided to retire from practice during the age of Covid-19. Personal meanings and style of work are accounted in an original way. Some typical themes connected to termination emerged: ambivalence, abandonment, anxiety, anger, regression, feelings of loss and lack, and for a couple of people, relief – finally they could fly from the nest. The year helped structure the work, resistances were lessoned as the clock kept ticking toward the end. The author's musings on the end of analysis, the nature of the client-therapist relationship, and the gift of mutual recognition are emphasized during the final session of therapy in an emotionally moving depiction of the termination process. During the final month, he accounts he had some beautiful interpersonal moments with his patients, reflecting on their life, growth, and their relationship, but he felt the final session produced the most moving personal experiences. All these 'goodbyes' occurring on the backdrop of the global Covid crisis.

Myths of Termination

There are many myths about terminating therapy with patients, such as a successful analysis leads to the resolution of clinical symptoms or internal conflict. Yeah, right. Another is you end up identifying with your analyst. Heaven forbid. And forbid the thought that you should be happy. As Freud reminds us, the most we can hope for is to turn neurotic misery into ordinary unhappiness. None of this is actually true, or if so, only in proportional ways. Analysis never ends even when therapy is over, because no human being can be fully self-actualized. That is another myth. So is achieving wisdom. Insight into oneself and life is a laborious process of becoming; just some of us are more successful at it than others. But even then, we all harbor anxiety – about our lives, careers, relationships, family, children, money, society, the state of world, and our own health as we face our being toward death. It is mainly for this latter reason that I decided to retire. Because I am going to die, I want to live my life more fully, richly, as every decision you make takes away from something else more meaningful you could

DOI: 10.4324/9781003266402-22

choose to do instead. I can already see myself on my deathbed staring back at me, a lifetime passed in a blink.

And what is "analysis" anyway? Who is analysing what, and who? Is this merely a pretentious word for what we do – think and talk? And the narcissistic cult of who deems you worthy to practice psychoanalysis or conveys such a title is another myth under the banner of exclusionary proprietary rights. How often do we hear colleagues' gossip about others, saying "He is not an analyst"? Here the frequency and furniture wars are no stranger to Jungians.

Those Who Suffer

In truth, I never referred to my clients directly as "patients," even though they suffer (*pathos*). In my private practice I never liked being so formal to present myself as "doctor." In fact, my typical dress was a flannel shirt, jeans, and a pair of Crocks. I never referred to them as "clients" either, just by their first name as individuals needing to talk about their troubles. The notion of "treatment" is even a misnomer. I never treated anyone. I just listened and engaged in dialogue. Listening, asking questions, communicating. A relationship would naturally ensue if they stayed with me.

But sadly, in my experience, most therapy is a commodity exchange. The public purchases your professional services like it were a consumer product, expecting to get exactly what they want, much like getting an oil change, only then to be surprized when no quick fix can be purchased or guaranteed. In these situations, there is little to no recognition of you as a person. Endings are rather informal, simply a business transaction despite being pleasant and perhaps showing some appreciation for your help. Having vain concerns over my narcissism hardly entered the picture. People paid me to listen and speak. When they felt they had gotten something from it, or when their symptoms became more tolerable, they left, unless their insurance ran out. Then they simply stopped coming. They ended the therapy. Here I provided a function: money is exchanged, and I am no more valued than what I can offer them that hour, like an expensive night out for dinner.

As a clinical psychologist, I saw over a thousand people in my career, in a variety of different settings and capacities. As a psychoanalyst, I had a small caseload in my later years. But when I decided to retire during the age of covid, I had only been seeing my long-term analytic cases, some for 20 years. Like most therapists, when the international lockdowns happened, we immediately shifted to sessions over the phone or by videoconferencing. For me, I preferred Zoom. In some ways that made ending more intimate yet surreal: virtual reality is not in the flesh, but when you are in the same boat together, we make due. In other ways, it also made it easier for some, as our virtual presence allowed for some emotional distance. But for other patients, I got the distinct feeling that we were both being robbed of something important. Discussing our mutual experience of ending this way was largely avoided. No one likes to face finality, even when seeing each other on a computer screen. We run from it whenever we can in order not to have to say "goodbye."

All of my patients had profound developmental traumas, most of them with entrenched character pathology, or they would not have likely stayed with me for so many years. Facing the uncertainty of when society would return to the new abnormal, I gave everyone one year notice of my pending retirement so we could work toward a proper termination. Given I have never done this before, and only having my own experience of ending my own analysis, I was surprised by some typical themes that emerged, which could have been out of a textbook. Ambivalence, abandonment, anxiety, anger, regression, feelings of loss and lack, and for a couple of people, relief – finally they could fly from the nest. The year actually helped structure our work – resistances were lessoned as the clock kept ticking toward the end. The work suddenly became more intense and deepened due to the call of finality. No patient wanted a referral: they had gone too far to start all over with a stranger, and they knew it would not be the same with a new therapist. "No one could replace you. Time to go it alone," as one of them put it, the culmination of their individuation process. Hearing that felt very satisfying, was natural, and in my opinion, healthy.

The Gift of Recognition

During the final month, I had some beautiful interpersonal moments with my patients, reflecting on their life, growth, and our relationship, but I felt the final session produced the most moving personal experiences for me. A psychoanalyst friend of mine Rick Hansen once told me that at the end of a more or less successful therapeutic collaboration, the patient should be able to realize and appreciate the burden that the analyst has borne during their work together. He told me of a severe borderline woman he had been seeing in analysis for 25 years who, following a tempestuous interchange, said spontaneously, "You know, I don't know how you tolerated me at times when I would go off on you. I would have thrown me out!" He said that he had rarely felt more loved and appreciated as an analyst in that moment.

There are instances of recognition that hardly ever happen where we truly feel valued as a person. His experience reminded me of when I once told a severely disturbed patient after being routinely verbally devalued, nearly every week, that "No one would put up with 4 years of emotional abuse from you than me." She immediately became remorseful and said, "I know, I'm sorry, thank you" and started to cry. Sometimes guilt inducement and shame are an unavoidable part of being human. This was a turning point in the therapy.

We as therapists bear the brunt of all of our clients' internal pain, trauma, acting out, aggression, and deprecation with affective costs to our own psyches and physical health. When patients are able to come to their own realization of what you have done for them and show gratitude, it produces a shared emotional joy in being recognized that is deeply affirming and validating, as is mirroring your appreciation for their recognition. I was grateful for these departing gifts.

The Final Session

Mitchell and all of his siblings were subjected to horrific developmental trauma as children at the hands of a sadistic father who was an abusive psychopath and who terrified the family during drunken rages. Mitchell had developed alopecia in elementary school and became the laughingstock of his class. He went bald rapidly and his father insisted he get hair implants, which made matters ripe for more ridicule. As the target of bullying, Mitchell had identified with the aggressor and developed a violent persona. He was constantly in fights and mischief. He soon became the displaced object of ritual beatings by his father for his oppositional defiance.

Generally you become unconsciously the very thing you think you have escaped from. Mitchell had become his father. By the age of 20, he was in Alcoholics Anonymous, had already slit both of his wrists, and ended up in a psychiatric ward. When he came to see me, he was in his 50s, had a volatile marriage, and owned a demolition business. He looked like Mr. Clean: completely bald, no eyebrows, and was a solid piece of muscle.

"I don't even have a hair left on my ass," he said acerbically.

Every other word that came out of his mouth was "fuck." His marriage was falling apart and he was involved in physical altercations with his teenage son who had become just like him. He knew he had become an unsavory person and had hated himself for it. He could not rid himself of that atrocious gap in being left at the hands of his father. He was tormented by the sundry traumas he endured during childhood including being forced to break the wings of a whole flock of ducks while his father watched howling in hysterical laughter with a beer can glued to his hand. Despite his own abusive tendencies and suicidal depression, Mitchell stayed sober, worked on his traumatic past, and improved his marriage. Over the years I watched as his business flourished and his son joined the company.

In our final session I asked Mitchell to reflect on the time in his life when he first came to see me and what had changed in his personality since then.

"I think I have become a better person, at least better than I was. I did so many awful things. I have more empathy for others now than I used to." He also unexpectedly added, "I want to thank you for putting up with all my bullshit over the years." We both smiled and laughed. Here he knew the stress I had to bear in working with him for so long.

I told him that I was glad to be a part of his life and he of mine. "You take care of yourself Jon."

Lily came to see me after she started to develop posttraumatic symptoms following being verbally harassed by her boss at work. Lily was repeatedly physically, verbally, and emotionally abused by her mother during her entire childhood. She was never shown love, recognition, or emotional warmth, physical affection or hugs, and was constantly subjected to her mother's verbal tirades, explosive rages, and physical beatings when she did not do exactly what she was supposed to do or in performing domestic tasks. Lily could never anticipate or know when her mother would become erratic: she would spontaneously fly into rages and start beating her with kitchen utensils or her fists, and was fond of throwing objects while in the kitchen. Lily was once taken to the hospital when she was hit in the back of her head with a knife her mother had thrown. She was forced to say she had fallen and cut her head.

Although Lily survived her childhood, it left an engrained, traumatized internal structure where she was prone to unpredictable rages, verbal devaluation of others, and unprovoked violence just like her mother. By the time she was an early adolescent, she had gotten involved in drugs, organized a small youth gang who broke into houses to get money, and burned down a lumber yard. After being convicted for arson, she stole her father's car and ran down the local prosecutor while walking on the street. She was sentenced to a youth corrections facility, where she resided until she was 18 years of age. She then was homeless, lived on the street, sold drugs, and "did anything to survive." In retrospect, Lily thought this was the only way she could escape her mother's constant abuse.

Remarkably, Lily was "saved" by the Salvation Army, was taken into their physical and spiritual care, educated, and went on to earn a graduate degree in one of their religious college affiliate institutions in the United States. She then returned to Canada as a professional adult and entered a successful career until the precipitating events with her boss brought on feelings of reliving her childhood abuse. Her conflicts at work started to trigger her chronic, complex unresolved trauma, which led to unrestrained swearing and devaluation of others, episodes of road rage, and the repeated physical battery of her husband, including even chasing him around the house with a knife – in the kitchen nonetheless, a return of mother.

Lily had seven miscarriages. She was never able to have children, which added to the void of her emotional pain. One included a tubal pregnancy where the fetus had died and required emergency attention, which she could not accept, hence necessitating a temporary hospitalization after becoming delusional. Then she got thyroid cancer. At this time, I began to see her 5 days a week. She eventually recovered after treatment and later retired from her job after winning a judgment from her workplace harassment complaint.

"I can never thank you enough." she said in our final session. "You are the only person in my life who was there for me. I want you to know that you really made a difference. I'll never forget what you've done," she continued.

"You are a beautiful person Lily" I replied, both of us looking at each other with tears in our eyes, "and I will always keep you close to my heart."

Three of my patients said that if it was not for me, they "would have committed suicide." I found this to be the ultimate form of confirmation and numinous experience of my career. Those few words seemed to instantly validate my existence and dissolve any ambivalence I had going into the profession. As one of them said, "I owe my life to you. I would have killed myself if it wasn't for you." This later brought me to tears thinking how I could play such a significant role in another's life, and also how sad that I was needed in this way. It is this type of obligation that is foisted on any therapist even unwittingly. I never presumed responsibility for others' lives, let alone being a lifeline or keeping them from killing themselves.

Bill came to me after having fantasies of putting a gun in his mouth. He was a career cop who felt persecuted at work and targeted by his superiors for his strong opinions, attitude problem, confrontational demeanor, and anti-social tendencies that led to him being disciplined and removed from his duties as a detective. Having been stripped of his professional identity and personal self-worth, he was contemplating murder-suicide.

Beneath the despair, helplessness, hopelessness, and need for revenge, was a sordid and traumatic past. Bill was unconsciously impelled to become a cop because his father beat his mother during drunken stupors in his presence, and he felt paralyzed as a little boy unable to protect his mother while witnessing such traumas unfold. But the dark side of Bill, the shadow of his father, left its own pathological debris.

Bill was twice divorced and estranged from his extended family, including his only daughter. He was emotionally stoic with a rigid moral outlook, especially during acts of dispensing justice. The public were treated by him in a criminal manner including physical abuse and threats of death and violence during police engagement. Plagued by paranoia, suicidal depression, and night terrors, he had done many terrible things and suffered from unconscious guilt and the need to be punished. Throughout his career he was in several high-speed criminal pursuits that led to many severe accidents including seven concussions, head injury, herniated discs, and a heart attack, hence necessitating the need to go on medical leave and enter into rehabilitative recovery several times. He was also shot at, survived a knife fight, and about got his head decapitated from a Samurai sword during an apartment raid on a domestic dispute call. Rather than talk to others about his symptoms and the effects of his trauma, an unspoken prohibition in police culture, he drank himself to sleep every night.

Seventeen years later, Bill is now retired and became a vegetable farmer living a quiet existence alone with his dogs in the country. Looking back at his life and our work together in our final session, he thanked me for saving his life.

"It's been a privilege to know you, Bill. You're a good man."

At that moment, I picked up a wooden pen off my desk and said, "Thank you. I'll never forget you."

When he saw the pen, one he made in his workshop and gave to me as a gift after first coming to see me, his face froze. He saw that I valued him and he knew that I knew; then tears came to our eyes. It was the first and last time I ever saw him cry.

"Goodbye Jon."

Chapter 14

Impact of the Pandemic on my Therapeutic Practice

Marianne Müller

In this chapter, Müller discusses her professional experiences as a psychotherapist during the acute period of the pandemic. In her practice, she experienced significant differences in how clients reacted to the new life situation with its restrictive conditions and the looming threat: many in the form of anxiety, stress, depression, addictive behavior, uncontrolled emotional outbursts, intensified inner and outer conflicts, and more. This depended on various factors, e.g. the economic situation or the housing conditions, but also on the inner psychological structure of the patients and their ability to deal with prolonged uncertainty, and on the available resources and how the person in question was able to utilize them. Her thesis is that the pandemic triggered many fears. She observed above all a greater stress-related tension, through which already existing deficits or disorders became more noticeable. Various therapy situations are presented. Emphasis is placed on issues of the setting and, in particular, on online sessions. She makes reference to the large number of younger clients who came into therapy during the pandemic. The impact of the pandemic on the therapeutic process is considered separately, as well as the question of the analytic attitude in this particular time.

As I write my contribution to this publication, we have been living with the pandemic for almost two years. The Covid-19 virus has put not only the physical health of humans at risk, but also their mental health, indeed it has hit them directly and hard. I experienced this first-hand and clearly in my psychotherapeutic practice. Not only was there suddenly a greater need for psychotherapeutic care, a much greater number of requests for therapy and analysis, but also a strikingly large number of young or even very young adults were seeking support and help.

I am now writing about my professional experiences as a psychotherapist during this time, and I am trying to place them in a larger context with a few general considerations.

Like hardly any threat before, the pandemic was a topic in all therapies, at the latest from the moment it reached our country and the state had taken first mild then drastic measures for the safety of the population. Most clients

DOI: 10.4324/9781003266402-23

felt safer and more protected, accepted the sometimes painful restrictions and were grateful that the state took responsibility and gave them guidelines on how to behave. In my practice, there were only a very few who rebelled against this and expressed this during conversations in therapy.

In the beginning, the pandemic was a great unknown, unresearched in its effects and extent. This caused fear, triggered stress and was very unsettling. Science was initially unable to provide any clear information, changed its assessment of the danger and nature of the virus, and therefore also of recommended behavior. Government measures, motivated by health, social and political factors and prioritised with different intentions and goals, also varied depending on the state and situation, and in our country partly depending on the canton or even region. This contributed to further uncertainty.

In my practice, I experienced significant differences in how clients reacted to the new life situation with its restrictive conditions and the looming threat. Although all were affected in some way, they showed different psychological effects, many in the form of anxiety, stress, depression, addictive behavior, uncontrolled emotional outbursts, intensified inner and outer conflicts, and more. Some were able to recover over time and adjust themselves to the new situation, finding support in inner strength despite external insecurities. Some even mustered the courage and strength to tackle something that was new for them. Others, on the other hand, were able to deal with it relatively easily at first, adapting to the changed situations. At the beginning, they appreciated the opportunity to retreat, to slow down and reflect on the essentials, but they were then caught up again by their personal disturbances at a later stage. This depended on various factors, e.g. the economic situation or the housing conditions, but also on the inner psychological structure of the patients and their ability to deal with prolonged uncertainty. It also depended on the available resources and how the person in question was able to utilize them. In many cases, the prolonged restrictions, the lack of social contacts and the continuing uncertainty caused additional stress. In short, this pandemic has been quite stressful and challenging for all of us in one way or another.

My thesis is that the pandemic triggered many fears. They were first of all a healthy reaction to a really dangerous situation. This natural fear reflex made it possible for individuals to take the necessary precautions in the first place. Fear was then also a topic in many therapies, but in the form of an anxiety symptomatology and corresponding pathology no more frequently than before. I observed above all a greater stress-related tension, through which already existing deficits or disorders became more noticeable. This also led to more and a different range of people coming into psychotherapy.

I will now describe in more detail the changed therapeutic situation as a result of the pandemic as I experienced it in Switzerland, on the basis of three factors: setting, topics, process. I focus here in particular on the changes in this regard due to the pandemic.

Setting

In Switzerland, it was possible to see patients in the practice and conduct face-to-face sessions throughout the pandemic. I provided this setting; only in Zurich, where I work one day a week, I offered only online sessions for six weeks. In summary, I can say that most of my patients made use of my presence offer and came to the practice. However, I always kept open the option of conducting the sessions online. I myself never explicitly stated that I preferred one or the other. In retrospect, I am surprised that almost all clients preferred the session in the office. This may also have something to do with the small size of Switzerland and the city of Berne. My practice is located in the middle of the city, it can be entered on the first floor, I always take a break of at least fifteen, often thirty minutes between two clients, so that they do not have to cross and meet each other. This way the clients felt safe and so did I.

I am aware that just by being open in my choice of setting, I made some impact on the patients. But in doing so, I also preserved a piece of normality. In addition, in my practice, masks were obligatory only from January 2021 until the end of June 2021. Before and after that, I left it up to the clients whether a mask was worn or not. Here, too, I certainly exerted influence by not insisting on mask wearing. Personally, I was very relieved when the obligation no longer existed. So, except for the six months, I worked mostly without a mask, but of course with a large distance between the chairs and always fresh air.

I would like to emphasize again that I always experienced the online session as a good alternative when face to face sessions were not possible. Indeed, there have been a few clients whom I have seen only online and with whom a helpful, supportive process was still possible. One pregnant client, with whom I worked only online, expressed great amazement but also gratitude in our last conversation before the birth of her child about what psychotherapy could do. Her strong emotional outbursts, no doubt exacerbated by the constraints of the pandemic, had brought her into therapy and compelled her to go through a painful but ultimately liberating process of coming to terms with herself. She had to deal with the background of her strong, uncontrollable emotions that had brought much suffering to her partnership. Through the intensive inner process it became possible for her to take more responsibility for her emotions, she learned to perceive them more consciously, to verbalize them as well, and thus gradually to regulate them better and better. Above all, she was able to place her strong emotional outbursts, which were not appropriate to the situation, much more clearly in her life history, and to unmask and recognize them in part as learned, inherited behavioral complexes. By understanding the function of the emotions more and more clearly, she was able to deal with them more consciously.

The process was accompanied by an intensive confrontation with her origins, from whose culture she had broken away after leaving her parental home for her studies. Previously, she had grown up in different cultures: until the age of 12, she lived in her distant country of origin, separated from her parents except during school vacations. At the age of 12 she moved to her parents and was transplanted into a completely different culture, whose language, values and code of conduct she did not know. She used all her energy to gain a foothold, but continued to live in the family in the traditions of origin. The various ruptures, which were also accompanied by violent conflicts and injuries in the family, now had to be explored and processed in therapy, if inner-psychic healing and reconciliation were to become possible.

The positive process was also astonishing for me and a new experience, especially since I had never seen the client in the therapy room. In the last session, she announced that she would come to my practice after the birth of her child. She was very much looking forward to that. For me, this statement was very understandable. For despite the positive progress, physical contact had been missing in this therapeutic work, so to speak. In my experience, for a deeper and more extensive psychological process, the shared physical presence in the same room is indispensable. It opens up another dimension to the encounter. Towards the end of our work, the client mentioned how it was fundamentally difficult for her to stand in front of someone, not to avoid them, and especially to be face to face with them. It was very enlightening for me that she expressed this and thus also the need for a direct, physical encounter, and also the desire to go one step further in the therapeutic process.

Recently, and especially since the pandemic, much has been written about the experiences and scientific findings of online therapies (Roesler, 2017, Merchant, 2021). These diverge and, in some cases, diverge quite widely. Some see a major shortcoming of online sessions in the lack of physical proximity, which complicates transference, unconscious communication, and countertransference (cf. Cwik, 2021, p. 415). Cwik himself sees telecommunications as a new form of therapy, with clear advantages and new possibilities, in which imaginative work plays an important role. He therefore resists a comparative approach with in-person analysis (Cwik, 2021, p. 416).

In this sense, the online sessions also had clear benefits for the previously mentioned pregnant client. With no direct or face-to-face confrontation she felt less inhibited. For her, the online sessions offered a new experience with new opportunities. They made it easier for her to enter therapy, as inhibiting patterns came into play much less for her in this setting. This shows the special character of online sessions, which are experienced very differently individually or depending on the interaction between analyst and analysand. In any case, they do not exclude the emergence of a therapeutic alliance that is so central to a positive course (Merchant, 2021, p. 8).

Basically, for me personally, the online sessions were easier with established clients who had come to my practice before, whom I knew, their physicality and their whole appearance and with whom I had already established a therapeutic alliance. I was better able to remember the online sessions with them and thus experienced more continuity with them as well. On the other hand, when someone I had initially only seen online for some time then came into my practice, I experienced this as a new beginning. Many of these clients then clearly preferred the sessions in the practice.

In general, I welcome the possibility of online therapy, as I said, whenever the real physical encounter is not possible and both conversation participants have a safe place available where they are not disturbed. Quite a number of clients wanted to come to the practice precisely because this condition could not be fulfilled for them, i.e. because they did not feel safe enough at home. For them, an online session was out of the question.

I remember a client who lived with her boyfriend in a two-room apartment where they both lived and worked during the lockdown. For her, an online session would never have been an option, partly because the cramped living conditions regularly led to conflicts in the partnership, so she did not feel safe enough within her four walls for a therapeutic conversation. For another client, an online session would have been out of the question because the entire family was home during the lockdown. For these people, the therapy room as a safe place had and still has a central importance, and this has become increasingly so. It was and is a place outside of the living situation, which no longer felt good due to multiple use. Some clients would have been undisturbed at home, but preferred to have another place for the therapy sessions and to leave the house for them. Surprisingly, this was also true for many people who basically like to retreat behind their four walls. Some had to protect this private space for themselves and struggled to provide insight in any way. This was especially true for analysands whose lives had always been strongly affected and also disturbed by fantasies. I am thinking of a patient who suffered from anorexia, or another who could get carried away with fantasies of jealousy and mistrust. They all needed the consulting room as a real safe place that only in this concrete form could also symbolically become a therapeutic container and field. I agree with Merchant's point that certain diagnoses are contraindicated for online therapy (Merchant, 2021, p. 13).

Topics

As I said before, the many clients who came to my practice during the pandemic came for just as many different reasons as before the pandemic. In contrast, I was surprised by the many younger people who suddenly appeared. They, too, brought their long-standing problems. However, because of the stresses of the pandemic, these came to the surface, distressed them, and needed to be dealt with. These were depressive symptoms, but also compulsions or eating disorders, some of which showed themselves for the first time in such severity or had recurred in a more acute form.

I had the impression that older clients were possibly more able to deal with the uncertainty of the pandemic due to their life experience. Younger people, on the other hand, were inhibited by it in their development, in that they could no longer casually meet with peers and have the vital social experiences appropriate to their age group. They felt reduced to the family environment from which they were about to break away.

The need for an emancipatory developmental step was even more clearly felt in the increased constriction. This was evident in the case of a young man in early adulthood who was still in apprenticeship and living with his parents. This was an extremely sensitive, introverted person, with hypochondriacal fears, but also social anxieties. These had led him to focus almost exclusively on education and his personal interests. Interaction with peers was minimal and even more limited by the pandemic, as the client was also required by his employer to work from home. It was finally his parents who asked him to take up psychotherapy because, as he himself said, he had become almost unbearable at home when dealing with his family. He himself was able to accept this challenge and engaged well in therapy. It even turned out that, due to his introverted nature, he felt comfortable and understood in an analytically oriented approach, because it was mainly about understanding and allowing needs, in great openness and freedom, without direct instruction in terms of behavior. His blockages could be released more and more and his individuality was given space to develop. The topics discussed in the sessions also occupied him between our meetings and enabled him to ask questions and to name and explore more and more openly psychological connections that he had been mulling over for some time. He became noticeably freer and his physical symptoms gradually changed as well. Despite the pandemic, he ventured to establish social contact with peers in a responsible manner, and was able to experience that other young people were dealing with similar questions and that he could even be an important discussion partner for one or the other with his thoughtful, sensitive manner. There were setbacks and self-doubts, as in every development process, but they could be discussed openly in the therapy.

What touched me most about this process was the fact that precisely because of the pandemic, a therapy became possible that mobilized deeper needs and allowed them to be implemented in life. This might have been more difficult to realize at a later point in time. By talking openly about his experiences in therapy, even with peers, this client motivated other young people to take their psychological problems seriously and to seek therapeutic help.

The impact of the pandemic was often particularly challenging for people with a low tolerance for fear and a high need for safety. For them, being uprooted from a familiar daily routine was particularly difficult. For them, the dangers of the pandemic were difficult to assess and contain; they mainly experienced the threat. I am thinking of a client who often wanted to know my opinion in therapy as to whether this or that behavior was dangerous or justifiable. Here it was particularly important to take the client's personal feelings and fears very seriously and also to elicit well the fantasies behind them. These usually led away from the concrete situation of the pandemic to the personal background. The fantasies and fears of familial catastrophe had already led in this patient's earlier history to great insecurity and readiness to conform. By re-experiencing the early distress and becoming aware of the connections, it was also possible to unmask the inhibiting fantasies and transform them into responsible, future-oriented attitudes. As a result, the client's thinking also became freer, less inhibited by anxiety, more inspired by future-oriented ideas and perspectives. This made it possible to act in a way that was appropriate to the situation, even during the pandemic.

The pandemic was particularly hard on people with a depressive disposition. This was often not apparent from the outset, and reactions were stronger or weaker in different phases. The home office mandate could even contribute to temporary relief from obligations at work, until a feeling of loneliness, isolation or abandonment took over more and more at home. Finally, there was a lack of regular social contacts, which had previously also often been experienced as exhausting. I witnessed that some clients were temporarily no longer able to cope with their daily work. They had to take sick leave and be treated with medication. In all of these cases, the effects of Covid-19, with its sense of insecurity and also stress, had exacerbated an already existing overload at work and, to some extent, they broke the camel's back. However, among other things, this also provided an opportunity to rethink the whole life situation.

Another client felt trapped at home with her family, having withdrawn from almost all social contact. In particular, she missed the exchange with friends and the family abroad, where she originally came from and where she used to travel regularly, which was now not possible. The longing for the culture of origin and its language, in which she felt at home, became almost unbearable. More and more, a feeling of foreignness set in, combined with the feeling of being enclosed, not free and almost imprisoned. Here, too, there were early personal experiences of abandonment and alienation in the background that went back a long way. It was a great challenge to take the current extremely difficult situation seriously in therapy and at the same time to relate it to the personal complex constellation and its history.

Death, which was so centrally present in this pandemic, also became a topic in my practice. Relatives of clients had died from Covid-19, and a close family member of a client had committed suicide during the pandemic. I will not dwell on this here, but note how central existential questions and the limitation of life were conjoined by the experience of the pandemic and had to become topics in a variety of ways.

Process

Did the pandemic affect the therapeutic process in any way? There were one or two clients who interrupted therapy with the initial lockdown. They came back to my practice at a later date. For one client, the realization that she was not really ready to enter into a therapeutic process clarified itself along the way. Some clients switched to online sessions at the first lockdown and then came back to the practice later. The therapeutic process could be maintained in this way, which was very valuable. The therapeutic field, the container, was also maintained in some way. I agree with August Cwik (2021, p. 415ff.) that with online therapy it became clearer how diverse the clients' co-creation of the framework for the analytic work was. They basically do this in every therapeutic process; however, the virtual insight of the online sessions into the client's life space makes this more conspicuous. This poses new challenges to the therapeutic interaction, which can also be understood as an imaginative process. Ultimately, however, there are many different reasons why some clients may feel comfortable in online sessions and others may not.

Some clients sought reassurance or help in making decisions about their behavior and living arrangements in therapy by asking questions, such as whether or not they could spend Christmas with their parents. Or they wanted to know in what form and under what circumstances they were allowed to meet with friends. I was assigned the role of the person in the know and an advisor. In these cases it was important to give space to the concerns and to look at the uncertainties without giving an answer, but to let the clients in their uncertainty find a way by themselves. Such reactions, often regressive, must and can be used for therapy, as can unconscious projections. Because dealing with transference and counter-transference is part of the important analytic tools even in these times, it is just as perceptible and applicable in online sessions (Roesler, 2017). At the same time, I too was personally confronted with the same questions as the clients. I could and wanted to relate not only to the transference situation, but also to contribute as a human being, as far as I considered this useful in the interest of the therapy.

Such an approach was particularly important with a younger client who was very insecure about her behavior during the pandemic. She did not want to endanger herself or others and therefore withdrew more and more behind her four walls. Among other things, she found it difficult to understand and accept when her boyfriend or other close caregivers behaved differently from what she thought was right. Strong emotions were aroused and first had to be understood and put in order in therapy. They had to do with their own insecurity and fear of making mistakes. She first projected these feelings onto others until she was able to recognize and admit their origin within herself. The clearer she was able to understand and put this dynamic in a context, the easier it was for her to take back the projections, to find her own point of view, and to deal with other perceptions. In our discussions, it also became clearer to her that, despite restrictions, everyone could and had to determine how they interpreted them and use their own sense of responsibility, even in the exceptional situation.

As a therapist, I, too, was naturally challenged to review my attitude again and again. I was aware that I represented a position simply by my behavior. So I made it clear that I had been vaccinated. At the same time, I relaxed the mask requirement again at the end of June 2021, after this was officially permitted, by initiating the discussion as to whether we wanted to continue wearing a mask during the session. Of course, I left the decision to the clients, but also made it clear that both were now possible and acceptable for me. It seemed important to me to address the handling of the pandemic in this way and also to look for a way together within the therapy hours.

I became aware that I had to examine my analytical attitude more carefully than usual. Of course, I was also affected by the pandemic as a human being, and it was sometimes difficult for me to maintain my restraint as a therapist, for example, when a denial of the pandemic became an issue. For more detail see my concluding remarks.

Mediation

Inner psychological pressure and the corresponding burden not only affected the state of mind of the individual, but also had a great influence on how people were living together. Since I myself am also a trained mediator, I received requests for family mediations in which dealing with Corona was the central topic. Here, too, already existing underlying tensions in the family led to explicit conflicts and the behavior which resulted, such as breaking off contact, refusing to talk, which made clarification with outside help necessary. For example, I experienced how in one family the different views on how to deal with the restrictive measures of the pandemic updated old feelings of being excluded, of not being respected, and triggered strong emotional reactions. In the mediation talks, the old hurts had to be named so that those affected were at all able to find a reasonable way of dealing with the current situation. Thanks to the willingness on all sides to listen to each other, the conflict was resolved within a foreseeable period of time. Of central importance was everyone's desire to place the family community on a new solid foundation, on which different opinions were permissible and a new culture of open exchange should and could be sought and cultivated in the future. Without mediation, an understanding of this kind would hardly have been possible.

It is well known how much events such as the Covid-19 pandemic also influences social coexistence. The personal assessment of the situation and the corresponding way of dealing with Corona differ from person to person, due to the personal attitude towards life, life experiences and other factors as unconscious inner-psychic conflicts, which become fixed in the outside. Polarizing and irrational opinions can endanger the harmonious coexistence and make an open discussion about the reasons for the personal attitude and thus also a mutual understanding impossible. However, as long as there is a desire for understanding, as in the example of the family mentioned above, ways can be found across seemingly unbridgeable divides. Behind the crises in family and partnership caused by the pandemic, there are always earlier injuries or ruptures. They must be listened to and taken into account in a mediation process. Finding solutions too quickly or even hastily often means that they are not sustainable.

Concluding remarks

I understand the therapeutic process as an interaction or, as Jung put it, a "mutual influence" (Jung, 1929, para. 163) between analyst and analysand. According to this, the therapeutic process unfolds between two subjects (cf. also intersubjectivity theory, Altmeyer and Thomä, 2010), who encounter and act on each other, with their conscious and unconscious parts. It is not a particular technique or method that is of primary importance, but what happens in the here and now. My attitude as an analyst is oriented towards this special interaction, taking into account transference and countertransference phenomena, and at the same time being aware of the asymmetry in this exchange, as well as the possibility of the analyst's fallibility. The whole process is oriented towards the well-being of the client. This extremely complex process has now been given a very special coloration by the pandemic.

As already mentioned, I as a human being was just as affected as my clients by the special situation of the pandemic. This was also reflected in the therapeutic interaction. I, too, was repeatedly faced with the question of how to deal with the current situation, for example, with regard to the setting. In this regard, there was room for maneuver that we had to clarify in therapy. Initially, it was the question of face-to-face or online sessions, later the wearing of masks, disclosure of the vaccination status or other things. There were no clear-cut answers. My guideline was to always critically observe and analyze my interventions. A few times, nevertheless, I found it difficult to maintain my restraint as a therapist to the extent I expected of myself, such as when pandemic denial became an issue.

I am thinking here of a client who had from the beginning been critical of the limitations due to the pandemic. He then became seriously ill with Covid, and also had to be treated in the hospital. Fortunately, he recovered. We knew of our different attitudes towards the government measures, but never returned to them after his illness. In one therapy session, he brought up the issue of vaccination on his own in a somewhat provocative manner. I showed astonishment that he was still unwilling to vaccinate, despite the serious illness, whereupon he went into a lengthy explanation and justification. I felt more and more uncomfortable with this and finally expressed my feelings. I explained that I respected his position and did not want to endanger our relationship by this conversation. Nevertheless, I would be very interested to know why he thought he had to take this particular position. Were there any reasons for this?

I had become very serious at that moment, I really wanted to understand. It amazed me then how he changed the level in the same seriousness and began to talk about the religious community to which he and his family belonged. Out of the experience of being met with incomprehension, he had increasingly avoided talking about it. Belonging to a minority, he often did not feel accepted and understood, neither by the majority of the population nor by the state. He and his community, however, would fully accept those who thought differently. He, on the other hand, had often felt unjustly treated.

I could now understand his position better, his remarks somehow made sense, touched me, especially the knowledge of his personal, painful experiences. Since his individual level could become the subject, a dialectical procedure in Jung's sense was also possible between us, "consisting in a comparison of our mutual findings" (Jung, 1935, para. 2). As a therapist, I was "no longer the agent of treatment but a fellow participant in a process of individual development" (ibid., para. 7). Now this was even more important in this case because the client was leading a rather conformist life. To try to normalize him in any way would therefore be, according to Jung, a "bad mistake" (ibid., para. 5).

What had happened? I had let myself be provoked by a statement of my client and lost the necessary reflexive distance for a moment. Checking my counter-transference feelings, I asked myself how I had allowed myself to get so involved. I sorted through my own parts. Through my client's response I became aware of the way in which I had also become a co-actor in his inner-psychic drama. He himself had been brought up very rigidly in terms of correct behavior, had always tried to be correct, and yet had developed unpleasant obsessive symptoms. Corona's restrictions had activated his authority complex, and with it his specific resistance to authority. After I had addressed my discomfort and formulated my real interest in wanting to understand him, something came into motion that allowed us to feel a new level of openness and closeness, which we had not yet experienced in our relationship, and which was not been able to foresee.

In psychology there are different terms for this happening: A synthesis, an "analytic third" (Ogden, 2010; Cwik, 2021), or a "moment of meeting" (Stern, 2005) can emerge through the encounter in the unconscious. These are moments that cannot be produced by technique or conscious attitude. They happen, present themselves.

Covid-19, in this as in other situations, has reinforced and made visible the divisive. Conscious and unconscious seemed to fall apart more and more in many places, became almost unbridgeable, as we see it in a neurosis. This dynamic of hardening and fixation on one side or the other is evident during the pandemic not only in the communication between people, time. In a therapeutic process, it is now precisely a matter of taking a look at this separating and diverging and making an effort to adopt an attitude that makes it possible for the unconscious to cooperate instead of opposing.

References

Altmeyer, M. and Thomä, H. (eds) (2010). *Die vernetzte Seele. Die intersubjective Wende in der Psychoanalyse*. Stuttgart: Klett-Cotta.

Cwik, A. J. (2021). The technologically-mediated self: Reflections on the container and field of telecommunications. *Journal of Analytical Psychology* 66 (3): 411–428.

Jacoby, M. (1993). *Übertragung und Beziehung in der Jungschen Praxis*, Olten: Walter.

Jung, C. G. (1921). *The Therapeutic Value of Abreaction*, CW 16. Princeton, New Jersey: Princeton University Press.

Jung, C. G. (1929). *Problems of Modern Psychotherapy*, CW 16. Princeton, New Jersey: Princeton University Press.

Jung, C. G. (1935). *Principles of Practical Psychotherapy*, CW 16. Princeton, New Jersey: Princeton University Press.

Merchant, J. (2021). Working online due to the COVID-19 pandemic: a research and literature review. *Journal of Analytical Psychologe* 66, 3, 484–505.

Ogden, T. H. (2010). Das analytische Dritte, das intersubjektive Subjekt der Analyse und das Konzept der projektiven Identifizierung, in Altmeyer, M. and Thomä, H. (eds), *Die vernetzte Seele. Die intersubjective Wende in der Psychoanalyse*. Stuttgart: Klett-Cotta.

Roesler, C. (2017). Tele-analysis: the use of media technology in psychotherapy and its impact on the therapeutic relationship. *Journal of Analytical Psychology* 62 (3): 172–194.

Stern, D. N. (2005). *Der Gegenwartsmoment. Veränderungsprozesse in Psychoanalyse. Psychotherapie und Alltag*, Frankfurt: Brandes & Apsel.

Chapter 15

Living in the Shadow of War

Ruth Williams

In this chapter the author looks at the unprecedented situation in which we found ourselves during a global pandemic from both a personal and global/ environmental perspective. She touches on the trauma of living in the period 'as if' it was a war. The daily grief at hearing of such enormous losses was traumatising. People have hunkered down and withdrawn into their small worlds, as they have had to, to keep safe and even alive. They shared copious newsfeeds and information about how to keep safe, cutting off from contact with nearest and dearest, with lives suddenly curtailed overnight. The trust in the politicians was daily challenged, as we were forced to witness their utter helpless/hopeless incompetence. Inevitably, the pandemic put us in touch with our own mortality as we have witnessed the daily rounds of death and lives transformed by the long-term effects which will remain. In addition, it has linked us to the wider climate connections to which the current generations have to wake up. Williams reviews some of the practical ramifications which have flowed from the shifts which have been thrust on to practitioners as well as ethical concerns.

I was born roughly a decade after the end of the Second World War, as a result of which my parents came to the UK as refugees. On one side my parent was a direct refugee from the War (about which I have written elsewhere in a chapter on the intergenerational transmission of trauma – see Williams, 2020). The War was therefore a frequent topic of conversation during my childhood and I recall clearly the dread and fear hearing about this period conveyed. I would often think to myself as a child – I hope to God I never have to live through a war.

Living through the Coronavirus pandemic has been like living through a war. Many of us have felt traumatised by the daily tally of deaths, by the 'rationing' at the beginning of the period when supermarkets were overwhelmed by people stockpiling toilet paper and such like as a way of coping with the shock we were forced to rapidly absorb. None of us alive today has ever lived through a pandemic. (There were of course outbreaks of Ebola and Sars in far flung places on the other sides of the globe which I am afraid just did not touch many of us in the industrialised West in such a personal way.) The daily grief at hearing of such enormous losses has been traumatising. I

DOI: 10.4324/9781003266402-24

cannot get away from that word. We have hunkered down and withdrawn into our small worlds, as we have had to, to keep safe and even alive. We shared copious newsfeeds and information about how to keep safe – whether we need to wash packages as they arrived at our doors, keeping a distance from delivery drivers and others, fearing any contact could be the source of a deathly infection. Cut off from contact with nearest and dearest, our lives were suddenly curtailed overnight. Our trust in the politicians daily challenged us as we were forced to witness their utter helpless/hopeless incompetence. (I am writing this from a UK perspective but few leaders have acquitted themselves terribly well although interestingly those led by women seemed to fair better, but that is a subject for another day.)

As many of us have worn out the path between desk and fridge, there has been time to contemplate. This piece is written from somewhere between the depressive position and the depressed position! (I hasten to add that this is said with humour.) So this is a rather sober account of events. The experience of the pandemic and associated lockdown has been depressing for probably most people I would hazard. The shock, the traumatic impact, the loss and more. This will almost inevitably lead to mental health issues which will be present in our practices for many years to come. In adults and children. In all of us who have lived through this period. It has led to some tremendous gallows humour which has rapidly circulated between friends, often multiple times a day, as we have tried to cope with the enormity of the situation.

Overnight our practices were turned upside down and our method of practice shifted to working online, something most of us would never have dreamt of doing previously. I did already work online with a number of people in distant countries but would never have contemplated seeing local patients and supervisees remotely and indeed would have been highly dubious of any supervisee who suggested doing so. And yet it has worked remarkably well. I have found the quality of the work to be consistent with face-to-face work on the whole. There are caveats to that claim. Coping with the shift to online working has been largely dependent upon psychological type with highly introverted individuals finding it really quite tolerable, even amenable. Some patients have even fared better online by which I mean that I have noticed revelations which have been enabled by the distance offered by remote working. And some patients who are challenged by the greater intimacy of face-to-face work, have felt able to open up and become more 'Relational' using the screen of the screen. I am thinking of one patient with autistic traits for whom this has been a real positive. I have also found some people have allowed greater access to the erotic transference online, perhaps knowing there is no possibility of this feeling eliding into physical acting out. This has been fascinating to witness and experience. How can there be a greater warmth with some people through a computer monitor? And yet, there it is. And I have found myself reciprocating, able to respond to that greater warmth in kind, not feeling so under attack at a distance and so the relationship has in some cases grown. I suspect we may revert to the familiar mode of relating once we – if we – return to face-to-face meeting. But even if that does happen, we will have gained an important insight into the mechanism of this relational dynamic.

One feature of this shift nearly all colleagues have noticed is the greater fatigue of working remotely. This has been quite a challenge which some have coped with by rescheduling appointments with greater gaps, or taking longer breaks or taking naps. Some of the issues have been highlighted in a recent article which has identified what it calls 'brain fog.' This is made up of forgetfulness, inertia, dullness of thinking at times. Sarner has gathered these symptoms together in a recent piece (2021) which lays out a recognisable pattern. Jon Simons, professor of cognitive neuroscience at the University of Cambridge, quoted in Sarner says: "There isn't something wrong with us. It's a completely normal reaction to this quite traumatic experience we've collectively had over the last 12 months or so." This may come as something of a relief. Fortunately it seems to be a fluctuating pattern so that many of us have also been highly creative and written books and films during lockdown. It may be that the initial burst of creative energy has given way over the interminable length of lockdown to the cognitive fog. We will all have had our own ways of coping with the trauma. Certainly it is doubtful that any of us have previously had to deal with such extended isolation (whether that has been *en famille* or in solitary confinement). It has been quite a year!

Practitioners have had to think about new boundaries and how to maintain a holding environment in the new situation in which we have found ourselves. An example is thinking about who sends the link to the online session. There are equally valid alternate views on this. Personally, I ask the person I am meeting to send me a link. I see this as analogous to coming to knock on my front door. Others opt to send the link to their patient/client. They see this as equivalent to providing the facilitating environment. Both these views have merit.

It is not always easy or practicable to replicate the exact environment the patient/client is used to experiencing in the room. When I work online, I sit at my desk which is in my consulting room but faces in the other direction so that the patient/client does not have the same 'view' as they are used to in the room. I know some people have set up a system so that they can sit in their usual chair which is more ideal but I have not found that physically so comfortable.

This new world of working online has also meant that we get to see into our patients' homes. This interrupts the transference with the reality of their environment. It is interesting to note whether this accords with or is at odds with our internal fantasies. We are sometimes visited by cats and dogs on screen which adds a whole new dimension, sometimes creating moments of intimacy when we share the enjoyment of the pet's visit. They are sometimes introduced like family members whom we have heard about.

Finding myself working in this unprecedented period has meant thinking about things I would never have considered before. In addition to offering the online option of having sessions (which everyone but one person took up), I have in one case offered to meet outdoors. This is a practice which has gathered momentum over about the last decade. It is still quite an experimental alternative but is gaining greater respectability as it is more deeply thought about and theorised. Rust has written about this and cites some wonderful examples of how she finds synchronicities tend to arise more often in the outdoors setting which raises interesting questions about why this might be. Perhaps being closer to our own instinctual nature in 'nature,' creates the conditions?

The very nature of clinical practice requires us to constantly assess ethical issues and this has been an essential matter during this year when 'normal service' has not been possible. I guess we could have stopped practice until it was possible to return to meeting face to face, but this seemed too rigid. And given how long the pandemic has lasted, would have been utterly impractical. I would question the ethics of withdrawing sessions on this basis.

Another changed feature of practice has been around billing. In usual circumstances, I would hand a fee note to patients at the end of the month. In Covid times I now do this by emailing the fee note with banking details and everyone pays online. This actually suits me better and is a very streamlined way of managing payments, although I know some colleagues not accustomed to using online banking have found this difficult.

We have truly been 'in this' together to an extent which is not usually the case. We have lived with the uncertainty, fear and vulnerability alongside our patients/clients and this has meant an increased 'reality principle.' I found that many people have tended (especially at the beginning of the pandemic) to ask me how I am at the beginning of a session. In normal times I would have shifted the focus back to the patient. However, given the hyper real situation in which we were meeting, I felt it was a genuine concern which I wanted to answer. At the early stages every cough and sneeze would create alarm and both parties would quickly reassure "it's not Covid!" We would both laugh at this at the same time as realizing this tension was all too real.

The pandemic has not solely been a purely personal experience for any of us. Inevitably it has put us in touch with our own mortality as we have witnessed the daily rounds of death and lives transformed by the long-term effects which will remain as a reminder of the horror we have endured forever. But more than that – or as well as that – it has linked us to the wider climate connections to which the current generations have to wake up. John Vidal, *The Guardian* newspaper's Environment Correspondent, established a link between the global, environmental and health issues. As early as 2004 he noticed that deadly diseases new to humans were emerging from biodiversity 'hotspots' such as tropical rainforests and bushmeat markets in African and Asian cities. He reported that a number of researchers today think that it is actually humanity's destruction of biodiversity that creates the conditions for new viruses and diseases such as Covid-19 (Vidal, 2020). He saw that, when we disrupt ecosystems, we shake viruses loose from their natural hosts. And, when that happens, they need a new host. We have seemingly become that host. And of course there are other viruses out there which have not yet made that transition into the human species. Not yet. Vidal quotes Kate Jones, chair of ecology and biodiversity at UCL, who calls emerging animal-borne infectious diseases an "increasing and very significant threat to global health, security and economies." Jones and her team (in 2008) identified 335 diseases that emerged between 1960 and 2004, at least 60% of which came from animals. Let me quote directly:

> Increasingly, says Jones, these zoonotic diseases are linked to environmental change and human behaviour. The disruption of pristine forests driven by logging, mining, road building through remote places, rapid urbanisation and population growth is bringing people into closer contact with animal species they may never have been near before, she says.
>
> The resulting transmission of disease from wildlife to humans, she says, is now "a hidden cost of human economic development. There are just so many more of us, in every environment. We are going into largely undisturbed places and being exposed more and more. We are creating habitats where viruses are transmitted more easily, and then we are surprised that we have new ones."
>
> (Vidal, 2020)

There is much to ponder as well as act on here.

What I have done here is look at the unprecedented situation in which we find ourselves from both a personal and global/environmental perspective. I touched on the trauma of living in the period 'as if' it was a war. I have also reviewed some of the practical ramifications which have flowed from the shifts which have been thrust on to practitioners. There are real ethical concerns at every turn when changing the mode of working and it has been enormously valuable to have colleagues with whom to think things through for which I am very grateful.

References

Rust, M-J. (2020). *Towards an Ecopsychotherapy*. London: Confer Books.

Sarner, M. (2021, 14 April). "Brain fog: How trauma, uncertainty and isolation have affected our minds and memory." *The Guardian*. Online at: www.theguardian.com/lifeandstyle/2021/apr/14/brain-fog-how-trauma-uncertainty-and-isolation-have-affected-our-minds-and-memory?CMP=Share_iOSApp_Other (accessed 14 April 2021).

Vidal, J. (2020, 18 May). "'Tip of the iceberg': Is our destruction of nature responsible for Covid-19?" *The Guardian*. Online at: www.theguardian.com/environment/2020/mar/18/tip-of-the-iceberg-is-our-destruction-of-nature-responsible-for-covid-19-aoe (accessed 18 May 2020).

Williams, R. (2020). "Intergenerational transmission of trauma in refugee populations: Misdiagnosis as Borderline Personality Disorder?" In Kiehl, E. (ed.) *Encountering the Other: Within Us, Between Us and in the World*. Einsiedeln: Daimon Verlag (eBook).

Chapter 16

Home, Sweet Home

Tine Papič

The chapter describes two specific phenomena that we encounter when doing analysis via video systems. The first phenomenon described is the issue of analytical setting when analysands' homes become part of the analytical setting. The author looks at what influence this aspect has on the process and how to work with it. The second phenomenon is the role of technology in analysis. Papič addresses the questions of how it influences the analysis and how to deal with the problems that might emerge while using video systems. It emerges that the right question is not if remote therapy is as good as the one in the classical setting but if it is "good enough." The author's position is that if it is done properly – if we do as much as possible to provide adequate experience, a "good enough" setting, and combine it also with sessions in person when it is possible – remote therapy can offer a lot. Thus, the relevant issue is not if we will provide therapy via video conferencing systems, but how we will do it in the future. On this issue, the time of the pandemic is a great teacher.

There are several phenomena that I encountered when doing therapy in the time of COVID-19 and they are all very interesting to discuss. However, due to space limitations I will look at two that I found particularly noteworthy.

In general, the biggest change that we encountered was the inability to meet our clients in person for a certain period of time. Here technology with video systems like Zoom and Skype came to our rescue. Writing on virtual interaction, Christian Roesler (2017, p. 376) claims that we can perceive virtual space as a sort of transitional space (based on the psychoanalytic theory of Donald W. Winnicott, 1971), due to anonymity and the so-called exit option. It is implied that one is anonymous in virtual space and the exit option means that one can always leave at a touch of a button, which gives one more psychological freedom to express oneself. This might be true for virtual spaces, such as computer games and forums, but it is different in the analytic setting. First, the anonymity – the clients are never anonymous, particularity if they have just moved from a standard setting to the virtual space. It is rather the opposite, as the goal of analysis can also be seen as the first of the Delphic maxims: getting to know oneself.

DOI: 10.4324/9781003266402-25

The idea of the exit option giving analysands more freedom in the virtual analytic setting, as they can exit anytime, is also questionable. We do not usually keep our analysands captive during therapy sessions, as they can always leave; it is rather the agreement between the analysand and the analyst that keeps us sitting there. Actually, with virtual space it is quite the opposite: it is not that one can leave whenever they want, it is that in a certain way one can never leave. In the next paragraphs I will try to explain why.

Home

He is happiest, be he king or peasant, who finds peace in his home.
                                                          – Johann Wolfgang von Goethe

One of the things psychotherapists take particular care of are our offices, where we practice. We do this for several reasons: one is how we present ourselves with narcissistically putting books on the shelves and diplomas on the wall, in order to look smart and to overcome our own anxiety, coming from questioning our capabilities and knowledge. A healthier reason is that the space needs to be safe due to therapeutic reasons. It needs to contain, to symbolically represent an analytical vessel, where in its safety and the seemingly hermetic seal the alchemical process of transformation can take place. What does that mean in practice? Analysands have to feel, not only know, that whatever they say will remain in that room. It is the feeling of safety and acceptance that does the magic trick, enables the patients to talk about things they were not even able to think about before, where the process of reverie can take place (Bion 1962). For this reason the place needs to be comfortable, where one feels well, at peace, safe; it has to be soundproof, a womb where time can stop and one can detach from everyday life, where a sort of sacred place emerges.

Then all of a sudden, because of the coronavirus pandemic, all our efforts to establish this safe, sacred space were in vain, as analysands could no longer visit us in person. We had to start using video conferencing systems, where they had to rely on the safety of their own homes. Here several problems emerge. Goethe was genius when he wrote "he is happiest who finds peace in his home," as he was aware that for most people this does not happen. There could be loud children rushing into the room as the little trickster archetype-driven complexes with their synchronistic precision, there could be partners, wives or husbands, somewhere in the house, listening to analysands, or at least that is what they imagine. Even if, for instance, the analysand's partner leaves the house, so that the analysand has peace and privacy, they mostly report that they still feel unsafe to talk about themselves, as if their partners were still symbolically present. I guess our complexes are unconsciously connected to a certain place, and since it is inevitable that our loved ones become the victims of our projections and of the play of transference, our complexes – from demons to angels, from dwarves to the ghosts of the past – will inevitably inhabit our homes.

There is also the question of coming to and going from the therapy session. Everyone who had the privilege of being in therapy is well aware that going to the session is analytic in itself. The analysands usually think about what they will say in therapy and are in process already. During the pandemic this was lost, one could argue that analysands think about the process all the time between sessions, which is partly true, but everyday activities usually take most of our time, consciousness and energy. Travelling to therapy, however, is already a reserved – dedicated time for analysis, for ourselves, our souls.

Another moment lost with the video conferencing systems is the fact that once we leave the therapist's counselling room, there is also a ritual in leaving this sacred space. The process is symbolically closed. This does not happen so clearly during video conferencing therapy. The computer is still there. The room is also still there. It is harder to get out of the complexes, to re-establish borders again with the unconscious, to bring back the defence mechanisms, which are there to enable our everyday living. Even if the analysands are not consciously aware of all of this, they feel unsafe. This tends to manifest in the fact that video therapy sessions usually tend to convert to small talk rather than deep analysis working on unconscious processes. For instance, every therapist knows the phenomenon of the last-five-minute revelation, when the analysands say something really important in the last five minutes, just before they leave. This does not happen so often in online therapy. The logic behind this is clear: to avoid pain, they drop the bombshell at the end of the therapy session and escape before the analyst could start drilling them with questions, which might be similar to the dentists doing that with a tooth.

It is a phenomenon especially frequent with beginners and tends to wear off with years of practice, as with years therapists spot faster through transference that the patient is carrying something hard to reveal. In my experience this phenomenon almost does not happen with video therapy, because, the ritual of leaving the sacred place, does not happen and the distinction between home and the therapeutic space is not present. One does not leave symbolically what was said with the therapist, to hold it and process it until the next session, but is left alone with it in the presence of one's everyday home. A situation one would avoid at all cost.

What can one do about the problem of being in analysis at one's own home? It is important to raise the question of safe space in analysis with the analysand in an analytic way, to bring the problems discussed before to consciousness, rather than giving advice. Some analysands will organise their hours accordingly with the loved ones so that they are not at home at the time of online sessions, others, who have more space, might organise a special room for therapy sessions. Some people will creatively find some other space to do it: in a local community center or at their place of work in the afternoon. Some will prefer to put therapy on hold.

Technology and Transference

Another aspect that I want to discuss concerning therapy over video systems is technology. There are several things to consider. We can get back to Roesler's (2017) idea of virtual space as a transitional space, where he is probably referring to Winnicott's idea of potential space (Winnicott 1971). An analytic setting with its safety, where fantasies can freely be expressed, already creates a transitional space. A virtual meeting is only a variant of it. Here Jung's view on perception becomes interesting:

> We perceive nothing but images, transmitted to us indirectly by a complicated nervous apparatus.
>
> (1935, par. 745)

We can look at technology as a sort of extension of this apparatus, so that we can perceive someone from afar. In this sense, we are not really in a virtual space as in computer games or similar activities, but rather in a real setting, where the perception of the other is enabled with technology, but also blurred due to its limitations. In the future, it is possible that there will be systems where such meetings will be almost indistinguishable from the real ones. Unfortunately, we are not there yet. At the moment, the picture on the screen is usually small, we do not see facial expressions in detail, we do not usually see the whole body, we do not smell each other. All of this transmits a lot of information at the unconscious level, which we do not fully understand. We just know from the phenomenological point of view that a lot is transmitted unconsciously, that ordinarily, during in-person therapy, we tend to feel the clients' feelings, even if they are not expressed verbally. We can feel their fear, anxiety, anger and joy; we can feel all sorts of feelings even if the analysand suppresses them. In a remote video session a lot of these channels of communication are missed. We do not see the whole body, consequently the analysand's body language is not perceived fully, consciously and unconsciously. We see only the face; facial expressions communicate a great deal of emotions, but the quality is again in question. There is the known phenomenon of the "moments of meeting," where we look into each other's eyes for a moment and a sort of unconscious conjunction happens, a moment of meeting, where one feels seen and understood (Stern et al. 1998). Can this also happen online?

In my experience, one of the most important channels of communication, which stays well preserved in video calls, is the sound of the voice. A lot of unconscious information is transmitted not only in the content of the language, but in the form of the voice. For instance, even if we do not understand a foreign language, we will usually still understand the feeling tone of communication. In my experience, I find it extremely important that I hear the analysand well, that in this way the analysand is psychologically closer. For this reason, I prefer to use a headset instead of speakers, which enables me to hear the analysands much better, and to cut the surrounding out. I can better concentrate on their voice, I am closer to them psychologically. The picture does not seem that important, as it might be problematic because of the setting – are the analyst and the analysand looking at the camera, where is the camera positioned, are they looking into each other's eyes? These are all problems that cannot be solved fully, but we can look at a relationship, a communication, as a sort of gestalt, a total experience, which consists of several channels of communication. These all build into something bigger, more functional, which can enable us a "good enough" analytical experience, where moments of meeting can happen (Stern et al. 1998). Not all channels of communication have to be perfect, as they never are, but they have to be good enough, where one channel can compensate for the other. We also know that when something is missing, our mind fills this lack with fantasy, projections, as we call them. This always happens and is a part of the phenomenon called transference. In this way, a virtual, video setting might even amplify such a process. Jung (1958) said that transference is always present. This is also true for video systems (Gabbard 2001).

Here I would like to discuss a specific problem, which does not appear in a classical setting, namely technical difficulties. One does not suddenly disappear from the room, it also does not usually happen that someone speaks, but the voice is not there. Such occurrences are, however, quite frequent in video calls. The question arises what to do with them. As Jungians we can always contribute them to synchronicity and not, for instance, to our stinginess when choosing the cheaper internet provider. I have a degree in Computer and Information Science and I actually believe that synchronistic events can interfere with technology. However, I will spare here the usual quantum physics explanation; I have an extended knowledge in physics, and it is always painful to listen to psychologists talking about quantum physics. I am afraid I would not do a much better job, so I prefer to skip the explanation and stay with the fact that I believe in the phenomenon, which is similar to believing in god, whereas the word believe in itself already implies a certain doubt.

How can we interpret such things? Usually we can look at them as an image (Cambray 2002), similarly to dreams, depending on what associations analysands have with the occurrence of technical problems, when our communication is somehow omitted. Some will curse the pandemic and the fact that they have to stay inside the house, and they are fed up with everything, others will see it as a repetition of their troubled relationship with their mother, where they were not heard or seen. We can look at it using the concept of the total situation (Astor 2001), where in transference the inner world is reflected in the current situation. Maybe one was not heard and understood at home, and here that dynamic is repeated again, not being heard or understood through technology. One could argue that this is simply not possible, a far-fetched idea, however, It is not really important if this is really a synchronistic event, where the total situation is reflected in technology, or just a coincidence. But it is much more important what is projected into the event, what part of our psyche resonates with it, what it is really about at the level of our psyche. For that reason, I believe that technical problems might well be interpreted through the lens of synchronistic event in the context of transference.

In conclusion, I propose that the question if remote therapy is as good as the one in the classical setting is wrong, because obviously it is not. The right question is, is it good enough? It is certainly better than nothing, especially in times like the Covid-19 pandemic, where other options are not possible. If it is done properly, if we do as much as possible to provide adequate experience, a "good enough" setting, and combine it also with sessions in person when it is possible, remote therapy can offer a lot. The Covid-19 pandemic is a tragic collective event, but also a collectively transformative event, which pushed us into virtual spaces and into the coming age of digitalisation. If digital technology was the domain of younger generations and IT enthusiasts before Covid-19, it has now become a reality for everyone. Like everything, it has its good and bad sides, however, there is no question if we should use it, as it is inevitable. Analysis via video technology has become a fact that will stay with us and spread even further. It will enable people to commute less, which has a huge environmental impact. It will enable people to get therapy in remote places, where this is not possible, and it will enable poorer people in more developed countries to get therapy from therapists from less developed and poorer countries, where living standards and prices of therapy are lower. Therapy will truly globalise. The question is not if we will provide therapy via video conferencing systems, but how we will do it. For this, the time of the pandemic has been a great teacher.

References

Astor, J. (2001). Transference the 'total situation'? *J. Anal. Psychol.*, 46 (3): 415–430.

Bion, W. (1962). A theory of thinking. *Int. J. Psycho-Anal.*, 43: 306–310.

Cambray, J. (2002). Synchronicity and emergence. *Amer. Imago*, 59 (4): 409–434.

Gabbard, G. (2001). Cyberpassion. *Psychoanal. Q.*, 70 (4): 719–737.

Jung, C. G. (1935). *Mysterium Coniunctionis*. CW 14. Princeton: Princeton University Press.

Jung, C. G. (1958). *The Practice of Psychotherapy*. Translated by R. F. C. Hull. Princeton: Princeton University Press.

Roesler, C. (2017). Tele-analysis: The use of media technology in psychotherapy and its impact on the therapeutic relationship. *Journal of Analytical Psychology*, 62 (3): 372–394.

Stern, D.N., Sander, L.CW., Nahum, J.P., Harrison, A.M., Lyons-Ruth, K., Morgan, A.C., Bruschweiler-Stern, N., and Tronick, E.Z. (1998). Non-interpretive mechanisms in psychoanalytic therapy. The 'something more' than interpretation. *International Journal of Psychoanalysis*, 79: 903–921.

Winnicott, D. (1971). *Playing and Reality*. London: Tavistock.

Chapter 17

The Expanded Container

Analysis in a Pandemic

Nancy Robinson-Kime

In this chapter the author uses personal experience and clinical examples to reflect on the process of working online both before and during the pandemic through a discussion of the analytic container. The relationship between outer and inner, the concrete-material and psychological is discussed in various contexts: the analyst's office which is created through a myriad of conscious or unconscious choices, the patient's home, patient information gained from interactions that are not face to face, and the technology itself. In linking outer and inner, our view of the analytic container expands from its concrete determinants into a psychological process of connecting and relating to psychic energy through whatever means possible. While there are instances in which working in person is necessary – there are times in which words do not yet exist and the body is the necessary vehicle of expression – in others, working "remotely" is a viable means for in-depth, transformative work, because it is experienced as an extension of the analytic container in a deeply intimate process of change.

Through the pandemic, much of the world moved into lock-down and much of analysis into a format that for many was unfamiliar – raising questions about the efficacy and desirability of working online. In reflecting on my experience of working remotely, I thought about the outer, concrete issues and how they are related to the inner, analytic process. Even before the pandemic, working online was not new to me. In 2009, I moved from Los Angeles to Switzerland – continuing to work with approximately half of my practice online. At the time, having worked with patients only in person, I did not know whether seeing patients remotely would "work" or work well.

The first issue that arose was the concrete container. In working in person, one creates, in a myriad of ways, the environment for the work: the privacy, the lighting (bright enough to see but warm, not glaring). I realized, on reflection, that in each of my different offices I have faced the window and placed patients with their back to it (for reasons of both confidentially and to reinforce interiority). One chooses the colors (of the carpet, furniture), the pictures, the books and objects one has in one's office. At one time, I had a ceramic Tarot tile of the Hanged Man (Nr.12) – deciding that Death (Nr. 13), while applicable to psychological

DOI: 10.4324/9781003266402-26

transformation, could be too overwhelming. Working online extended the work-space from one's own environment to that of the patient – in instances requiring an explicit statement about the need for a private, calm space in which to work. Excluding public spaces such as coffee shops, speaking while driving in one's car, or the possibility of being overheard by family members underlined the value of inner work, its difference from a call to a friend, through defining the concrete outer space. The regularity, the dedicated time and use of headphones (even when the patient lived alone) supported the containing quality of the experience.

But the question remained: would it work? One loses, concretely, the body: the way the person walks into the room, sits, nervously moves their foot; how they smell, how they are in their body. Two things compensated, in different ways, for this loss. As in a Bergman film, the focus shifted from being across a room to a close-up of the patient's face, eyes, mouth, eyebrows. The analytic frame was in a way more focused, more intimate, and simultaneously enlarged by including a wider range of personal expression through the environment. One was brought into the physical reality of a patient's home: it was cluttered, sparse, cold, cozy. What pictures (or lack of) did they have on the walls; what colors had they chosen for their home? What kinds of things were in the room – stuffed animals, technical equipment, an unmade bed. Like three-dimensional picture inter-pretation, one pondered the symbolic significance of the images in relation to the individual psyche not simply as a static picture but as a series of images that could subtly change from week to week – or not. An older man initially descri-bed feeling ashamed of having been fired from his last job but noted that he had been unhappy at work the last few years. Ultimately, he felt relieved since being fired had indirectly given him what he wanted. One day I asked him what the blanket behind him on his left was covering. He laughed and said that it was a pile of boxes from his last job he had angrily left there and covered when he was fired. As directions (right – left, in front of – behind) are themselves symbolic, we could say that behind his apparent acceptance, he covered not only his anger but a core theme in his life. The covered pile of boxes he had not yet gone through visually represented an underlying complex in which he was an unlucky (or in other instances, lucky) recipient – someone to whom things happened – rather than an active agent in his life.

Even without the presence of the patient in the room, psychic energy is ubi-quitous – constellating in whatever way it can. An interesting story I heard about the use of very simple materials (sticks, leaves, stones) for sand tray work in South Africa contrasted with the proscribed necessity of having a comprehensive col-lection of figurines. The point was that the psyche uses whatever tools are avail-able. Even when working in person, one pays attention to information from sources other than the face-to-face interaction: the first phone call or email con-tact is formal, overwhelmed, clear or confused. What is the quality of the voice? What is the counter-transferential response? What images, feelings, thoughts come up? Does the person remind you of someone – real or fictional? Like a first dream, you pay attention to whether the person is late, gets lost on the way.

The psyche unconsciously constellates in a myriad of ways. When an intern at the Jung Institute Los Angeles, I spoke to Edward Edinger about doing my Ph.D. dissertation on the projection of evil. He cautioned me against it, saying that one needed to be very careful since what one writes about gets constellated in the psyche. So too in group supervision where the psychic material of the patient gets constellated in the room – both in the analyst and other group members. If the analyst is experiencing a particularly strong maternal countertransference with a vulnerable child-like patient, someone in the group inevitably experiences the opposite side of the mother archetype. The psyche manifests in order to become conscious – at least potentially.

In working with patients online, the technology itself can become another expression of psychic energy – a part of the analytic field. Variability with the internet may at times *not* be meaningful (a cigar being simply a cigar). There are other instances, however, in which the connection (or lack) adds to the clinical picture. One session in working with a patient, the lighting in her room kept changing – one moment light and the next shadowy; the internet disconnected several times and had to be restarted. That session, the patient seemed scattered – describing feeling unmotivated and loafing on her job which paid the bills – nicely – but wasn't interesting. In parallel, her creative writing in the evenings had devolved into playing on the computer. Her tone was one of amused and superior cynicism. In this instance, the disjointed light and technical disconnection mirrored her symptomatic state: her creative ability reduced to playful indulgence; genuine pride, to superior conceit. She seemed to be on the wrong side of the problem of her own creativity – unconsciously acting out a raw, undeveloped version of the energy (like the *prima materia* in Alchemy) that was the seed of her future potential self. With another patient, the actual sound quality was not only choppy but tonally distorted in a way I had not previously experienced – like voices in a horror film. As the patient history unfolded, she talked about her experiences of having grown up in a schizophrenic family.

While technology can be both a tool for and expression of psychic energy, it is not viewed unbiasedly. On-line work is described as working "remotely." Computers/technology can carry the projection of being an inanimate, inhuman and at the same time potentially sentient force capable of overthrowing or undermining our humanity. And as a knife (in contrast to a spoon) has certain real attributes that lend it to being weaponized, so too there are real, concrete attributes of computers and technology which can be used destructively: superficial sound bites can reduce our tolerance for complexity; anonymous posts of unmitigated primal affect can increase disconnection – an anonymous mob replacing individual relationship.

But the tool is not the same as its effect. Even technology's attributes of distance and disconnection can be destructive or constructive depending on the context and use as I was surprised to discover in my first year in Switzerland. One of my patients preferred working over the phone rather than with video. While I initially thought that such an additionally remote way of working would likely not be fruitful, in trying it, I found the opposite. The patient with whom I had worked for a number of years was intensely sensitive to others, including me when face to face in my office. He wanted to work on a Freudian couch (frustrated by my two-person sofa) and considered changing to a Kleinian analyst. Unexpectedly, working together over the phone simulated a neutral environment that, like the psychanalytic couch, allowed him to focus on his internal perceptions without the distraction of seeing the analyst.

Analysis involves a process of separating an "entity into its constituent elements"[1] through objectification. While working online (like an unknown person writing for help) may be "remote," the means or way in which the material comes up is not necessarily the key issue. Of more importance is the creation of an analytic attitude which I discovered in my own work over the years. Having been interested in Analytical psychology from an early age – initially doing symbolic interpretations of literature as an undergraduate English major – I have experienced different phases of the work, different relationships to the psyche over time. I completed a traditional Clinical Psychology Ph.D. program as a precursor to Analytic training – interning at the Jung Institute of Los Angeles for two years from 1986–1988 where I took classes and had individual and group supervision. Before starting the Analyst training program a number of years later, I wondered whether formally training as an analyst would fundamentally differ from being a Jungian oriented Psychologist since, in the intervening years I had continued to take classes at the Jung Institute, been in Jungian group supervision, and personal analysis.

What surprised me once I began training was that doing so created a temenos in which everything that happened during that seven-year time-frame – in classes, my analysis, inner and outer life – were a part of the process of becoming an analyst. The vessel both expanded and at the same time became more focused. Why was the seven years of training different from the preceding years? A concentrated and consecrated analytic space had been created – an analytic attitude of relatedness, connectedness, and integration. Through whatever means or tools – psychic energy constellates. The task is to create links between the inner and outer reality of the patient, environment, and ourselves, between the unconscious and consciousness.

There are, as well, limitations to working online. The loss of the bodily reality of the patient was not as noticeable in my first years of working remotely since I had previously worked with my patients in person for a number of years. We had a visceral sense of one another as a base to the relationship. However, with my growing practice in Switzerland, coupled with teaching some on-line courses at the Jung Institute, Zürich, I had occasion to begin working analytically with patients who I had not met, at least initially. With all of the information that working remotely can provide, I was nonetheless surprised by some unexpected differences on meeting the individual in person. A young woman who was struggling with social anxiety presented online as cheerful and intelligent, with a wry sense of humor. On meeting her in person however, one experienced more directly her lack of understanding of social cues and personal distance. Seeing her in a social context highlighted others' conscious efforts to include her coupled with their instinctual desire to get away from her.

While I continued to work remotely with some former patients, the majority of my practice in Switzerland was again face-to-face until the pandemic. When the pandemic required that the work move into an online format, two factors influenced the ease of doing so. I was again shifting the format for patients with whom I had worked in person. My patients were also individuals who for the most part had secure, well-paying jobs from which they could work remotely during the pandemic. Neither they (nor their families) suffered in direct response to the pandemic apart from being unable to travel to see their families of origin during this time due to travel restrictions across countries.

This is to say, that the specific patient population with whom I work did not suffer great losses or anxiety during the pandemic; the virus was not a predominant focus of the work. These circumstances impact my impressions of working remotely to the extent that the lack of a physical presence was for the most part mitigatable by the psychological containment of the analysis. For other patient groups, however – ranging from schizophrenics, anxiety disorders, and children to those suffering trauma and loss – the need for the concrete bodily presence could be arguably more paramount. The one instance in which I hugged a patient was a spontaneous response to the painful death of the patient's father. Another related instance occurred when I was teaching a class in person at the Jung Institute Zürich on archetypes – material which could be difficult and activate the unconscious. Before one class, a student told me an upsetting dream she had had in response to the material. As she spoke, I reached out and put my hand on her arm. Nothing was explicitly said. It was a calming, bodily reaction through touch. In Greek mythology, Theseus' response to Hercules (suicidal after awakening from a state of madness in which he had murdered his wife and children) is to take Hercules' hands in his own.

Analytic work is never simply intellectual and verbal (whether in person or online); there is rather a psychic stratum that underlies the words which is the focus of the work. There are, however, instances – with certain patient populations, diagnoses, and techniques (body work, sand tray) – in which the bodily presence would be important and working online would be counter-indicated. Analysis works at a number of levels with different emphases resulting from both the patients' needs and an analyst's strengths – the way in which s/he works best. While there are times in which words do not yet exist and the body is the necessary vehicle of expression, there are as well instances in which working online is experienced as an extension of the analytic container in a deeply intimate process of change.

Note

1 www.dictionary.com

Image from the Manly Palmer Hall collection of alchemical manuscripts, 1500–1825, used with permission from The Getty Research Institute, Los Angeles.

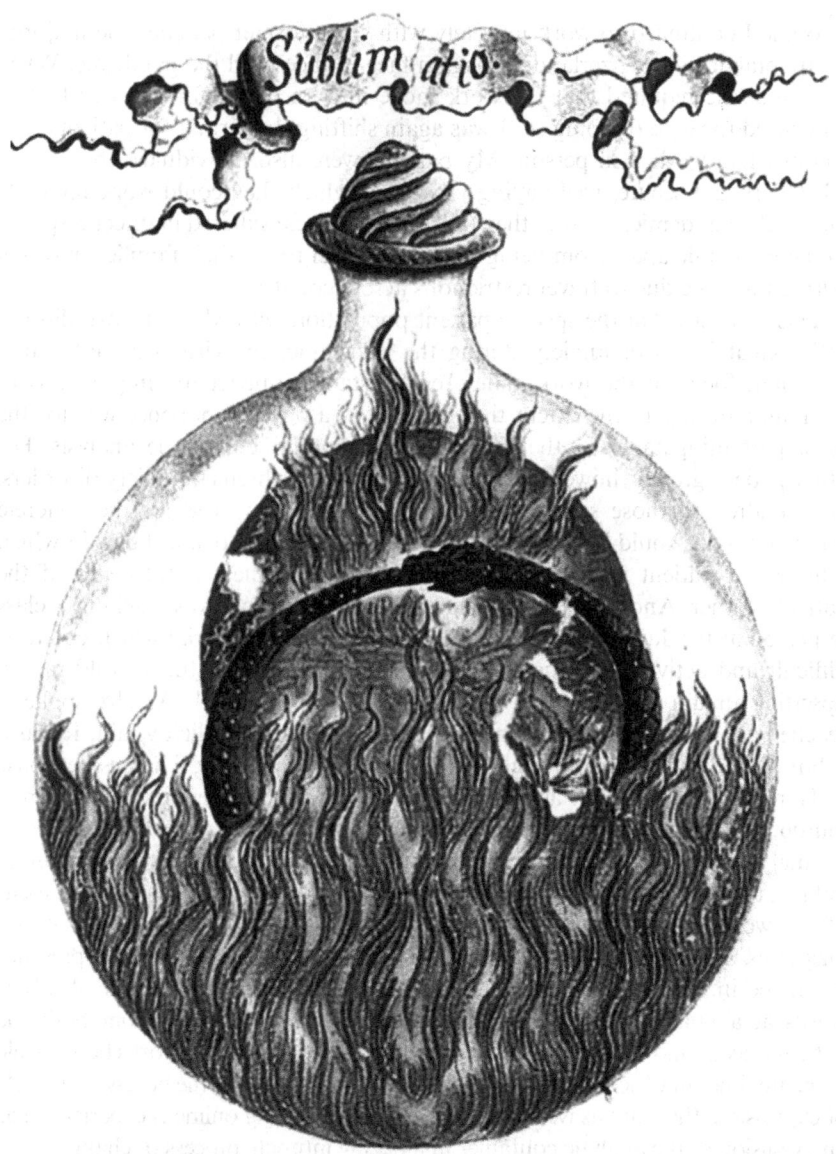

Chapter 18

Facing Suffering, Compassion and Transformation

Heyong Shen

The Covid-19 epidemic affects the entire world, has caused so many people to lose their lives, leaving behind the grief and suffering we have to face. "The Garden of the Heart & Soul 2020 Online" is a project aimed at providing psychological aid for the people of Wuhan, for the frontline medical staff and volunteers, patients, early suspected patients and their families. Thousands of people were visited and according to the researches and the experience of our work, "general anxiety" is the most prominent psychological response to the impact of the epidemic, and related depression, fear, and anger. Behind the anxiety and depression, the shadow of death is stirred; there may also be unexpressed sadness and unfinished mourning behind it. The author tries to use the I Ching images and the images of Chinese characters as threads, to analyze the meaning of "suffering" and "anxiety," "compassion," and "transformation." Language is the soul of a culture. Chinese characters contain readable prototypes, the way and the method for depth psychology, such as their pictogram, ideogram, and combined ideogram. More importantly, the Chinese characters for the words compassion and love, healing and transformation, contain clues about how to do that.

In 2020, the year of the Gengzi in the Chinese Lunar Calendar, the epidemic of Covid-19 suddenly came and gradually affected the entire world.

On January 26, 2020, we launched the "The Garden of the Heart & Soul 2020 Online,"[1] which is a project aimed at providing psychological aid for the people of Wuhan, for the frontline medical staff and volunteers, patients, early suspected patients and their families. We provided professional one-to-one psychological counseling services, and organized Jungian analysts to give a series of related lectures.[2] Thousands of people were visited and got help from us. Later, our group participated in similar work with IAAP and an Italian group of Jungian colleagues that set up an emergency project to provide psychological help during the pandemic.[3]

According to the researches and the experience of our work, "general anxiety" is the most prominent psychological response to the impact of the epidemic, and related depression, fear, and anger. How do we understand

DOI: 10.4324/9781003266402-27

that? Behind the anxiety and depression, the shadow of death is stirred; there may also be unexpressed sadness and unfinished mourning behind it.

We all know that this epidemic has caused so many people to lose their lives, most of them because of respiratory failure, passing away alone, no family members with them, and even no farewell ceremony; how many people are heartbroken and how many families have been fragmented; leaving behind the loneliness and pain that survivors cannot express; leaving behind the grief and suffering we have to face; this all related to the "general anxiety." The existence behind it requires our understanding and reflection.

As "general anxiety" is the highlight of the psychological distress affected by the epidemic, so let's take a look at the image of the two Chinese characters of "anxiety," and to feel the meaning, inspiration, and thread for healing in them.

The Chinese characters for "anxiety" is "jiaolv" (焦慮), the first character of jiao, is based on the image of suffering of a "bird"; the upper part is a symbol of bird (隹), the lower part is a symbol of fire. According to the Chinese five elements theory, the image of fire is related to the heart; this is not just a coincidence. There was an ancient form of the character of jiao, three birds above, and the fire below: 㷱; "three" as a symbol means many; maybe it is to express collective anxiety and suffering.

"Anxiety" is actually related to "suffering." The Chinese character of "ku" (bitter, also means suffering), the upper part of the symbol is "grass," and the lower part is "gu" (ancient), carrying an image of "ancient herbal medicine." Since there is sadness, sorrow, anxiety, and suffering, there should be healing. Therefore, the word "ku" (bitter, suffering), originally has the meaning of healing from "bitter" and belongs to a kind of herbal medicine. According to traditional Chinese medicine, ku begets the heart, so there is the principle of nourish the qi (energy) with bitterness and nourish the heart with bitterness.

The second character of suffering in Chinese is "Nan" (難, difficult), also related to the image of the bird, like the Chinese anxiety. In ancient times, the "Nan" was combined with the image of the heart below: 戁.

This reminds me of the hexagram of 36 in I Ching (the Book of Changes): "Ming I," Darkening of the Light, ䷣. At such a moment, it is appropriate to persevere in the right way in difficulty. Just as the image suggests: the sun sinking into the earth symbolizes the darkening of the light. It is as if a man were yielding and obedient in appearance but virtuous and brilliant inside. In this way he can get across great disasters (Fu Huisheng 2008, pp. 205–207). Six in the fourth place of the hexagram means: he penetrates the left side of the belly, that is, he finds out the inmost sentiment of the heart. Richard Wilhelm explained the meaning of the image: "Thus does the superior man live with the great mass, he veils his light, yet still shines" (Wilhelm 1967, p. 332).

The philosophy of "suffering" in Chinese, just like the Chinese "crisis" (危機), carries the special meaning of "danger and opportunity coexisting." While putting our "anxiety" and "suffering" into images, it already contains clues to coping and healing. This is also the basic idea of the psychology of the heart: the

Chinese characters not only present vivid images but include also "methods," that is how to do it; in this sense, Chinese characters can be called "readable archetypes." That's C.G. Jung's understanding and expectation of archetypes (Jung 1973, pp. 584–585).

So for "compassion," in its Chinese symbolic characters, contains the way and method for how to face suffering, and as well as for healing and transforming.

We have two characters for "compassion": Ci-Bei.

The character of "Ci" is a picture of growing (increasing) on top of the heart: 慈 , carrying the meaning of love. The character of "bei": 悲 (grief, suffering), which combines "no" and the heart, has the meaning of "without heart," or "lost heart."

So, when "Ci" combines with "Bei" they yield a special term: "Ci-Bei" (compassion). Integrating Ci and Bei together, the word looks like two sides of a whole, and a new meaning emerges. When we hold and contain love and grief together, within the free and protected space, like in our Garden of the Heart and Soul, then we have the chance to experience the transcendent function and compassion. As it could be seen in Delphi's motto: the suffering, and the knowledge that derives from it; "Ci-Bei" in the Chinese (and also used in Buddhism), conveys the meaning of the Great Love.

It is true that, in the Chinese dictionary, Ci-Bei, compassion, is also "love." Sigmund Freud agreed stating that love and work ... work and love, that's all there is. The concept of love has a deep meaning and inspiration, such as the image of Psyche and Cupid, in psychoanalysis, analytic psychology and depth psychotherapy.

The archetypal image of love in the oracle bone script form is expressed in the following manner: 愛 . The upper part of the character is the symbol of trust and sincerity. In the I Ching this symbol is precisely the image for hexagram 61, the Inner Truth. The second figure in the middle is a symbol of protection, giving the image of the womb, the mother's or the Great Mother's womb. The third lower part is "hand in hand" and means support and harmony. At the center or core is the image of the heart.

Language is the soul of a culture. Chinese characters contain readable prototypes, the way and the method for depth psychology, such as their pictogram, ideogram, and combined ideogram. More important, Chinese characters, such as the Chinese characters of compassion and love, contain clues about how to do it.

I have always believed that the real healing factor lies in the heart of the client, and the real healing power is also in the heart of the client. Based on the established therapeutic relationship, to awaken the healing factors and healing power in the heart of the client, is the basic principle and method of psychology of the heart. Then, with "compassion" and "love," as Jungian analysts, we can take it into our practice, to give play to it and reflect its meaning in our work. At the same time, each of us, also need compassion and love to face our own suffering and grief, and use the same compassion to establish a relationship with our own inner suffering. Only with compassion and love we can play the role of container and healing.

This is the image of the Chinese character for "healing": 療 . The upper part of the character refers to the image and meaning of how to make a boat or a canoe. For making a boat or a canoe, the most important thing is that it is empty and steady or in equilibrium. This equilibrium rests on the philosophical as well as physical level and also on the psychological (or psychotherapeutic) level. The lower part of the character of healing is the image of the heart. This Chinese image for healing, "the boat on the heart," offers a special image to reflection. With the image of the Chinese character for healing and the psychology of the heart, there must be something inspiring for our Jungian analysis and depth psychotherapy. As the old Chinese proverb says: "Boat supporting/benefiting the world" (Fu Huisheng 2008, pp. 412–413). For therapy, or therapy with healing, as Jungian analysts and depth psychotherapists, we should remember this image and the meaning, to find, or to construct the "boat on the heart" with our clients. Or, remember the old Chinese that says: (about being a therapist or analyst) the Heaven/God is using you as a boat, as an oar and a row.

Facing suffering and grief, it is, first, an attitude, which requires courage and wisdom at the same time. As far as I understand it, love and compassion can endure everything; only love can endure, tolerate, and contain. If we want our species to survive and discover the meaning of life, the meaning of every creature that lives in the world, love and compassion is the way, for healing, and transformation.

Notes

1 We, Oriental Academy for Analytical Psychology, China Society for Analytical Psychology, and China Society for Sandplay Therapy, organized several hundred certified psychological counselors for this task.

Our team, the volunteers of the "Garden of the Heart & Soul", participated in the psychological counseling of the Wenchuan Earthquake (2008) and Yushu Earthquake (2010). We have established more than 80 workstations in orphanages in the mainland of China for the last ten years, to support the psychological development of orphans.

2 The lectures were given by Andrew Samuels, John Beebe, Luigi Zoja, Harriet Friedman, Robert Bosnak, Martin Schmidt, Brian Feldman, Joan Chodorow, Riccardo Bernardini, David Rosen, among others.

3 "Reaching out the wounds of health professionals and population: An online psychological support in the current COVID-19 crisis".

References

Huisheng, F. (trans.) (2008). *I Ching, the Chou Book of Changes*. Changsha: Hunan People's Publishing.

Jung, C.G. (1973). *C.G. Jung Letters. Selected and Edited by Gerhard Adler and Aniela Jaffé*. Princeton: Princeton University Press.

Wilhelm, R. & Baynes, C. (trans.) (1967). *The I Ching, or Book of Changes*. Princeton, NJ: Princeton University Press.

Chapter 19

Online Therapy
The New Normal?

Pia Skogemann

Since 2020 the author has been working online more than before as the country shut down but kept the practice open. She was already comfortable with online sessions, having used it for years, and did not think of it as a problem, if the analysand and the analyst have already connected based on a physical presence. After the second shut down in December 2020, all but a small handful of clients went online. Much more complicated was how to handle the teaching of the candidates; learn how to use Zoom for teaching purposes and adapting the day schedule. In February 2021 a new training group started online. We worried, but it went very well. The participants as well as the teachers had a whole year behind them where they had to adapt to the Covid-19 situation. The pandemic has brought irreversible changes, but not in the quality of the therapeutic work. It is a collective situation and as analysts we are as much a part of it as everybody else and have to adapt.

On March 11, 2020, the Danish premier minister Mette Frederiksen closed the country. She appeared dressed in black with a tight hairstyle and a very grave tone of voice. Kids should stay home from school; their parents should work from home. Only food stores should keep open, and one should keep a distance while shopping. We should see as few people as possible and preferably meet outdoors. Of course, I had been following the spreading of the pandemic in the world on the news, so I was relieved that she took this step. I think it was wise, and it has later been confirmed that it was just in time.

Then I realized that there was a lot of fuzz in the psychotherapeutic world around me. The psychologists were recommended by their organization to shut down their practice or at least be outside – do walk and talk therapy. There were meetings in the Psychotherapist Association where some of the groups were in a panic – they stopped their training programs altogether. For some, online meetings were unthinkable. We were also recommended to follow the same principles as the psychologists in our practices.

I did not get it, really. I felt I took good care and did not run any risk with the practice habits I already had. I work from home. I have a spacey consultation room that can easily be aired. I do not give hand at the door. We sit

DOI: 10.4324/9781003266402-28

two meters apart. I bought hand disinfection and cleaning wipes, of course. So, I kept my practice open for those who wanted to come. However, I offered those of my clients who used public transportation an online solution, which they took. No one stopped.

The major difference was only that I now had much more online work than before. Maybe the difference between me and many other therapists is that I did not see that as a problem in any way. I have been using Skype for more than ten years, so I was already comfortable with that. I just bought a better Zoom connection. I can't even remember how I began using online sessions. Maybe it was with the American client, who had been living in Denmark for some years, but now married and moved to another country – and did not feel like ending the therapy. Or maybe it was with the Danish client whose physical condition made it more and more impossible for her to come in person. In any case, gradually it became natural to work online with clients and supervisees who live far away and for whom the traveling time would diminish the frequency of our meetings.

I have on and off thorough the years been in discussion with more hesitating colleagues about the use of online sessions, and I have always stated that if it is a question of keeping up a frequency or keeping up at all, surely it is the better choice. In the old days I used the telephone occasionally, and compared to that, it is so much better to see each other's faces. But I don't think of online sessions as a poorer solution. According to Merchant (2021) this is backed up by evidence.

> In my experience it is probably a question of whether I and the client already have formed a connection based on the physical presence, and then the relation does not need to suffer. That is the real test. Everything that happens in the chair can also happen online
>
> (Merchant 2021, p. 491).

Only once I made an exception from beginning with the physical meeting – I was contacted by a young Danish man, living in Iran. Obviously, he would not be able to come. I said to him that we could give it a try, but that I was not sure it would work. After a handful of sessions or so, he decided to stop. He felt I was not active enough, he said. For me, I rather think that because we did not have had the personal, physical contact, he was not able to read me enough. Of course, this is no proof, as it also happens that clients stop after a short time under normal circumstances, but I do think it is an indication.

But what about all the times when clients with several hours of travelling time have described the journey as part of the therapy itself – both as the preparation and the slow working through afterwards? Covid-19 certainly put a stop to that kind of process for those using public transportation and especially if they crossed a border – it is not so unusual for people living in Sweden to come to Denmark for analysis or supervision. I did not have such cases at the time when the pandemic broke out, and only time will show if that frame of mind returns, when another option is easily available. A couple of months ago I was called by a new client living in Northern Jutland who already in the beginning of the talk asked me: "Do you give online sessions?" That has never happened before Covid-19 – over the years, when I have had clients with many hours of travelling time, I have noticed than when we got closer to terminate the therapy, one of the sure signs was that they began to be bothered or bored by the long journey.

After all this have been said about the benefits of online sessions, I should also mention that a small handful of patients have kept coming in person – during the whole time and even after the second lock down before Christmas, when all the rest were going online, while we were waiting for the vaccinations. I had my first prick in April and the second in the beginning of May. I kept the online practice until the summer vacation. When I began again in August 2021, most of the clients went back to physical sessions, because the infection rate was low, and the majority had been vaccinated.

With one of these few exceptions, a long-time client, himself a psychotherapist, the possibility of online sessions was never even discussed between us. He simply appeared after the Christmas holidays wearing a transparent face mask and sat down wiping his hands in the sanitizer as the very first thing and wiping the arms of the chair when he got ready to leave. Not that we did not talk about Covid-19, we did (as I have been doing endlessly with all clients as well as with everybody else) – his ex-wife was infected and one of their children, too. However, his wordless signal was clear enough for me to refrain from suggesting any online sessions.

With other three clients, all women, I discussed the online possibility. All of them spent about an hour in their cars to my house back and forth, but they clearly expressed that they preferred that. We tried, though.

One of them, also a long-time client, was visibly uncomfortable during the online session. I also felt that our rapport was not as it usually is. We discussed it and agreed just to go back to normal, so that was it. It was a clear example of what have been described by online skeptical colleagues!

The second women, a psychotherapist, had never tried an online session before, and she expressed that it felt strange. She had been infected before Christmas together with her husband and daughter, so our risk was very low, and we went back to physical meetings. However, she herself asked for a single online session later in the spring because she was feeling a little sick and did not want to miss a session. This time she expressed gratitude that such an option existed!

The last woman, a senior candidate at our Institute with a growing practice, did accept a few online sessions in the beginning of 2021, mostly because her husband is a surgeon, and as such worked in the front line. But after he got vaccinated, she went back to our physical meetings, simply because she preferred it.

Much more demanding than the question of online sessions to me was how to handle the teaching of our candidates; that was a completely new thing. I had done online teaching only once – where somebody else handled the practical things. Now I had to learn how to use Zoom for teaching purposes, and after the first seminar which was conducted with the same time schedule as we used to, I realized that both I and the candidates were completely exhausted. We had to adapt with a long break for lunch, and alternately use zoom rooms with small groups of three to five people and presentations from teachers. Merchant (2021) refers to the issue of online exhaustion (p. 487), but not in relation to teaching.

Still, the candidates were not happy about the online teaching, they complained a lot. They sadly lost a teacher to Covid-19. They missed being together and they missed the place where we usually meet. They also missed sorely the yearly residential weekend which we use to have every March.

The epidemic became less threatening over spring and summer 2020 and in October we managed to conduct a two-day conference with an American guest – with face masks and distance and much caution. But then the infection sky-rocketed again, and in December, everything was shut down for the second time. That was harder. One had to look forward to several dark month of wintertime.

In February 2021 we were starting a foundation course with 19 new participants from Denmark, Norway, and Sweden, and we had only two options – to cancel or to go online. We chose the last option but were worried about how it would have been. Interestingly, it went very well. There were several reasons for this. The participants were prepared that at least some months of the course would have been online, and they had a whole year during which they had to adapt to the situation in their respective workplaces. And we – the teachers – had also been learning through 2020 how to do it in a way that could still be rewarding and make the group feel together. We had become much more professional. We hired a technician to help with the practical things. For instance, at the beginning of these foundation courses, we usually ask the participants to present themselves with a piece of music. It quickly became clear that they could not use their own sound devices so that we all could hear properly. But our technician found out to play the pieces from You Tube, which was very satisfying, even moving, together with the narratives that went with the music.

The group met for the first time in May, still with a handful of participants online because of the travel restrictions from Norway and Sweden.

Covid-19 has brought irreversible changes – but not in the quality of the therapeutic work, I think. And if there had not been a digital option, we would all just have been out of work, and our patients and trainees would have been left to themselves. The world has changed, and we have had to adapt. It is a collective situation, and as analysts we are as much a part of it as everybody else.

References

Merchant, J. (2021). Working online due to the COVID-19 pandemic: A research and literature review. *Journal of Analytical Psychology* 66 (3): 484–505.

Chapter 20

Is the Genie Out of the Bottle?

The Impact of the Pandemic on Analytic Process and Analytic Training

Mark Winborn

This chapter examines the rapid expansion and acceptance of computer-mediated technology for the provision of analysis and analytic training during the Covid pandemic. The author takes the title of this chapter from the recurrent figure of the genie in Persian fairytales, such as Aladdin and the Wonderful Lamp. In these tales, the genie is a mischievous spirit with magical powers who often is reluctant to return to the lamp once it has been released. He proposes that the increased reliance on computer-mediated platforms for the conduct of analysis and analytic training during the pandemic has resulted in a similar "release." The implications for the future of psychoanalysis and analytical psychology are explored. This chapter proposes that computer-mediated technology introduces a variety of distortions to the interactive field and interferes with channels of implicit and unconscious communication normally utilized during in-person analysis and analytic training. It also highlights the alterations that occur in the field when physical bodies are not mutually present, as well as highlighting the reduction in analytic ritual and frame that occurs when analysis is mediated via computer. The negative impact of these developments on future psychoanalysts and therapists is also addressed.

Introduction

I take the title of this chapter from the recurrent figure of the genie in Persian fairytales, such as *Aladdin and the Wonderful Lamp.* In these tales, the genie is a mischievous spirit with magical powers. Often the genie is reluctant to return to the lamp once it has been released. In our common use, the phrase, "the genie is out of the bottle," refers to something that has been done or created which cannot be changed or stopped, especially something which some people regret. A similar theme can be found in the myth of Pandora's Box, in which Pandora's curiosity leads her to open a container left in the care of her husband, thus releasing a variety of physical and emotional curses upon mankind. I propose that the increased reliance on computer-mediated platforms for the conduct of analysis and analytic training during the pandemic has resulted in a similar "release."

DOI: 10.4324/9781003266402-29

The Sequela of the Pandemic

In late February 2020 I returned to the United States from a teaching trip to Zurich and Moscow. I had heard the early news reports of the coming pandemic prior to my departure but the full extent of coming pandemic was quite unclear at that time. By the time of my return, it seemed the world had shifted on its axis. Within two weeks after my return, my analytic practice had shifted from eighty percent of the sessions being in-person and twenty percent on-line (or phone) to one in which eighty-five percent of the sessions were on-line (or phone) and only fifteen percent were conducted in-person. I never fully closed my practice to in-person sessions; taking appropriate precautions, I permitted my patients to choose what format they were comfortable continuing in. All my teaching activities and presentations were either cancelled or shifted to on-line platforms. I continued in this mode for the next fifteen months.

After twelve months (March 2021), I noticed I was experiencing significant somatic disruption which I associated with the large number of hours spent in front of a computer screen. I began to develop regular headaches, pain in my neck and back, dryness of eyes and eye strain, and increasing fatigue, particularly at the end of the day, leaving me with little energy to engage with life in the evening. Adjustments to my sitting position and placement of my computer screen brought some small, short-term reduction in my symptoms, but inevitably I quickly returned to previous levels of discomfort. Many of my colleagues reported similar somatic responses. Empirical research emerging from the pandemic now confirms that almost everyone experiences a heightened degree of eye strain as hours spent in front of a computer screen have increased. This emerging research also confirms that we tend to move less when seated in front of a screen, thus increasing musculoskeletal symptoms. Finally, this research indicates that we have to "work" much harder to discern and process social cues during onscreen interactions than during in-person interactions.

It was clear some of my patients enjoyed the convenience and ease of simply logging onto their computers rather than having to drive to my office for their sessions. However, during our sessions, I noted a mutual decline in emotional/affective engagement and focus. I noticed, for my patients and myself, how easy it was to become distracted by incoming emails, on-screen notifications, the intrusion of unsilenced phones, or family members and pets entering the visual field. One day I became aware that I could not continue in this fashion indefinitely; I decided in late March to give my analysands who live in the local area a firm deadline to return to my office by June 1, 2021. Most of my patients were already vaccinated (vaccines had become widely available in the Memphis area beginning in January 2021). The timing of my deadline allowed eight weeks for my unvaccinated patients to obtain vaccination, if they wished, prior to returning to in-person visits.

What Do We Lose in Computer Mediated Therapy and Analysis?

Commentaries and Research

As Essig (2019) points out, computer-mediated therapy is not the same as in-person. He says, "One cannot simply assume all the research and clinical wisdom acquired over decades of physically co-present psychotherapy can be directly applied to technologically mediated simulations of traditional psychotherapy via video technology" (Essig, 2015, p. 691). Essig (2019, par. 3) further asserts that computer-mediated therapy creates, "a culture of artificial intimacy." Essig (2019) cites research indicating that in-person therapy has better treatment outcomes, regardless of theoretical orientation, when compared to computer-mediated therapy. He also highlights research which indicates that patients involved in computer-mediated therapy remember less of the content of their sessions than patients being treated in-person. In addition, research indicates that the more time someone spends interacting with computer screens – whether it be for therapy, work related meetings, making phone calls, or reading – there is an accompanying increase in anxiety, depression, and loneliness. Essig also indicates that trust in the therapeutic relationship is more difficult to establish in computer-mediated therapy. Essig (2019, par. 1) summarizes his position, "Everyone, from patients to providers to payers, would be wise to keep in mind that sometimes the most helpful, innovative development is recognizing there's no substitute for being bodies together, even when all you're doing is talking."

In examining the impact of computer-mediated interaction on analysis and psychotherapy, Russell (2015) ventures beyond psychoanalysis into the fields of neuroscience, communication studies, infant observation, cognitive science, and human–computer interaction. Research from these fields provides insights into the ways that embodied interactions differ from computer-mediated ones. Russell's approach is not anti-technology so much as it is advocating for maintaining the minimal conditions necessary for analysis and psychotherapy to occur. In summarizing her research, she says,

> I discovered that because screen relations eliminate co-present bodies, they limit psychoanalytic process to 'states of mind,' rather than 'states of being.' It became impossible to ignore the fact that analytic couples need the traditional experience of presence, and not just technologically simulated presence, to deepen the psychoanalytic process.
>
> (Russell 2015, p. xvii–xviii)

Lyons (2020) focuses on the fate of the body and affect during on-screen analysis, emphasizing the dilemmas posed in the work with erotic transference when the transgressive excitement of possibility (i.e., actual erotic contact between analyst and patient) is absent. She also addresses the impact of computer-mediated communication on the analytic frame and analytic process, as well as elaborating on the limitations experienced in the phenomenology of the clinical moment. Given these influences, Lyons articulates concern about on-screen treatment with dissociated and traumatized patients and highlights the likelihood that the move to on-line analytic interaction potentially reinforces defenses of dissociation and disconnection, rather than promoting an experience of intimacy.

Relying on contemporary communications models for support, Brahnam (2017) points out that computer-mediated platforms significantly attenuate and distort the implicit communication avenues ("channels") that psychoanalysis relies on heavily for the understanding of unconscious communication; channels vital to entering states of reverie[1] essential to the conduct of analysis. Brahnam (2017, p. 153) also indicates that, "Perceptual asynchrony artifacts, such as misalignment of audio and visual cues, are confusing to viewers, they also elicit negative emotions." As several of the authors cited above point out, the positioning of video cameras precludes the possibility of direct eye contact while fostering the illusion of direct eye contact, thus introducing significant interpersonal/interpsychic distortion when conducting analysis via computer-mediated platforms.

Ritual

The process of analysis is embedded in an analytic ritual which we refer to as the analytic frame. The external aspects of the analytic frame include the well-sealed vessel (*Vas Bene Clausem*) meaning a closed, protected space in which confidentiality is maintained. The analytic frame also includes other features, such as how often and when sessions will occur, how fees will be paid, whether the analysand will use the couch or chair, general guidelines as to how the participants will interact with each other, and so on.

As Joseph Campbell points out, ritual is mythology in action (1988, p. 82): "A ritual is the enactment of a myth. And, by participating in the ritual, you are participating in the myth." Part of the ritual of analysis involves the time and effort spent going to and from the analyst's office. These periods of reverie, psychological preparation, and integration are an important part of the analytic ritual. This time of coming and going introduces a liminal state – the threshold state of betwixt and between identified by Victor Turner (1969). The coming and going also involves sacrificing time from work, family, or leisure, yet many things worth experiencing often involve some degree of sacrifice. In the shift to on-line training and therapy there is a reduction in the libidinal investment in the process. There is little "skin in the game."

The appeal of convenience is seductive. As Modell (1989) points out, the analytic setting and frame are not just a set of guidelines for conducting the physical characteristics by which analysis takes place. The analytic ritual is also the conduit by which multiple levels of reality are passed through – including ordinary reality, the reality of the analytic stage, the specific analytic stage of the transference-countertransference matrix, the unfolding of the archetypal drama within the analysis, and states of regression encountered in analysis. However, in computer-mediated analysis, most elements of the analytic ritual are diminished, eliminated, or become distorted. There is little ritual involved when the analysand only has to stop the activity they are currently engaged in and log onto their video platform for their session. Then they are able to return immediately to their previous activity after the session ends. While a few analysands may create space for reflection before or after computer-mediated sessions, my experience is that many do not.

Finally, we might wonder what happens to the patient's experience of the analyst's office as "container" (Bion, 1994) or "holding environment" (Winnicott, 1965), especially when the patient has never physically entered the space. Can the patient internalize the analyst's office as "environmental mother" (Winnicott, 1965) if they have never been *inside*? Is there an experience of the *vas hermeticum* if the analytic experience is virtual?

The Body

Well over one hundred years ago, Williams James highlighted the importance of the body as the center of our experience (1890, p. 154),

> The world experienced comes at all times with our body as its center, center of vision, center of action, center of interest. Where the body is, is 'here'; when the body acts is 'now'; what the body touches is 'this'; all other things are 'there' and 'then' and 'that'.

Years later, in seminars offered between 1934–1949, Jung (1988, p. 396) made a similar observation,

> The difference we make between the psyche and body is artificial. It is done for the sake of a better understanding. In reality, there is nothing but a living body. That is the fact; and psyche is as much a living body as body is a living psyche: it is just the same.

The importance of the body as an extension of unconscious and implicit experience has taken on heightened recognition in recent years. Authors such as McDougall (1989), Sidoli (2000), Sletvold (2014), Van der Kolk (2015), and Dunlea (2019) have all written in depth about the essential importance of recognizing and integrating the bodies of the patient and the analyst or therapist in any depth work. The analyst's body is a tuning fork that establishes an empathic resonance with the body of the patient. Can we register and integrate the body (soma) into our work as analysts if we are dis-embodied by virtue of computer-mediation, or if we are relying on a virtual experience of bodies separated by screen and geographic distance?

In computer-mediated analysis, it is primarily the visual and auditory senses that come most actively into play. With in-person analysis, all sensory modalities are engaged – visual and auditory, but also olfactory, kinesthetic, tactile, and sometimes even gustatory. Smell is particularly important to the experience of being in one's body and the experience of the other, yet it is completely unavailable in on-screen sessions. As Sarafoleanu, Mella, Georgescu, and Perederco summarize (2009, p. 196),

> Olfactory sense is, in terms of evolution, one of the oldest senses, allowing the organisms with receptors for the odorant to identify food, potential mating partners, dangers and enemies. For most living creatures and for mankind smell is one of the most important ways of interaction with the environment. In humans, olfaction…plays an important social and emotional part…. The most significant role of olfactory signals in humans appears to be the modulation of their behavior and interpersonal relationships.

I once had a patient who was a senior cardiologist. He indicated that he could diagnosis a variety of cardiovascular conditions simply by smelling the patient, but he bemoaned the fact that younger residents no longer cultivate this capacity because they have been taught to rely on "objective" testing in their medical training.

Do not the emotional fields constellated in analysis also have a smell? If we are interacting through a screen, how will we know if the musky aroma of arousal has entered the field? How will we know if the acrid smell of fear has filled the air? How will we know if the acidic stench of envy has entered our space? Or whether the sulfuric odor of anger is rising from the seat opposite ours? Where do these scents reside when we go on-line and what impact does it have if we are not both present in our bodies to smell them?

Is Analysis an Art that Deserves a Body?

I find most in the Jungian and psychoanalytic communities have significant interest in the arts. Would any of us say that seeing our favorite musicians perform via a live video stream is as rich, exciting, entertaining, or enjoyable as seeing them perform live? The same could be said for live theatre, dance, or opera. If we are honest, isn't the experience of these art forms richer when experienced in-person? If we are physically present in a venue, with our bodies, we experience the performance in a much more vital (even magical) manner. I believe most would also say that standing (i.e., embodied) in the Rijksmuseum before a painting by Rembrandt is a completely different experience than looking at the same painting in a book. Should we be willing to relegate our analytic art form to computer-mediated platforms just because the technology permits it?

The Impact of Computer-Mediated Learning on Analytic Training

As Caratanuto (1991) says, Jungian analysis is a "difficult art." But there is difficulty, not just in the process of analysis itself, but also in the process of training to become an analyst, which involves significant focus, expense, sacrifice, and dedication to complete. How much more arduous does the task of learning "the difficult art" become if a significant portion of that formation takes place through distance learning?

Consider specializations in medicine, such as heart surgery or neurosurgery. Would we choose a surgeon to cut into the delicate tissues our bodies who received significant portions of their training through the internet? Music provides another example. Would the cellist Yo-Yo Ma or the pianist Vladimir Horowitz have become such masters of their instruments had they received instruction through the internet rather than through years sitting physically beside their teachers; teachers who could see, feel, and hear the way they were breathing, moving their arms, and carrying the rhythm in their bodies? Doesn't the practice of psychoanalysis and psychotherapy also require the cultivation of nuanced, complicated, and sophisticated skills, capacities, and knowledge which are more effectively acquired in embodied encounters?

During the pandemic, the training society to which I belong, shifted entirely on-line. Naturally, we had no other choice given the severity of the pandemic. By the time this is published, the business meetings, analytic conferences, admissions, evaluations, and graduations will have been conducted on-line for over two years. Our last in-person meeting was October 2019, and we likely won't resume in person meetings until April 2022. I am aware of similar situations in Jungian and psychoanalytic institutes around the world.[2]

As we begin to emerge from the limitations of the pandemic, already there is a push from candidates and institutions to hold onto some of the conveniences of distance learning. For the institutes, many of which are experiencing a declining pool of applicants, I can see why the opportunity to offer their programs to a wider geographical group of potential is enticing. However, if we follow this path, I believe we will be training a group of future analysts who do not know the full depth of our profession, because they have not learned it as embodied experience. I know personally, from hours of teaching conducted on-line, that the dialogue with students is significantly reduced during on-line seminars. Dialogue is one of the most important ways we digest and integrate the concepts and methods of analytical psychology. Also, my sense of how participants are reacting to the presentation is greatly diminished, particularly when the seminar is more than about eight or ten participants. In person, even in a large class, it is possible to notice and engage with participants who appear confused, lost, uncertain, shy, or upset by the material. This is nearly impossible in larger on-line classes.

In reflecting upon our current situation and the impact on analytic training, I am often drawn back to Plato's Allegory of the Cave from *The Republic*. It is written as a dialogue between Plato's brother Glaucon and his mentor Socrates. In the allegory, Socrates describes a group of prisoners who have lived inside a cave all their lives, chained, facing a blank wall. The prisoners watch shadows projected on the wall from figures passing in front of a fire behind them. The shadows (two-dimensional figures) are the prisoners' only known reality, but the shadows are not accurate representations of the real world existing outside the cave. The inmates of the cave do not even desire to leave their prison, for they know no better life. However, if they did make their way out of their limited environment, they would not be able to function in the outer world which requires the capacity to navigate the world in three dimensions. I am concerned for the future generations of analysts (and their analysands) if a significant portion of their analytic training and personal analysis has occurred on-line. It seems unlikely they will recognize or fully register certain elements of the analytic encounter because, like the prisoners of Plato's cave, they have not had previous experiences of them.

Conclusion

Prior to the pandemic, I was concerned about the future of analysis and analytic training, largely because of the aging of our teaching analysts, the increasing age of admission of candidates into analytic training, a cultural immersed in technology and immediate gratification, and the proliferation of various short-term psychotherapies which do not have sufficient depth to engage the whole person. Now, the seductive convenience and the illusion of connection offered by computer-meditated analysis and training has become a greater and more immediate concern. Speaking to this dilemma, Russell (2015, p. xviii) indicates,

> Psychoanalysis faces a profound irony in the second decade of the twenty-first century. Increasing mobility, the emergence of modern economies, and fast-paced lives are accelerating demand for 'screen relations' based treatment. In response, many psychoanalysts are embracing technologically mediated treatment. However, this comes at a time when authorities on how technology shapes relationships are voicing serious concerns about the damage technological mediation does to both intimate connection and reflective solitude.

I have been surprised to encounter many colleagues who are excited about the possibility of continuing to work exclusively on-line after the dangers associated with the pandemic have largely been mitigated. The reasons reported often focus primarily on finances (being able let go of the cost of office space) and convenience (working from home and being freer to travel), but those reasons have little to do with cultivating the optimal environment for the engagement of unconscious processes and the facilitation of transformation.

Naturally, there are good therapeutic encounters and good analytic training experiences that can occur on-line. On-line therapy and training are certainly preferable when no other options are available. But I do not believe on-line and in-person experiences are equivalent. I believe an open embrace of on-line technology is a greater threat to the survival of in-depth psychological work than all the other societal pressures currently confronting the analytic field.

In *The Red Book*, Jung (2012, p. 119–120) said, "The spirit of this time would like to hear of use and value.... The spirit of the depths took my understanding and all my knowledge and placed them at the service of the inexplicable and the paradoxical." I pray that those of us involved in the world of analytical psychology and psychoanalysis will continue to harken to the spirit of the depths, rather than to succumb to the spirit of these times. I pray the future generations of would-be analysts do not become imprisoned in Plato's cave. I pray we are able to get the genie back in the bottle.

Notes

1 For a Jungian perspective on reverie, see Winborn (2014).
2 Even prior to the pandemic, in the United States, several distance-learning analytic training programs have sprung up that require little, if any, in-person instruction, analysis, or supervision.

References

Bion, W. (1994) *Learning from Experience*. Northvale, NJ: Aronson.

Bomba, M., Alibert, J-F., & Velt, J. (2021) Playing and virtual reality: Tele-analysis with children and adolescents during the COVID-19 pandemic. *International Journal of Psychoanalysis*, 102 (1): 159–177.

Brahnam, S. (2017) Comparison of in-person and screen-based analysis using communication models: A first step toward the psychoanalysis of telecommunications and its noise. *Psychoanal. Persp.*, 14 (2): 138–158.

Campbell, J. (1988) *The Power of Myth*. New York: Doubleday.

Carotenuto, A. (1992) *The Difficult Art: A Critical Discourse on Psychotherapy*. Wilmette, IL: Chiron.

Dunlea, M. (2019) *Bodydreaming in the Treatment of Developmental Trauma: An Embodied Therapeutic Approach*. London: Routledge.

Essig, T. (2015) The gains and losses of screen relations: A clinical approach to simulation entrapment and simulation avoidance in a case of excessive internet pornography use. *Contemporary Psychoanalysis*, 51 (4), 680–703.

Essig, T. (2019) What to expect from psychotherapy on screen. *Wall Street Journal*, online at: www.forbes.com/sites/toddessig/2019/02/26/what-to-expect-from-psychotherapy-on-screen-a-consumers-guide/?sh=c25b7165ea8e

James, W. (1890) *The Principles of Psychology*. New York: Henry Holt and Co.

Jung, C. G. (1988) *Neitzsche's Zarathustra*, Vol. 1. Princeton, NJ: Princeton Univ. Press.

Jung, C. G. (2012) *The Red Book: A Reader's Edition*. New York: Norton.

Lingiardi, V. (2008) Playing with unreality: Transference and computer. *Inter. J. of Psychoanalysis*, 89 (1): 111–126.

Lyons, L. (2020) Can I touch you through a screen? *Psychoanalytic Dialogues*, 30 (3): 365–372.

McDougall, J. (1989) *Theaters of the Body*. New York: Norton.

Modell, A. H. (1989) The psychoanalytic setting as a container of multiple levels of reality: A perspective on the theory of psychoanalytic treatment. *Psychoanalytic Inquiry*, 9: 67–87.

Russell, G. I. (2015) *Screen Relations: The Limits of Computer-Mediated Psycho-analysis and Psychotherapy*, London: Karnac.

Sidoli, M. (2000) *When the Body Speaks*. London: Routledge.

Sletvold, J. (2014) *The Embodied Analyst*. London: Routledge.

Sarafoleanu, C., Mella, C., Georgescu, M., & Perederco, C. (2009) The importance of the olfactory sense in the human behavior and evolution. *Journal of Medicine and Life*, 2 (2): 196–198.

Turner, V. (1969) *The Ritual Process*. Middlesex, UK: Penguin.

Van der Kolk, B. (2015) *The Body Keeps the Score: Brain, Mind, and Body in the Healing of Trauma*. New York: Penguin Books.

Winborn, W. (2014) Watching the clouds together: Analytic reverie and participation mystique, in Mark Winborn (Ed.), *Shared Realities: Participation Mystique and Beyond*. Skiatook, OK: Fisher King Press.

Winnicott, D. W. (1965) *The Maturational Process and the Facilitating Environment*. London: Hogarth Press.

Chapter 21

Accelerations and Decelerations
Individuation at Pandemic Speed

Luciana Ximenez

The author is inspired by the peculiarities of Brazilian cities, each city's rhythms of life. On February 2020 these different cities suffered the same impact by the coronavirus, which hit not just Brazil, but the entire world. Covid-19 started to show its face. Each mayor and governor tried to manage the crisis according to the needs and uniqueness of their cities, which came to have very similar external rhythms. What has changed with the advent of the pandemic? Not much, the author states: cities decelerate, but social demands – from social networks, from internal expectations, pressure from work, family, online classes, livestreams, books we haven't yet read, newly-released articles – have kept us at an accelerated rhythm very similar to the previous one. On top of that, some professions simply couldn't consider deceleration in moments like these. And what can be said about how fast it spreads? Or about the deaths, or the mutation of the virus? Apparently, the quarantine imposes a mandatory slow down it interrupts us, puts us in an inward and downward movement, an opportunity for us to go into the transformation cave. But wouldn't the demand for slowing down and deceleration also be a form of pressure by similarity?

Brazil, with its countless discoveries, never ceases to bring me inspiration and reflection. This time, my attention is drawn to the peculiarities of each city's rhythms of life. Observing São Paulo – a completely different capital than Rio de Janeiro, which can't be compared to Porto Alegre, which in turn, contrasts with Belo Horizonte, and even more with Salvador or João Pessoa – is fascinating. Imagine, then, passing through Lajedo de Pai Mateus – a district in a city called Cabaceiras – Cambará do Sul, Sete Cidades, Novo Airão, Algodoal or Goiás Velho.

On February 2020, however, these different cities suffered the same impact, which hit not just Brazil, but the entire world. Covid-19 started to show its face. As the months passed, it showed more and more of its effects. Closed schools, postponed events, closed businesses, delivery-only restaurants, movie theaters? Absolutely not. Everything had changed. That's when an infinite amount of reflections came to me, and I ruminated on them, wrote them down, discussed them and observed them. Early in the quarantine, each city

DOI: 10.4324/9781003266402-30

was affected differently. Each mayor and governor tried to manage the crisis according to the needs and uniqueness of their cities, which came to have very similar external rhythms. However, the rhythm of a person born and raised in Lajedo de Pai Mateus will never be the same as that of someone born and raised in São Paulo.

This was the picture as we entered this period of isolation: all or most of us were taken by this new way of life which was almost mandatorily packaged with acceleration. What has changed with the advent of the pandemic? Not much, I'd say.

The acceleration is beyond the rhythm of the external world's impositions. Cities decelerate, but social demands – from social networks, from internal expectations, pressure from work, family, online classes, livestreams, books we haven't yet read, newly-released articles – have kept us at an accelerated rhythm very similar to the previous one.

On top of that, some professions simply couldn't consider deceleration in moments like these: doctors, biomedical scientists, delivery people, journalists, nurses, psychologists, IT workers. And what can be said about how fast it spreads? Or about the deaths, or the mutation of the virus?

Some people couldn't handle it. They can't handle it. They become depressed, anguished. The quarantine practically imposes a mandatory slow down. The quarantine interrupts us, it puts us in an inward and downward movement, matching what Vannoy Adams described (2020, during his talk on Thiasos, a shared imagination workshop, in content not yet published) as the "great introversion," an opportunity for us to go into the transformation cave. But wouldn't the demand for slowing down and deceleration also be a form of pressure by similarity? Here I am, in solidarity to those who can't or won't, for various reasons, decelerate. Could they be going the opposite way? And is going the opposite way necessarily against individuation? Is decelerating or slowing down the only way of coming into contact with the great introversion, the one that brings us into the cave of dreams, of fantasies, of images?

I hear things like: "I'm loving this deceleration!" or "It's so good to be able to avoid the traffic in São Paulo!" or "I want my life back!" It's not my intention to generalize everyone's relationship with acceleration and with their need to decelerate the rhythms of their lives on account of the isolation. But from my perspective, the acceleration remains as present in our lives as before. What changes is how it acts. This is not criticism, but an observation. This isolation makes it possible for each of us to find our rhythm. Those who are accelerated remain accelerated, and the decelerated have a chance to decelerate.

The worlds each individual lives in become their scenery, their landscape. A scenery for their lives, to find singularity, for "soul-making," according to a major line of archetypal psychology. In this sense, soul-making is based on the relationship each person establishes with internal and external objects. The city, the environment, the rhythm, the time, the speed of the world that surrounds us are inevitable. We have a certain autonomy – not much – to choose our scenery. However, given this scenery, our work is to establish an erotic relationship with it, whether it is sunnier or cloudier, greener or greyer, with or without water, accelerated or decelerated.

Francisco Bosco, in an article written for *Observatório da Imprensa* (2013), states that

> the technological acceleration and the predominance of the private sphere gave rise to a new problem, a new entanglement of individuals, this time with products, techniques, languages and services that threaten to steal all their time and transform their lives into the management of these acquisitions.

In other words, the compulsion for growth and innovation accelerates life. Hyperconsumerism. Consumption all the time: leisure, culture, material goods, technology. Modern society's desire makes us dependent on the market. Byung-Chul Han (2015) understands that to escape routine, to escape emptiness, we consume more and more new stimuli, new emotions and new experiences.

The German contemporary philosopher Hartmut Rosa (2019) defines a society as modern when it can only find a certain dynamic stabilization, when it is systematically disposed toward growth, toward increased innovation and acceleration. Acceleration comes with the definition of modern society. It uses terms like: compulsion to grow, compulsion to increase, to become faster and be capable of transforming.

A few feelings walk hand-in-hand and are even confused for the accelerated demand of modern society. I've picked two – angst and anxiety – because these two feelings are so present in this pandemic time. These affects might be confused for acceleration, especially anxiety, and they can often bring acceleration as a defense or escape to avoid the emptiness these feelings generate. These affects do not allow us to identify a specific cause, they are shapeless.

Angst, according to Freud (2014) is a reaction to a dangerous situation; the self spares itself of a situation interpreted as dangerous, developing a feeling of angst. Angst, therefore, signals a situation of significant danger, and arises as a reaction to that situation. It emerges when one of these states presents itself. It is that which cannot be named. It harkens back to an absence, which tends to be filled quickly with addictions and compulsions; to an emptiness, which can easily be filled with an excessively accelerated life.

Anxiety, according to Hillman (1980), has already been recognized as Chaos, faceless and nameless, a terrified and mad movement of the soul. The foundations of anxiety reside in need itself, a subjective need, which constellates and terrifies, precisely because of an unidentifiable and unavoidable need, which imprisons and subjugates the Ego to its fate. The relationship between need and the human condition is evident. A need for another, for an external object to fill the emptiness. Either you dive into this emptiness or you avoid it through symptoms and defenses. Here, we can find acceleration as a symptom.

There's a connection between angst, anxiety and acceleration. The soul wants, the soul fears, and ego hurries to try and evade suffering. And so, acceleration can arise as defense or escape, from demands for performance, which prevents a dive into real needs and wants.

The question to be asked is: in the name of what or whom does this acceleration insist? Symptom or not, this is an undeniable fact, and the great challenge is to individuate yourself "in" the acceleration. Not "in spite of" the acceleration. It is necessary to undo the myth that a process of deceleration is necessary for individuation to occur.

Still in the definition of Hartmut Rosa (2019), it's not "walking faster" or excessive work that cause disorders like burnout, but the yearnings of individuals for meaning, a horizon, a direction; or for relationships, resonance, connection. What is exhausting is running faster and faster only to remain in place.

One accelerates to search something. Just as a search for deceleration carries a request from the soul, a search for acceleration carries it too. Different cities, different rhythms, different wants. The eccentricity of people and cities, in this never-ending path called individuation.

Three stories, three images for us to rethink acceleration, this time not as a defense, but as a way of being, in an accelerated world.

The first story begins with this sentence: "You have to answer faster." What to do upon hearing that sentence, so often heard in corporate, virtual, school environments?

In the case in question, it was heard by a young adult woman who recently had entered the job market. An engineer and economist, she works with company purchases, sales and mergers. Despite the excessive work, early on she started finding – with hard work – her visibility, her skills, her competencies and her way of living amid the acceleration of daily routine. That sentence, however, coming mid-quarantine, when she's working from home – company demands were apparently under control, allowing her to work in a more convenient schedule – sounded bothersome. It gave rise to questions like: I like what I do, I belong here, I like the work and I like the people. But what's the point of me not being able to work late at night and replying the next morning? Why not – instead of asking me to be faster – call me or schedule a meeting to learn how we've been feeling during the pandemic?

Because of those questions, without turning her back to the acceleration imposed by her company, she took risks in other positions. She was able to question, reflect and fight for more humanity in her work

The second story begins with this sentence: "I can't take it anymore, being criticized for always being accelerated."

That sentence was spoken by a 48-year-old woman before the quarantine. People complain that she speaks too fast and never lets people finish their sentences. So she questioned why, if so many people have complained about it her whole life, can't she change? Is that her burden? By reflecting on it, she reaches an interesting question: can we maybe say that acceleration is the same as anxiety? Would that be her glory and her ruin? This expression that Hillman (2001) develops in his book *The Force of Character* makes me think whether acceleration is just a cultural demand or if we could think of it as a daimon.

I think the two aren't mutually exclusive. Archetypes are only accessible through an archetypal image, and it is known that an archetypal image is updated according to its culture. Besides, in mythology we can find stories that explain existential themes. And in mythology we can find the image of Hermes, the god of speed, with winged feet, invisibility helmet and winged thoughts. The only one who can move through Olympus, the world of the living and the world of the dead. Hermes, the god of acceleration.

Lastly, the third sentence was said by a 42-year-old journalist. "The fact is that this isolation has accelerated many processes."

The journalist recognizes this period of the pandemic as a historical moment. This would be the journalistic coverage of his lifetime. Intense workdays and angst facing the episodes he's forced to come in contact with at his job. In addition, an intense questioning of shared values, of what he accomplished in his life over so many years of hard work, and what he can still become, besides a journalist. He loves his profession and the rhythm of his life. In this time of the pandemic, he's taken several decisions he'd been postponing for years: professional, family and personal decisions.

When I came across these images, two points in common drew my attention: compulsion and questioning. It is impossible not to relate these images to the god Pan, son of Hermes. Pan rapes. When he rapes, it shows nature's compulsive need. He rapes nymphs, which have a form of consciousness that is undefined, incorporeal, out of contact and imperceptible. In these beings, feelings and thoughts are still cold, remote and reflective.

Here, two sides of the same archetype are identified: matter and spirit; instinct and metaphor; Pan and nymphs; the instinctive nature of the relationship with fear and the imaginative way with which ego relates to it. Jung (2000) placed instinct and image in the same continuum, thus offering a new entry into the world of Pan.

Hillman (2015, p. 74) reminds us that "behavior is also fantasy, and fantasy is also behavior." She is also physical, "a way of being in the world. [...] We can't move, talk or feel without representing a fantasy." Besides, following the line of thinking of imaginal ego, it is understood that behavior is always guided by imaginal processes. "Behavior is always metaphorical."

Going back to the myth, we find nymphs as characters of fundamental importance in Pan's relationships. They are opposite beings: body and instinct on one side, imagination and reflection on the other. Instincts form images, and images trigger actions. Any transformation of image affects behavior, and vice versa. Therefore, nymph and Pan belong to the same nature, and thus, are similar beings.

And where would be the resemblance of these two mythological beings? Nymphs, like Pan's drive, are nameless figures, impersonal objects, obscure and unknown. However, they promote a very interesting activity in Pan: reflection. Pan was in the habit of raping his nymphs, which evidences his compulsion. Its violent penetration into the nymph's virginal consciousness brings a reality never before experienced. It inserts it into instinctual life and introduces it into matter. The terror generated by the presence of Pan manifests itself through the flight of nymphs. And the escape, psychologically, can become reflection because it provokes a departure from the emotion of the stimulus, being analyzed indirectly, via thought.

Jung writes:

> Owing to this interference, the psychic processes exert an attraction on the impulse to act excited by the stimulus. Therefore, before having discharged itself into the external world, the impulse is deflected into an endopsychic activity. *Reflexio* is a turning inwards, with the result that, instead of an instinctive action, there ensues a succession of derivative contents or states which may be termed reflection or deliberation. Thus in place of the compulsive act there appears a certain degree of freedom, and in place of predictability a relative unpredictability as to the effect of the impulse. [...] This may take place directly, for instance in speech, or may appear in the form of abstract thought, dramatic representation, or ethical conduct; or again, in scientific achievement or a work of art.
>
> (Jung 1916, par. 241, 242)

With the evolution of the myth, Pan's objects of desire get their names. And from that point, reflection starts to become part of the experiences of this god, putting brakes on his compulsiveness, his literalized need, which becomes symbolized, sublimated, metaphorized...

What does the myth teach us?

It teaches us that acceleration requires reflection, otherwise it becomes empty, compulsive, purely defense or escape. As it becomes reflected or metaphorized, acceleration can be a style, it can be individuated at the speed and singularity of individuals and their sceneries.

But there's work to be done. This reflection does not happen automatically, because acceleration swallows us up. Each of us will need to build and reflect on our own way to individuate acceleration. Or, once we find our own decelerated style, find ways to exist facing an inevitable acceleration.

Pan's compulsiveness decreases when symbolized. Byung-Chul Han, in an interview about his new book *The Disappearance of Rituals*, defines rituals as symbolic actions that generate a community with no need for communication. He believes community is disappearing, especially due to hypercommunication, which generates communication without community, a cult, a worshipping of the self. Alienation.

Zoja (1992, p. 47), in his book *Nascere Non Basta* writes that the pre-fabricated life we insert ourselves in lacks soul. Hence, it requires this soul from us. And he suggests that society does not currently provide structures that could offer paths to rites of initiation. In his understanding, man is already born too close to civilization, to the collective, to culture and society, and rites of initiation have to adapt to modernity, because "the man of today feels dropped, as if by accident, into a specific culture and society which don't inspire any sacral respect." The author understands that contemporary rites of passage are not as clear and well-defined as in primitive societies, or even the Middle Ages, favoring a blunt and sudden passage.

However, neither myself nor any of these authors preach a return to the past, a rescuing of the rituals that were so useful in traditional society, or in ancient times. A rite is anything that distances us from our ego and connects us with the Other, whether it's an internal and external other. The psyche has endless resources to imagine new symbolic forms, new forms of collective actions that are realized beyond ego.

Let's return to philosopher Hartmut Rosa (2019), who uses the term resonance. Resonance can be a possibility in rediscovering forms of ritualization. Resonance, more than knowledge, is a relational mode, in which subject and world put themselves in a responsive relation. In love, in friendship, in democratic political action, modern subjects can initiate relations of resonance. Could relations of resonance be possibilities of finding new rites in modern society, despite the acceleration?

The utopia we wish to pursue is that we are able to respect and live with differences and singularities. Individual and cultural differences. What we can aim for is a certain friction between various peoples and cultures, with no attempt at colonization or erasing differences, finding a way to respect the self and the other. This is individuating. Individuating, respecting earth, nature, cities and other ways of life.

References

Bosco, F. (2013) O público e o privado. *Observatório da Imprensa*. Online at: www. observatoriodaimprensa.com.br/educacao-e-cidadania/caderno-da-cidadania/_ed770_ o_publico_e_o_privado_iv/

Freud, S. (2014 [1926–1929]). *Inhibitions, Symptoms and Anxiety*. O.C. 17. São Paulo: Cia das Letras.

Han, B. (2015) *The Burnout Society*. Petrópolis: Vozes

Hillman, J. (1980). Athene, Ananke, and the necessity of abnormal psychology, in *Facing the Gods*. São Paulo: Cultrix/Pensamento.

Hillman, J. (2001). *The Force of Character*: And the Lasting Life. Rio de Janeiro: Objetiva.

Hillman, J. (2015). *Pan and the Nightmare*. São Paulo: Paulus.

Jung, C. G. (1970 [1916]). *The Nature of the Psyche*. In CW, 8/2, Transl. H. Read, M. Fordham, G. Adler. Princeton: Princeton University Press.

Rosa, H. (2019) *Social Acceleration: A New Theory of Modernity*. São Paulo: Editora Unesp.

Zoja, L. (1992). *Nascere Non Basta. Iniziazione e tossicodipendenza*. São Paulo: Axis Mundi.

Part 3

Chapter I

Me and My Therapist are Bodies in Space

Embodied Sliding on the Ego-Self Axis

J. F.

In this chapter the author interrogates herself about the reason of her feeling comfortable with online therapy. How does it come that she had no creative complaint about being stuck in a flat, living her life off a screen? Exploring the wonders of online therapy, she focuses on embodiment and our ability to phantasize and float comfortably in space. Inspired by the song Ladies and Gentlemen and Garders philosophical novel, Dreaming Dakini suggests that for Jungians the perilous expedition to the outermost reaches of language and existence is the everyday endeavour of sliding on the ego-self axis. The author shows how she draws on body memory and the power of imagination when relating to the image of her therapist on a screen. Comparing this to active imagination, and spiritual practices in Christian and Buddhist tradition, i.e. talking with St Teresa and The Great Mother Prajna Paramita, she argues that in such moments she is floating in her Self and in the shared, collective unconscious. Concluding that her therapist on a screen functions as a symbol and a bridge to The Good Enough Mother to her Self.

I could write: "Online therapy works for me and my therapist," and add: "It mostly also works for me and my clients," which would be true, short and boring. A story needs a problem. My problem is, that I do not have one.

So I asked myself, why could I not join the choir of suffering comrades, who felt online therapy to be various degrees of intolerable? How does it come that I had no creative complaint about being stuck in a flat, living my life through a screen? And I wondered: Was it because the arrangement suits my lazy bone? Or my willingness to be afraid, very afraid of catching a Covid on a train? Or is it simply that my therapist and I date back to a long time ago?

Whereas all of this may be true, I believe the matter boils down to other things, that is our ability to be in our body, to phantazie and to float comfortably in space. I will tell you why.

As I wondered about the wonders of online therapy a song line flew into my mind and settled on replay. "Ladies and Gentlemen," it sang, "we are floating in space." It's from English space rock band, Spiritualized's 1997 album, and refers to a philosophical novel, *Sophie's World* by Gaarder. He writes:

DOI: 10.4324/9781003266402-31

Only philosophers embark on this perilous expedition to the outermost reaches of language and existence. Some of them fall off, but others cling on desperately and yell at the people nestling deep in the snug softness, stuffing themselves with delicious food and drink. 'Ladies and Gentlemen,' they yell, 'we are floating in space!'

(Gaarder 2010, p. 37)

With their song the space rock band seems to suggest that any spiritualized person, not just philosophers, embark on "this perilous expedition to the outermost reaches of language and existence." I agree. Jungians even make it their business. And occasionally do it without the desperation and the clinging. It is an everyday endeavour. Sliding on the ego-self axis, exploring the vast unconscious realms, the Self as Jung called it. Meditators call it to rest in space.

Embodied

Me and My Therapist Go Online

I do not recall it being a big shift. Just a moment of awkwardness on my part the first time. Then I plunged into the talking and it was business as usual. I blur, she listens, nods, makes invisible (not to me!) facial and bodily moves. I refer to it all; her moving body, her facial expressions, her tone of voice. Just like I did when I sat opposite her in a brown leather chair some 24 minutes train ride south of Copenhagen.

I don't know if the number of times I refer to my own body has increased or decreased. I know I do. Every time. While talking to her on the screen, I experience energy moving in my body and body memories appear, just like when I was in her room. For instance, Snuden, the little animal peeking out of my solar plexus when the coast is clear. Or my clubfoot. It is activated when certain tense emotions arise in me. It's a fantasized foot. You can't see it, but I can feel it. It's real to me. As real as she is on the screen. The foot is related a memory of my mother in fur believing herself to be the queen of Sheba. When I told this to my therapist, she replied that the queen of Sheba actually had a club foot, a goat's hoof.

I draw on body memory when we meet in space. Do you see? We know each other very well, me and my therapist. As embodied beings. And as I sit here, writing and looking at the letters on the screen from where she too appears, I sense her presence in the room. And in me, as bodily sensation.

Things I Miss I: The Blue Carpet

The things I miss are all related to embodied memory; my experience of being some-body in her room with her as Mother body.

I miss lying on the blue carpet between our identical leather chairs. Occasionally, I lie there to get out of my head into my body-mind. The ritual arose out of the blue. One day I expressed the longing to lie and she said please, go ahead. It is a bit like the famous couch. Or a cradle. Only I am floating on a blue ocean by her feet. She looks at my face, I sense the garden behind the glass door, close my eyes and drift off into space. *Ladies and Gentlemen, we are floating....* Our voices are an umbilical cord. The ego-self axis on which my awareness moves smoothly.

We also lay out papers I bring for the sessions on that blue carpet, drawings and stuff. Incidents, thoughts, memories, sensations, feelings. One day I saw how I place the Lego of my life on that carpet and then we play. Moving pieces, putting them together in new ways, adding new, taking away old. We tear down and construct my life worlds. Mandalas. Now we do it in space.

Things I Miss 2: The Chinese box

I also miss the Chinese box in which she keeps napkins. It lives on the little table next to my chair. It is a ritual. I arrive, bike-nose or not, lift the lid and read the inscription on the inside, neatly printed in italics by her maternal grandmother.

Things I Miss 3: Her Husband

One day I found a new cover for my bike saddle in my basket with a note: "Please use if you can." Only later did I realize, he does not even know my name. To him I am the Wednesday 10.05 session with the rotten saddle. And maybe she scorned him afterwards for doing what a therapist should not and would not do; exchange gifts with a client. I also miss seeing him in the garden. Or waving to me from his car as I arrive and he leaves.

Out of these tiny often wordless meetings, arose my transference of the good parents unto them. For a time I would often, shyly talk about my fantasies of being a well-loved child in this loving home. I would say: "I know, you are not old enough to be my mother," and she would smile and nod the "Go on" and we would Play House; work with the transference, Jungians say. "So you were the mother and I was the child" as Danish children say to indicate play time.

Symbols at work in body-memory

I use her husband, the Chinese box and her grandmother as symbols. They have become part and parcel of my healing process. Her grandmother is The Great Grandmother, the one who never fails you. And I have an embodied memory of how it feels to be held in her gaze when she smiles at me from the painting on the wall. As I leave, feeling warm, safe and well enough loved to go out and do my thing. Online Grandmother smiles at me all the time, from the wall behind my therapist.

Evidently, I have a lot to build on when I meet her online. And you might think all this missing of mine is put forward in favor of physical meetings, in rooms that give away traces of ordinary human life. But I have no complaints. I miss the good way, as my young children said. No feeling is final, Rilke said. The symbols are working in me.

Fantasizing

Teresa Goes Online in 1555

I was gazing out of my window into a cloudy sky, wondering why I so readily accept meeting my therapist on line, when Teresa appeared. I was looking for similar experiences, asking myself; where do I know this from? And there she was. *"Anda, hija,"* she said, *"me ves o no?"* Come on, girl. Do you see me or not? Quite like the deceased grandmother in Almodovar's film *Volver*. What could I say? No?

Relating to the image of my therapist on a screen, as if she was real, is like seeing Theresa of Avila who died centuries ago in Spain, outside my window, down town Copenhagen. I accept both as real.

I know Teresa quite well. We meet and talk frequently. Teresa used to be a Spanish noblewoman, but opted for convent life in 1535 and ended up a saint, one of the great mystics within the catholic tradition. God spoke to her, Jesus came for tea and once a nasty fellow speared her heart and brought about a huge shift in her understanding of pleasure and pain. Her visions of the inner-most secrets of the soul are in no way inferior to those of Jung. In her auto-biography Teresa describes her speciality – *oración mental* – what we today would label meditation or contemplative prayer and Jung would call Active Imagination. *"Contemplative prayer in my opinion is nothing other than a close sharing between friends. It means frequently taking time to be alone with Him whom we know loves us."* (Teresa of Avila 1976 p. 67). He was no more physi-cally present in her room than my therapist in mine during online therapy.

Being a long-time practitioner of so-called solo-meditation-retreats accord-ing to Vajrayna style, I have enjoyed the company of many deities, while supposedly being alone in a cabin. More than once have I offered *tsok*, the sanskrit word for a gay gathering of spiritual friends with good food, mantra recitation, song and dance. I have warm memories of a cold January on the Black Mountain north of Barcelona setting daily lunch tables for invisible (not to me!) guests; the Great Mother, wrathful protectors and mountain spirits a like. Never was I more sociable.

The power of imagination

Theresa of Avila used the image of watering one's garden as a metaphor for mystical prayer. Another gardener, the French impressionist Claude Monet said that while painting he entered into a state of mind close to prayer. Likewise Jung in his *Red Book* period found challenge and consolation in the inner world: He called his technique of conscious dialogue with the unconscious Active Imagination.

My point is that some of us have long accepted that just like a nightly dream, a vision of someone who is not physically present may feel real and have lasting consequences. Jung kept coming back to Philemon. Teresa was devastated when she did not hear from God. Active imagination can be life changing.

My therapist on a screen is as good as any vision of any deity from any religion. Mind you, I am not saying my therapist is God or The Great Mother, though sometimes it may feel like she is The Good Mother incarnate. Or the opposite, when I project the devil onto her and she is the intensely Bad Mother. I am just saying; the reality of it remains the same to me.

We are Floating in Space

Speed pilgrimage

I have tested ways of arriving to the meeting with my therapist online: wearing work clothes, wearing jumpsuit. Full makeup, no makeup. Sitting quietly for a few minutes, jumping straight from vacuum cleaning. I have simulated the train ride, going down my kitchen stair, and up my front stair. None of this impressed me much.

One day I understood why. That was when she had the time wrong.

I usually call and she picks up. Just like I ring her door bell and she opens the door. Only once did she call me. That was when she had the time wrong, and caused me the curious experience of watching my mind do a 15 seconds speed pilgrimage, travelling from my normal ego-awareness into a state of mind that may very well be likened to prayer. I felt/saw the effect from a row of neatly positioned black domino pieces, as they feel, one by one in an organic, smooth silent move. The defence wall came down, I settled into open space. Like a time traveller transported into another realm.

In the Buddhist tradition, The Great Mother Prajna Paramita symbolizes an open state of mind, referred to as emptiness. The emptiness out of which everything is born, arise and dissolve. Jung called it the Self. We usually think of it as a place of healing we go to alone, in our mind. In the Dream Matrix a whole group embark on the journey together. In therapy I go with my therapist *on this perilous expedition to the outermost reaches of language and existence* exploring unknown feelings and sensations.

In such moments I am floating in the Self, not mine, not hers, but the third, shared one – the collective unconscious. And she is with me. So what keeps me safe, grounded, connected? She does. She is earth control. Actually neither nor. Both and. Like the Self. Both center and circumference. One foot in space, the other in some soil south of Copenhagen. One day my body mind will take over.

Dreading the day I leave home

Every couple creates a ritual, going in and out of the Room. In her house she walks me to the door. She sways slightly on her feet, watching as I put on my coat in the entrance and try not to bogart her time, asking beggar questions like: do you think me an idiot? The online goodbye is more abrupt. My resistance more evident. I practice being adult with a jolly "Goodbye!" before I click the button.

Can you hear it too? I start to sound like a child who has been left home. A dear home. A well-loved child, with the Sunday blues. The sweetness of a melancholy moment. I dread the day I will not come to sit with her by the blue ocean. I apparently expect to do it again. And if online therapy was to last, I would mourn the loss of the last good bye. Her home and the hours well spent there will be part of the loss. "The art of losing isn't hard to master," the American poet Elizabeth Bishop lied.

My therapist on the screen is a special and good enough bridge to The Good Enough Mother, bringing "Her" closer to home, in a double sense. She is in me in a way, she was never before. Covid brought me closer to her in me and to a more flexible sliding on the ego-self axis. Occasionally more comfortable knowing that we are indeed floating in space.

So what was the question, again? How do I experience online therapy? Well, as I said, it works for me and my therapist.

References

Almodóvar, P. (2006). *Volver.* Spain: Warner Bros.

Teresa of Avila (1976). *The Collected Works of St. Teresa of Avila*, vol. 1. Washington, DC: Institute of Carmelite Studies.

Bishop, E. (1983). "One Art." *The Complete Poems 1926–1979.* New York: Farrar, Straus and Giroux.

Gaarder, J. (2010). *Sophie's World.* London: Weidenfeld & Nicolson.

Chapter 2

Coming and Going

K. E. K.

The approach to and departure from the analytic hour is a ritual integral to the therapeutic phenomenon that shapes the analytical experience. This essay explores how this ritual "frames" what occurs in therapy and helps facilitate what desires or is waiting to emerge in each session. The need for analysts to move analysis online, occasioned by the global pandemic, has seriously disrupted the typical ritual framework. Therefore, the essential value of this framing has become more evident through its absence. After establishing a definition of "ritual," a detailed personal account of an analysand's pre-Covid ritual is provided. The narration of the analysand's experience puts a spotlight on what is missing from online analysis, which seems not sinking in and taking root in his psyche the way in-person sessions do. He wonders if a lack of ritual accounts, in part, for this difference. This reflection leads to a deeper understanding of how one approaches, enters, and leaves the analytical hour has an impact upon the therapeutic experience as a whole.

Like many, my experience of the pandemic has been apocalyptic. By apocalyptic, I have in mind here not the word's popular (and grossly distorted) associations, but the core meaning of *apocalypsis* understood as "revelation." An apocalypse is an act of disclosure, like pulling back a curtain and unveiling what stands or exists behind it. It's a moment of insight and illumination that reorients one's life.

After more than eighteen months of analysis online, one thing that has become clear is the importance of the weekly ritual that used to frame my analytic "hour" before the pandemic. My analyst offered online sessions before Covid-19, but only when our respective schedules made meeting in person difficult. Throughout the pandemic, I have come to see in a new way, and appreciate, how ritual, specifically my ritual, plays an essential role in the therapeutic/analytic process. Ritual has a way of "framing" what occurs in the analytical hour and helps facilitate what desires to or is waiting to emerge in each session. What happens leading up to and following the hour is also part of the therapeutic phenomenon and shapes the analytic experience.

DOI: 10.4324/9781003266402-32

Ritual. From the Latin *ritualis* and *ritus*. Related to "rite." Often associated with religious ceremonies, "rite" has an older Sanskrit origin meaning "trend," "disposition," or "custom."[1] At its root is the prefix ri-, which mean "to go" or "to flow" ('river' has the same root). A ritual or rite is a custom, as it were, a habit, a meaningful ordering of time and actions. A rite or ritual can easily become an end-in-itself, empty of meaning or purpose, through overuse or mindless practice, absent of intention. With a proper intention, however, rituals and rites can provide the means through which something is allowed to come into being or awareness. The ritual anticipates the "flow" to occur and helps to channels the "flow." Ritual becomes a conduit, allowing for the flow and unfolding of insight, meaning, emotion, spirit, energy, life (both *bios* and *zoë*), libido, as well as the Holy. In this sense, all that one might experience in a religious ceremony or worship setting could be similarly experienced in (or on the way *to* or *from*) the consulting room.

Arnold Van Gennep (1960) first, and later Victor Turner (1995), demonstrated that rites and rituals are essential for personal and collective transformation. In his paper "Concerning Rebirth," first published in 1940, C.G. Jung too, highlighted the importance of a ritual for inducing (not producing) experiences of transformation and renewal (1940, para. 177). Through participation in sacred rites and rituals, mystery-dramas of transcendence that are different from ordinary experiences, an initiate can be conveyed into a deeper awareness of knowing and being known. And these rituals are more than internal processes or processions; they have external or social dimensions.

Here is a description of the pre-Covid ritual that framed my weekly analytical experience to make this more concrete. I live in Baltimore, Maryland. My analyst's praxis is in the Dupont Circle neighborhood, in the heart of Washington, DC. While the distance between Baltimore to Washington is only 35 miles (56km), it could take almost 90 minutes to get there by car, depending upon the time of the day. My appointment time is at 4 p.m., so late in the afternoon. I usually allow ninety minutes, not to be rushed. I use the time in my car to prepare for the session, often in silence or listening to classical music. I think about the previous week, reflect upon my dreams, and get a feel for what I need to bring into the session. Driving south from Baltimore down to Washington, I often take the same route. I exit off the Washington I-695 beltway, then drive down the length of 16th Street, turning right on New Hampshire Avenue, a left on 18th Street, and then a left on N Street, where I usually find a place to park. I love the energy of the city, the stately architecture, the rhythm of the traffic. With my black leather journal in hand, I pick up a cup of coffee (if I have time), look over my notes, and then walk to analysis with a sense of anticipation for what is about to be revealed.

My analyst works in the lower (basement) level of a beautiful nineteenth-century brownstone, the upper levels of which house the Embassy of the Dalai Lama. I walk down several steps to enter the building. The hallway has the scent of sandalwood. It's quiet (except for the hum of the white sound machine), calm. Alchemical prints line the corridor that leads to the waiting area. The lighting is soft. The space is welcoming. A silkscreen labyrinth hangs from the wall near the fireplace. In time, my analyst comes out to meet me and escorts me into the consulting room. Also this latter is very calm, welcoming, comforting. There are books on the shelf. The smell of wax is in the air. Candles are often lit in the fireplace hearth beside a small easel holding a print of the Annunciation. There's a sofa and across from it is the analyst's chair. And we begin.

When the session is over, I walk down the corridor past the Alchemical prints and exit through the same exterior door I entered. I cross the threshold, walk up the steps, and re-enter the rhythm and buzz of Washington. I often need to walk after a session. I like to wander over to Dupont Circle, sit near the fountain, watch people, and write in my journal. Sometimes I go to a bookstore or café to write. When the time is right, I get back into my car and drive back to Baltimore, reflecting upon the day.

Week after week. Over many years. Leaving "business as usual" in Baltimore and going south, going "down" to Washington, down the steps into the *temenos*, down into the depths. Then out of the depths, up and out into the city crossroads. In many places, Jung often talked about the significance of *rites d'entrée et sortie*. My approach, arrival, entrance, departure, and return are all part of the analytic experience. The ritual invites me, allows me to flow into a liminal space, a suspended place betwixt and between. In the analyst's *temenos* I am suspended in time, moving through time past, time present, with glimpses of time-to-come. And my body, too, is suspended in this space. A body that moves through space and time to dwell in a particular place. I enter in and fill that space with my body, in the presence of an *other*, another body that also takes up space. The ritual sets the stage for an embodied, felt experience, open to what is emerging into the light of consciousness, open to what desires to come to life in me and through me, open to the flow and unfolding of insight, meaning, emotion, spirit, energy, life (both *bios* and *zoë*), libido, the Holy.

After the session, the ritual helps me digest, metabolize, and integrate the analytic experience into the rest of my life. The ritual continues to serve as a conduit that moves me, shows me the way back, returning, like the Magi in Matthew's Gospel, "by another road," changed (if ever-so-slightly), transfigured, and sometimes transformed.[2]

Sitting in a chair at my desk at home, turning on the computer, clicking on a link that takes me to a screen that shows my analyst sitting, not in her praxis, but in a different chair, in a difference space, a more personal space – all of this pre-empts, undercuts, short circuits, and blocks the ritual flow aspect of analysis. Time and space are distorted. I am plopped down into something that, after more than 18 months, still seems odd. I can see into the home of my analyst. The analyst sees where I live. There's something nice about this. It's certainly convenient. I don't have to leave my home and contend with traffic. But then I don't get to leave home. And isn't analysis, in many respects, about "leaving home"? An online platform is just a part of my ordinary life, not very different from every other online meeting I attend throughout the week. It's not set apart. It's an extension or part of a daily norm. With a click of the mouse, I enter a different kind of space, and then with a click of the mouse, in a split-second, I'm out of that space and thrown back into my day and all the work on my agenda. There's no suspension betwixt and between, no hiatus, little sense of the liminal. There's no ritual. I often try to be quiet and reflective about thirty minutes before clicking on the Zoom link, but it's not the same. It's too easy for me to work on other things right up to the time for analysis and then jump back into work when the session is over.

Yes, I miss the therapeutic ritual. There's a place for digital therapy, of course, but I look forward to when my analyst and I can be in the same physical room, sharing the same space. I can't say that I haven't had intense, meaningful, productive sessions online over the past 18 months because I have. Looking back, these significant sessions, however, feel more like interspersed and scattered isolated events. It's more complicated, more challenging, threading them together and integrating the experience into my life. Although often meaningful, online sessions don't seem to take hold of me in the same way. They can feel disembodied. Online therapy doesn't sink in and take root in my psyche the way in-person sessions do, sessions that are framed by the benefit of an extensive framing ritual. They don't tap into my internal root system the same way and, perhaps, are less effective over time. And I wonder if a lack of ritual accounts, in part, for this difference. Maybe I need to develop a different ritual for online sessions. Perhaps. Or may I'm old school. I know what my soul prefers.

Notes

1 Online Etymology Dictionary: www.etymonline.com/word/rite
2 The Gospel According to Matthew (2:12), *The New Oxford Annotated Bible with Apocrypha: New Revised Standard Version* (New York: Oxford University Press, 2018).

References

Jung. C.G. (1940). Concerning rebirth. In C.G. Jung, *Collected Works*, 9, I. Princeton: Princeton University Press, 1980.

Van Gennep, A. (1909). *The Rites of Passage.* Chicago: University of Chicago Press, 1960.

Turner, V. (1995 [1969]). *The Ritual Process: Structure and Anti-Structure.* New York: Aldine de Gruyter.

Chapter 3

A Personal Experience of Therapy during the Covid-19 Pandemic

M. S.

Living at the border between Slovenia and Italy the author describes his personal reaction to the lockdown measures due to the initial spreading of Coronavirus in Italy. He describes his passage of gradual exit from a state of denial while adjusted to the new situation. The chapter focuses on his personal analysis, especially on transference dynamics when switching to online mode, and on a different meaning connected with the process taking place in the unconscious. The experience of online therapy offered the opportunity of realizing the void connected to a traumatic past, as if the screen mediated a possibility of connection with the feeling of void, especially when the screen froze or the connection was lost. Paradoxically, this facilitated to think the unthinkable, developing a safer attachment within the therapeutic relationship. The author believes it could not be done in any other way. It was an opportunity to become aware of the symbolic value of the process happening in transference in analysis and is very grateful for the experience and the lessons learned.

I remember it was late February and I was on a short spa vacation in the region of Ptuj in Slovenia. We followed the news about Europe on television and witnessed the Italians locking down one city at a time, slowly stopping the flights, then closing the borders. It was very surreal, as if it was happening to someone else, I remember I felt intense fear and anger, and the sense of absurdity and denial. How could this be happening in the twenty-first century? The images from Wuhan were like pictures from a sci-fi movie, to say the least. Could this be happening in Europe, as well? Europe seemed like a safe place.

When the pandemic started, I was already in my fourth year of analysis. I had also just begun my studies in Analytical Psychology at the IAAP and had started working with my first clients as a router. I live close to the Italian border, on the coastal part of Slovenia, so I watched the news with great concern. My small village lies exactly on the Slovenian-Italian border; if one takes the road down the hill one reaches Botazzo, the beautiful Canyon of Val Rosandra near Trieste. For us living here, the border is an important symbol of freedom, of two worlds coexisting. The fact that one can pass it daily unobstructed gives us the freedom of thought, which we consider culturally

DOI: 10.4324/9781003266402-33

very important. And this is why the shock was even greater when the Italian government decided to close the border between the countries. "Are they really going to do that?" It was as if plunging down back in history, it was like going back to 1947 when the border was strictly closed and dangerous. At the time it was still the border between Italy and Yugoslavia.

My analysis was filled with the same amount of fear, rage and disbelief at the beginning of the first lockdown. I remember thinking that my analyst was probably paranoid due to the gravity of his reactions toward the situation. However, with the first lockdown starting in March 2020, it became clear that the virus was spreading worldwide, with no exceptions, and that it was the beginning of a different world for all of us. Something that we have never imagined was starting to become real and a part of our everyday lives. The change of the setting in analysis and moving our sessions online was not such a big problem for me, because I had been used to working online via Skype already. The greater change was in my social life becoming restricted and that all social interactions were transferred online.

It was the beginning of a strange, yet very interesting year. Somehow, I felt safe at home. Being an introvert, staying indoors was not causing me a lot of problems; I liked the fact that I could organize my life during the day with long walks in natural surroundings. I live in a natural park area of amazing beauty, so the possibility of going for long walks was very refreshing and it gave me a greater sense of stability. It was also beneficial to my health and it became, for some time, a part of my new, healthier routine. It was basically something I have always dreamed of – working from home with the freedom of having time for myself as well.

However, analytically speaking, there was another anxiety that I noticed later in the new online setting that was perhaps deeper and more unconscious. Having already experienced quite a few problems with understanding a safe attachment due to a transgenerational trauma, with the sessions online I felt a certain void surfacing between me and my analyst. It was as if the screen was enabling me to get more in touch with this feeling. Sometimes this literally meant that the internet connection became slower and weaker, and the words we were speaking became lighter and unspeakable. Sometimes the connection was lost or the image froze. It was bizarre, like being in a place that was "neither here or there," it was like being in a void.

Alessandra Cavalli explained the concept of the void in beautiful words in her article about transgenerational trauma: "When the environment is not able to fulfil a containing function, it leaves a void, an irrepresentability. This void is felt as deadly, and has a traumatic value because it generates anxieties which have no name" (Cavalli, 2012, p. 601) Those moments were very frustrating, though sometimes funny, but it was as if the situation in analysis was revealing that I had to trust that the connection was safe, as though the setting was really disturbed by "unknown" digital interferences. And as we started to analyse the exact moments when this happened, it became clear that the digital disturbances were part of the process and my analysis. We started to "digest" the void in the way that we began adding meaning to it. The processing of the unthinkable was slowly gaining shape and I began to realize that my patterns of emptiness were constantly re/enacting the same feelings of deprivation and loneliness that were making me feel "a deadly desert and alone." The void was actually helping me to act differently this time, to feel more secure, because, objectively, I felt secure and that feeling gave me the power to understand the symbolic value of the process happening in transference and analysis.

As I write about this now, I think that the therapy was very intense in that period, because of the fact that the analytical setting enabled me to get in touch with a very vulnerable part of myself. I believe it could not be done in any other way and I am very grateful for the experience and the lessons learned.

References

Cavalli, A. (2012). Transgenerational transmission of indigestible facts: From trauma, deadly ghosts and mental voids to meaning-making interpretations. *Journal of Analytical Psychology* 57 (5): 597–614. doi:10.1111/j.1468-5922.2012.02005.x

Index